I dedicate this book to my staff at the UCSF Memory and Aging Center who support me every day in my work. Special thanks to Caroline Latham, Rosalie Gearhart, Anna Karydas, and Leslie Goss. Similarly, I have eternal gratitude to my patients and their loved ones, who are a constant inspiration and source of joy.

Preface

This book tries to capture the rich and quickly changing landscape of frontotemporal dementia (FTD). I became interested in this disorder in 1983 (called Pick's disease at the time) while working as a fellow with D. Frank Benson and Jeffrey Cummings, two extraordinary mentors, who taught me how to evaluate patients with dementia. Frank and Jeff correctly believed that frontotemporal dementia could be diagnosed and separated from Alzheimer's disease during life, although at that time the dictum was, "don't pick Pick's disease." This pithy statement suggested that Pick's disease was rare and impossible to diagnose.

Frank's passion for understanding how the frontal lobes worked was infectious, and Jeff had just returned to the University of California, Los Angeles (UCLA) from England, where he helped to define the clinical features of five pathologically proven cases of Pick's disease. They correctly posited that first symptoms, clinical course, and the cognitive pattern of deficits in a patient with a degenerative dementia allowed accurate prediction of the neuropathological subtype. Soon afterward, I met Arne Brun and Lars Gustafson, a brilliant neuropathologist and neuropsychiatrist team from Sweden who began their studies of FTD in the mid-1970s. Arne, Lars, Frank, and Jeff's encouragement were a strong impetus to work in this field, and with their help, I began to organize a large population of patients with FTD.

Soon I realized that FTD was a unique biological condition that offered an opportunity to understand how slow, progressive atrophy of the frontal lobes would subtly influence the personality, behavior, and cognitive abilities of a previously healthy individual. This led me to begin a "bionarrative" approach to the study of FTD that involved carefully documenting a person's life story, strengths, weaknesses, and eccentricities, in an attempt to understand when the disease began, and how its onset changed a life's trajectory. Through these narratives I began to realize that FTD's course was often long and complex and, in turn, I was forced to reconsider many of my ideas about social behavior, language, and creativity. Rather than a story of relentless decline, in some patients the disorder began with genius in business, athletics, or the arts. Even once the illness was well established, visual creativity could be maintained, particularly in patients with asymmetric left-sided disease. The experiences that I had working with my remarkable patients and their families are the inspiration for this book.

For investigators of the late twentieth century, the biology of FTD seemed impenetrable; clinical methodology for understanding FTD was sadly deficient, and the absence of cases (in clinical settings every dementia was called Alzheimer's disease) stymied systematic efforts to study the illness. Yet, the intellectual landscape surrounding FTD has changed dramatically in recent years, and there are few areas in medicine with so many advances and so many opportunities. The change was precipitated in 1998, when Michael Hutton and colleagues reported that exon and intron mutations in the tau gene were responsible for many familial forms of FTD. Suddenly, the rich biology of tau, already studied intensely by neurobiologists interested in Alzheimer's disease, was directly linked to a neurodegenerative condition. The importance of the work of scientists like Virginia Lee, John Trojanowski, Maria Spillantini, Kirk Wilhelmsen, Ken Kosik, and Dino Ghetti, who studied the relationship between genes, tau, and FTD came to the forefront of research into dementia. This work also brought FTD into the center of the world's dementia community. This "tau-centric" approach to FTD brought many advances at the clinical and basic level, but the focus on tau tended to ignore the 50% of cases with FTD in whom not tau, but ubiquitin-staining, was evident in neurons.

In the second half of 2006, four new discoveries were reported, generating further excitement and new hope for patients with FTD. First came the finding that missense and null mutations in the progranulin gene were a cause for autosomal dominant forms of FTD, a finding reported simultaneously from the research teams of Michael Hutton and Rosa Rademakers in the United States and

Christine van Broeckhoven in Belgium. These mutations appeared to cause a haploinsufficiency syndrome so that loss of progranulin production from the bad gene led to frontally predominant neurodegeneration. Progranulin's dual role as a growth factor and a molecule involved with inflammation, stimulated new ideas for FTD-related therapies. Within a month of the progranulin discovery, Manuela Neumann, working with John Trojanowski and Virginia Lee at the University of Pennsylvania, showed that FTD patients with tau-negative inclusions usually had neuronal inclusions that contained a DNA-regulating protein, TDP-43. This finding divided FTD into tau positive and TDP-43 positive subtypes. In late 2006, Seeley and colleagues at the University of California, San Francisco (UCSF) described the selective vulnerability of von Economo neurons in both the tau and TDP-43 forms of FTD. These ontologically and phylogenetically new neurons, found only in large-brained social mammals including great apes, humpback whales, and elephants, were selectively decimated in FTD, even in patients relatively early in their disease course. Finally, in 2011 Rosa Rademakers and Bryan Traynor led an international team (that included UCSF) that discovered that most cases of familial FTD-ALS were caused by a huge hexanucleotide repeat that caused an RNA-mediated neurodegenerative disease.

In this book I describe FTD and related disorders from clinical syndrome to basic biology. I hope that this will serve the needs and interests of specialists in neurology, neuropsychology, geriatric medicine, and neuropsychiatry, while bringing in a new audience of readers who are fascinated by the unique biological, psychological, and philosophical perspective offered by FTD.

I was inspired to write this book by many people too numerous to name, in particular the whole UCSF community where science and clinical care are carried out at the highest possible level. For basic science inspiration and friendship I particularly thank my mentors Stanley Prusiner, Stephen Hauser, Lennart Mucke, and Dan Geschwind. Howard Rosen, Joel Kramer, Rosalie Gearhart, Joe Hesse, Jennifer Merrilees, Robin Ketelle, Cindy Barton, Anna Karydas, Marilu Gorno-Tempini, Bill Seeley, Kate Rankin, Gil Rabinovici, Adam Boxer, Lea Grinberg, and Giovanni Coppola work with me daily on finding better diagnoses and treatments for FTD. My wife, Deborah; daughter, Hannah; son, Elliot; and mother, Harriet give me daily joy, and my father, Milton, inspired me to become a physician. The NIH has wisely counseled me on my work, and I am particularly grateful to Tony Phelps, Neil Bucholtz, and Nina Silverberg for seeing value in what I do. The philanthropy from the Consortium for Frontotemporal Dementia inspired by Robin Richards Donohoe and the Tau Consortium inspired by Richard, Todd, and Matt Rainwater have transformed the basic science of FTD. Finally, it was the daily generosity, good spirit, editing, writing, research, and work with figures from Caroline Prioleau Latham that made this book possible. She is one of a kind.

Contents

FRONTOTEMPORAL DEMENTIA

Chapter 1

History and Nomenclature

The birth of neuropsychiatry arrived in Europe around the turn of the nineteenth century. Case histories from Arnold Pick (Pick 1892, 1905), Alois Alzheimer (Alzheimer 1899), Alfons Maria Jakob (Sammet 2008), Carl Wernicke, and Friedrich Lewy (Kawamura et al. 2012) remain fresh and modern, a century after they were written. These early neuroscientists were talented observers who meticulously described the history, mental status, and basic neurological findings of their patients during life, while using new neuropathological techniques to understand the anatomical and histological substrates of the disorder that they had studied while the patient was alive. Findings from these clinical and neuropathological cases were placed into the context of what was known about the brain and helped to further understanding of the anatomy of movement, language, and behavior.

Between the years 1892 and 1922, Pick, Alzheimer, and Pick's students Gans, Onari, and Spatz (Gans 1923, Onari & Spatz 1926) defined the clinical and pathological features

1

of what is now called frontotemporal dementia (FTD). Later, Delay, Brion, and Escourolle in France (Thibodeau & Miller 2012) and Constantinidis from Switzerland brought refinement to our understanding of the differences between Alzheimer's disease (AD) and the frontotemporal dementias. Yet, further advances regarding these conditions stalled until molecular probes for the pathological and genetic substrates of FTD became available in the 1980s. In this chapter I describe the evolution of a nomenclature related to FTD, beginning with Pick's original paper (Pick 1892) (Figure 1–1).

PICK'S DISEASE: THE CONTRIBUTIONS OF ARNOLD PICK

Czech neurologist Arnold Pick (Figure 1–2) first described the clinical syndrome that is now known as FTD. He witnessed a fascinating language syndrome in patients with progressive neurodegenerative disease. In two seminal papers written in 1892 and 1905 (Pick 1892, 1905) Pick outlined a progressive neurodegenerative syndrome in patients where the atrophy was predominantly localized to the anterior temporal lobes (left more than right). Pick's patients suffered from slowly progressive language and behavioral disorders, and he concluded that dementia could be focal and begin with fluent language syndromes. Most of the patients originally described by Pick would be classified today as suffering from the semantic variant of primary progressive aphasia (Gorno-Tempini et al. 2011).

His most prototypical case, Josefa Valchar, was first seen in November 1901. Ms. Valchar was a 58-year-old woman who suffered a 2½-year history of progressive linguistic and behavioral decline, which led to the loss of her job in a tobacco factory. Yet, Pick's patient remained good with arithmetic. She began to bring home objects that she had taken from stores and falsely stated that her long-dead parents were still alive. Although navigational and memory deficits were evident, Pick was particularly impressed by his patient's language disturbance.

Josefa had fluent empty speech, verbal stereotypies, and a profound anomia. For the word "onion" Josefa stated, "that is something to put the potatoes in," and for "head" she noted, "I always forget that." Over time her disorder worsened, and she was rarely able to describe an object unless it was highly familiar. In February 1903 she still knew her first name, Josefa, but could no longer state her surname, Valchar. By autumn 1903 there was no spontaneous language, and word deafness was evident. Josefa died bedridden in December 1903 (Pick 1905).

At autopsy, focal atrophy was seen in the left and right anterior temporal lobes in the second and third temporal gyri. Pick suggested that these regions of the temporal lobes were critical for Josefa Valchar's language syndrome. A fastidious scientist, Pick cautioned that the paucity of similar cases diminished certainty that these specific regions of the temporal lobes were truly critical for aphasia. He hypothesized that Josefa's muteness came from atrophy in Broca's area. Pick's other cases were more elusive, complicated by presentation later in the course of the illness or associated with superimposed vascular events.

In 1911 Alois Alzheimer added a histological perspective to Pick's clinical and anatomical descriptions. He noted the presence of silver-staining "argyrophilic" cytoplasmic inclusions within neurons (Alzheimer 1911).

> Sections prepared with Bielschowsky method show small pyramidal cells containing an argyrophilic, sometimes structure-less ball near the nucleus, whose size varies from half to twice that of the nucleus. The inclusion is either above or below the nucleus, which is displaced accordingly downward or upward. Fibrillary changes are absent in the rest of the cell, the protoplasm and the axonal process are partially visible. (Alzheimer 1911)

In 1922, Gans (Gans 1922) suggested that this focal neurodegenerative condition should be called "Pick's disease." Pick's students Onari and Spatz (Onari and Spatz 1926) expanded on Alzheimer's findings by delineating two distinctive types of inclusions. The first type was round, well delineated, and cytoplasmic and did not alter the structure of neurons. For these inclusions they suggested the term "Pick bodies." For the large blob-like inclusions that filled the neuronal cytoplasm and distorted the

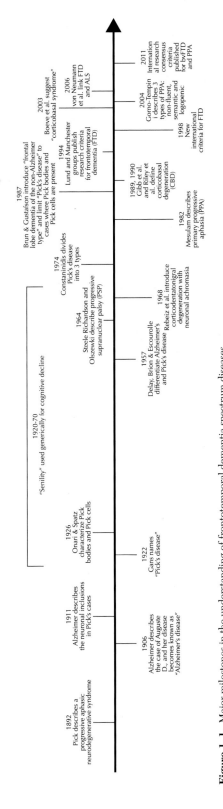

Figure 1–1. Major milestones in the understanding of frontotemporal dementia spectrum diseases.

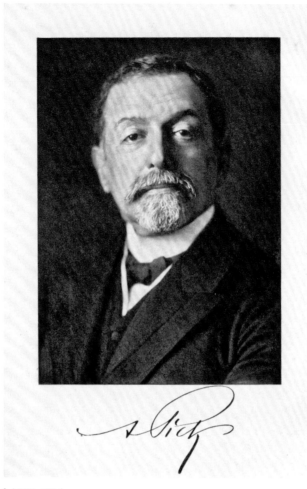

Figure 1–2. Arnold Pick (1851–1924).

neuron's structure they suggested the term "Pick cells" (Figure 1–3).

Sadly, little was added to the pathological description of Pick's disease until the 1990s, when it was determined that the Pick body and the related inclusions seen with corticobasal degeneration and progressive supranuclear palsy had, as the major constituent, the microtubule-associated protein tau (Dickson et al. 1996). Although Pick never emphasized the importance of the histological features of the condition that he originally described, by the 1980s, the silver-staining inclusions discovered by Alzheimer became required for the diagnosis of Pick's disease. The term "Pick's disease," which was meant to be used to describe all clinical and pathological forms of focal frontotemporal neurodegenerative conditions without Alzheimer pathology, became restricted to only cases with classical histological findings of Pick bodies and Pick cells (Dickson et al. 1996). Ultimately, this diminished Pick's seminal contributions to this field and also led to a splintering into multiple subtypes of what was once a unified disorder.

MAINTAINING EARLY TRADITIONS AND REFINING DIAGNOSIS—DELAY, BRION, ESCOUROLLE, MALAMUD, AND CONSTANTINIDIS

The years between 1920 and 1970 were "dark ages" for dementia. The clinical, anatomical, and pathological patterns defined at the turn

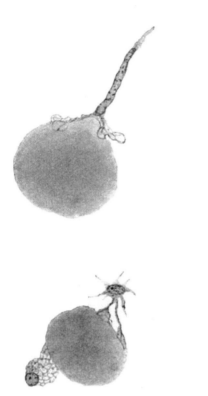

Figure 1–3. Alzheimer's drawings of the silver-staining "argyrophilic" cytoplasmic inclusions within neurons that came to be called "Pick bodies" and "Pick cells" (1911).

of the 19th century for the diagnosis of Pick's disease (and AD) were lost, while "senility" became the overriding term for patients with progressive cognitive decline, whatever the pattern. In Europe the separation of presenile (under 60) and senile dementia was retained, although in the United States this age-related distinction was blurred and eventually lost (Harvey & Rossor 1995). Alvarez and others proposed a vascular (arteriosclerotic) etiology for dementia, and senility became synonymous with a generalized dementing process caused by ministrokes and diminished cerebral perfusion (Jellinger 2007).

When I finished medical school in 1978, I was taught that most dementia in the elderly was arteriosclerotic. The concept of focality in the setting of dementia had largely disappeared!

Yet, the lessons of Pick were not entirely lost. Accurate clinical and pathological diagnosis of Pick's disease and AD was maintained in a few centers. Nathan Malamud in San Francisco collected a neuropathology series of Pick's disease and suggested that some cases were passed

from one generation to the next (Malamud & Waggoner 1943). Sjogren (Sjogren 1951) confirmed this genetic observation that many patients with Pick's disease came from a family where this disorder appeared to be inherited in an autosomal dominant fashion.

In the 1950s, French investigators Delay, Brion, and Escourolle (Delay et al. 1957) reemphasized and refined the clinical and neuropathological similarities and differences between AD and Pick's disease. They held the broad concept of Pick's disease that had been abandoned and included patients with predominantly behavioral, language, cognitive, or extrapyramidal syndromes within the inclusive category of the frontally predominant set of disorders that they called Pick's disease. While 59% of their cases had neuronal swelling, only 20% had classical Pick bodies. Anterior atrophy was the defining feature of this disorder. In contrast to AD, there was an absence of agnosia or apraxia in their patients, while at postmortem plaques and tangles were absent (Thibodeau & Miller 2012).

Constantinidis and colleagues (1974) in Geneva, Switzerland, were strongly influenced by Delay, Brion, and Escourolle, for whom they credited the differentiation of AD and Pick's disease. They divided Pick's disease into three major subtypes. Type 1 was frontoinsular predominant, and many of the cases had classical Pick bodies. A second subtype attacked the frontal convexity, pallidum, substantia nigra, and white matter. Clinically, patients with Pick's disease type 2 exhibited frontal amnesia, gluttony, and stereotyped behavior. Often, extrapyramidal and pyramidal symptoms and dysarthria were seen in this group. They had neuronal swellings but no argyrophilic inclusions. In retrospect, many of those patients would be classified as corticobasal degeneration today. Finally, Pick's disease type 3 had prominent temporal lobe involvement and no neuronal swelling or inclusions. Many of these patients would be called the semantic variant in modern terminology.

Hence, these authors used Pick's disease as an inclusive term that captured patients with frontal, anterior temporal and basal ganglia clinical presentations, in whom AD-pathology was absent. Pick's disease type 1 had Pick bodies, Pick's disease type 2 had neuronal inclusions but not classical Pick bodies or cells, and Pick's disease type 3 exhibited only gliosis and neuronal loss. Unfortunately, this elegant schemata was ignored and quickly forgotten.

SPLINTERING OF PICK'S DISEASE INTO MULTIPLE SUBTYPES

Corticobasal Degeneration (CBD) — Rebeiz, Gibbs, Riley, and Lang

The first entity that was stripped away from the inclusive concept of Pick's disease outlined by Constantinidis was Pick's disease type 2. Rebeiz and colleagues from Boston, Massachusetts (Rebeiz et al. 1967), introduced the term "corticodentatonigral degeneration with neuronal achromasia" to describe what they believed was a novel neurodegenerative condition. The authors described patients with focal parkinsonism, dystonia, and myoclonus. Although they suggested that the patients had "relative sparing of mental facilities," they did not comprehensively assess cognition or behavior. At autopsy there was gross atrophy in the right frontoparietal regions and microscopically swollen neurons that stained poorly. Rebeiz and colleagues called these poorly staining neurons, "neuronal achromasia." They proposed that, "the pallor and swelling of the nerve cells in the cerebral cortex and subcortical structures are reminiscent of the neuronal changes of Pick's disease, but the other features of the disorder are wholly inconsistent with that condition." Whether or not the authors were aware of the work from Escourolle is unclear, but, in retrospect, the entity that they created would have been characterized as a variant of Pick's disease (Pick's disease type 2) using Constantinidis's nomenclature.

Initially, CBD was characterized within the movement disorders community, who emphasized the parietal and movement features of this disease, although few of their patients had CBD confirmed with an autopsy. Gibb (Gibb et al. 1989) and colleagues and Riley, Lang, and colleagues (Riley et al. 1990) defined CBD as "cortical sensory loss, focal reflex myoclonus, alien limb phenomena, apraxia, rigidity and akinesia, a postural-action tremor, limb dystonia, hyperreflexia, and postural instability." Asymmetry was emphasized.

While these criteria proved to be robust for capturing a group of patients with a specific clinical phenotype, the emphasis on parietal findings and asymmetry has ended up describing a mixed cohort, many of whom suffered from AD (see Chapter 6: Related Disorders: Corticobasal Degeneration and Progressive Supranuclear Palsy). Recognizing the limits of this asymmetric extrapyramidal and parietal syndrome for predicting CBD pathology, Boeve and others suggested using the term "corticobasal syndrome" (CBS) for clinically diagnosed cases. At the same time it became apparent that many of the patients who presented with the non-fluent/agrammatic variant of primary progressive aphasia (nfvPPA), and some patients with the behavioral variant of FTD (bvFTD), had CBD. Hence abandonment of Constantinidis's category of Pick's disease type 2 splintered off a Pick's disease subtype while simultaneously blurring the diagnosis of AD and Pick's disease.

Frontal Lobar Dementia of the Non-Alzheimer Type, Dementia of the Frontal Type, Frontotemporal Dementia, and Frontotemporal Lobar Degeneration—Brun Gustafson, Neary, Bowen, Snowden, Mann

The 1970s and 1980s were a time when "dementia" became synonymous with "Alzheimer's disease." The robust correlations between plaque load and dementia in elderly nursing home patients shown by Gary Blessed, Martin Roth, and Bernard Tomlinson reinforced the concept that the plaques and tangles described in early-age-of-onset patients with AD were responsible for dementia in patients over the age of 65 years as well. Similarly, a 1975 landmark paper by Robert Katzman, a neurologist at Albert Einstein School of Medicine in New York, suggested that AD was an epidemic, inferring that the most common cause for dementia was the disease that Alzheimer originally described in patients with presenile dementia (Katzman 1976).

The aging field was presented with two paradigm shifts. First, the vague concept of senility was replaced by a disorder with specific clinical and neuropathological correlates, AD. While this represented a real advance in the field, an unexpected consequence of this shift was that many, particularly investigators in North America, came to believe that there was only one cause for dementia, AD. Pick's disease was ignored, and the phrase "don't pick Pick's disease" was coined, based on the misconception that Pick's disease was rare and indistinguishable from AD during life.

In opposition to this trend, investigators in Lund, Sweden, and Manchester, England, began to systematically characterize large dementia cohorts both clinically and pathologically. This work began in 1957 with Lars Gustafson, a neuropsychiatrist, and David Ingvar, a radiologist (Ingvar et al. 1968; Gustafson et al. 1970), who began a prospective study on dementia using clinical and cerebral blood flow measures to characterize their patients. Soon afterward, Arne Brun, an imaginative neuropathologist trained in Boston by the Russian embryologist Paul Yakovlev, joined Drs. Gustafson and Ingvar. Their findings, first presented in 1974 at an international neuropathology meeting in Budapest, were followed by their first major publication in 1987. Brun and Gustafson found that 20 of 150 consecutive patients evaluated in Lund had a frontally predominant disorder with precentral frontal atrophy. The clinical features of this frontal group included overeating, mental rigidity, childishness, apathy, and social withdrawal. Blood flow studies showed severe hypoperfusion in prefrontal cortex (Brun 1987).

At pathology, while 20% of these patients had classical Pick type changes, 80% had neuronal loss and gliosis, but no Pick bodies. The authors introduced the term "frontal lobe dementia of the non-Alzheimer type" for these patients and suggested that the Pick's disease term be reserved for those patients in whom Pick bodies and Pick cells were present.

In the early 1970s, David Bowen from London, England, began a prospective neurochemical and neuropathological study of patients with presenile dementia. David Neary from Manchester, England, characterized the patient populations with neurobehavioral reports and SPECT imaging. Although the Bowen studies were initially focused around AD, Neary commented on the patients in whom neuropathology showed non-Alzheimer-type changes, approximately 15% of this early-age-of-onset population. Neary, with Julie Snowden, a neuropsychologist, and David Mann, a neuropathologist, organized a large cohort and described the semantic variant of FTD. Working together, the Lund and Manchester groups organized the first research criteria for FTD in 1994. Four years later, an international conference was held outside of Toronto, Canada, where the term "frontotemporal dementia" (FTD) was proposed for the clinical syndromes and "frontotemporal lobar degeneration" (FTLD) for the neuropathological subtypes.

The Lund and Manchester groups played a major role in the history of dementia, formulating large and well-characterized cohorts of patients with a frontally predominant, neurodegenerative disorder. The work came at a time when most investigators were focused around AD, and Pick's disease had been dismissed as rare and impossible to diagnose. Their work showed that Pick's disease and related disorders could be separated from AD both during life and at autopsy. They proved that the use of CT, MRI, and cerebral perfusion along with modern neuropsychiatric and neuropsychological approaches could greatly improve the diagnostic precision for dementia patients during life. They replaced the term "Pick's disease" with "frontotemporal dementia" (FTD) and suggested that Pick's disease be restricted to the patients in whom Pick bodies and Pick cells were present. Finally, they began to formally link amyotrophic lateral sclerosis to FTD.

Primary Progressive Aphasia (PPA)—Marsel Mesulam, Norman Geschwind, John Hodges, Julie Snowden, Karalyn Patterson, and Marilu Gorno-Tempini

By 1972, Norman Geschwind was aware of an aphasic disorder of the temporal lobe that was associated with profound semantic deficits. He elegantly documented such a case in the Yakovlev brain bank in Washington, DC. Yet, to our knowledge, Dr. Geschwind never described his knowledge of semantic dementia in a clinical report. Similarly, in *100 Years of Solitude*, Gabriel García Márquez beautifully wrote about a patient who suffered from a degenerative neurological condition with remarkable parallels to semantic dementia. His book was published in 1967, years before semantic dementia was described in the modern neurological literature.

The first modern neurological report on progressive aphasia came from Marsel Mesulam in 1982 (Mesulam 1982). He described six right-handed patients with a slowly progressive aphasia syndrome for which he coined the term "primary progressive aphasia" (PPA). The initial difficulty was anomic aphasia in five and pure word deafness in the sixth. These patients' predominant atrophy was left perisylvian. A cortical biopsy in one patient showed no neurofibrillary tangles, amyloid plaques, or neuronal inclusions. The research definition for PPA required the presence of a progressive degenerative disorder with selective involvement of language for at least two years with relative sparing of behavior, cognition, and daily function. PPA represented a condition that was distinct from AD.

The groups from Manchester, England, led by Julie Snowden and David Neary (Snowden et al. 1992), and Cambridge, England, led by John Hodges and Karalyn Patterson (Hodges et al. 1992), helped to delineate two major PPA subtypes, one a nonfluent syndrome and one a fluent disorder with prominent semantic deficits. In 2004, Marilu Gorno-Tempini and colleagues at University of California, San Francisco (UCSF) (Gorno-Tempini et al. 2004) reported that there were three major variants of PPA: nonfluent/agrammatic, semantic, and logopenic. They suggested that the nonfluent/agrammatic variant (NFV) and semantic variants (SV) of PPA were true FTD subtypes, while the logopenic variant (LV) was a subtype of AD.

Work from Keith Josephs demonstrated that many patients with the nfvPPA had CBD or progressive supranuclear palsy (PSP) pathology (Josephs et al. 2006). By contrast, recent research has demonstrated that the svPPA nearly always showed TDP-43 pathology. Finally, most of the lvPPA patients have AD neuropathology (Gorno-Tempini et al. 2011).

Progressive aphasia, a syndrome that captivated Pick, now carries the formal name of PPA. PPA is now subtyped into at least three major variants, two of which are associated with non-AD pathology—svPPA and nfvPPA, while the third—the logopenic variant, lvPPA, is usually an asymmetric left, posterior temporal parietal subtype of AD.

UCLA and UCSF Studies

In 1981, Jeffrey Cummings published a paper on the "Human Kluver Bucy Syndrome" based on a clinical review of five patients who died with Pick's disease (Cummings & Duchen 1981). This represented a new behavioral approach to dementia that had all but disappeared in the United States. Encouraged by Drs. Cummings, D. Frank Benson, and Arne Brun, I began systematic studies of FTD while a junior faculty member at University of California, Los Angeles (UCLA), in the mid-1980s in collaboration with neuropsychologist Kyle Boone, psychiatrist Ira Lesser, and SPECT expert Ismael Mena. We studied the clinical and imaging features of FTD versus AD and delineated the anatomical underpinnings for the behavioral and cognitive changes seen in FTD (Miller et al. 1991). Dan Geschwind and Kirk Wilhelmsen helped to expand the scope of this work at a biological level.

More recently, Howard Rosen, David Knopman, and Brad Boeve began important longitudinal and biomarker studies on patient cohorts with FTD. This work is preparing the field for treatment trials that use biomarkers as outcome measures (Knopman et al. 2008).

THE BIOLOGICAL REVOLUTION

Genetics

TAU

The genetic basis of Pick's disease, previously noted by Malamud and Sjogren, was confirmed when Wilhelmsen and colleagues linked a small region on chromosome 17 to the clinical phenotype of FTD (Wilhelmsen et al. 1994). Soon afterward investigative teams from Seattle, Cambridge, UCSF, UCLA, and the Mayo Clinic showed that tau gene mutations caused chromosome-17 linked familial FTD. One truly novel aspect of these findings was the discovery of Michael Hutton and colleagues (Grover et al. 1999) that intron mutations adjacent to exon 10 could lead to abnormal splicing of tau and an excessive concentration of 4R tau in neurons and glia (Figure 1–4). This demonstrated at a mechanistic level how a tau mutation could lead to neuronal degeneration. Studies from John van Swieten in Holland and the Mayo Clinic team found that tau mutations accounted for approximately one-quarter of all familial forms. Family cases were similar to what was seen with sporadic forms of FTD; presentations in familial cases ranged from classical FTD to PPA, CBD, and

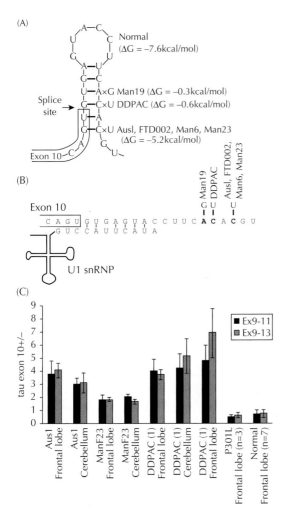

Figure 1–4. The splice site in **(A)**, the predicted stem–loop structure, and **(B)**, the linear form. Mutations are marked and the predicted free energy of the stem–loop is indicated. Predicted binding of U1 snRNP to the 5′ splice site is shown. **(C)** RT-PCR analysis of the molar ratio between tau mRNA with and without exon 10. RNA from frontal lobe (4 cases) and cerebellum (3 cases) from FTDP-17 brains with splice mutations (DDPAC (2), ManF23 and Aus1) has ratios >1.6 (left, 14 bars): RNA from frontal lobe of normal brains (n = 7) and P301L mutation brains has ratios <0.8 (right, 4 bars). Analysis of total tau mRNA revealed no significant differences. (Hutton et al. 1998.)

PSP-like syndromes. Amyotrophic lateral sclerosis (ALS) was rarely described.

PROGRANULIN

Tau mutations proved responsible for many of the familial forms of FTD, but some chromosome 17–linked families were found in whom no tau mutations were present. Six years after the discovery of mutations in tau, two different scientific teams, one led by Michael Hutton at Mayo Clinic (Baker et al. 2006) and the other by Christina van Brookhoeven in Belgium (Cruts et al. 2006) reported on mutations in progranulin, a gene adjacent to tau on chromosome 17. Progranulin mutations proved to be as common as tau mutations, accounting for approximately one-quarter of all autosomal dominant cases of FTD and nearly 5% of all FTD. When these mutations in progranulin were reported, little had been written about this molecule, but it was known that progranulin had both cell survival and inflammation-related functions.

Unlike tau, where the mutations led to excessive aggregation of phosphorylated forms of this protein, progranulin mutations work via a haploinsufficiency mechanism. Nonsense, frameshift, and promoter mutations in progranulin cause one chromosome to underproduce progranulin, and this decrement in brain progranulin triggers abnormal aggregation of the TDP-43 protein within the neuronal nucleus and cytoplasm.

The clinical phenotype of progranulin was similar to what was seen with tau with FTD, PPA, CBD, and PSP-like presentations. How the deficiency in progranulin leads to cell death is still under active study, but it appears that the whole progranulin molecule has growth and anti-inflammatory effects, while the granulins that are cleaved from progranulin are pro-inflammatory (Ward & Miller 2011). The exact contribution of the growth, anti-inflammatory, and pro-inflammatory aspect of this molecule is under study (Figure 1–5).

C9ORF72

This is the most recently discovered and most prevalent FTD gene. In 2000, Hosler and colleagues led by Bob Brown at Harvard (Hosler et al. 2000) linked a familial form of FTD and ALS to a region on chromosome 9. Subsequently, many other families with varied mixtures of FTD, ALS, or both FTD-ALS were linked to this same region. In late 2011 two international consortia simultaneously reported on finding a large hexanucleotide repeat mutation expansion in the non-coding GGGGCC repeat in gene *C9ORF72* (Figure 1–6).

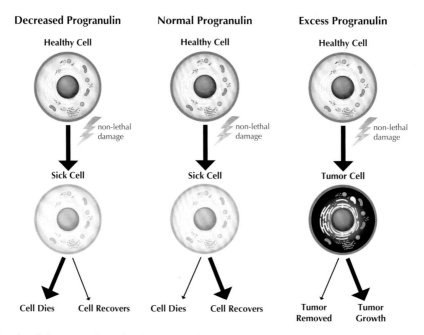

Figure 1–5. The whole progranulin molecule appears to have growth and anti-inflammatory effects on cells.

The expansion in the open reading frame is very large (over 400 repeats), and it appears to cause disease via RNA-mediated neurodegeneration leading to toxic gain of function. Other diseases with a similar mechanism are myotonic dystrophy and fragile X-associated tremor/ataxia syndrome. With those diseases, these large mRNA segments cause transcriptional alterations, appear to sequester mRNA-associated protein complexes, and disrupt transcription of multiple proteins. This mutation is found more commonly at UCSF than all of the other FTD mutations combined. While the phenotype associated with this mutation is still being determined, many of the cases present with a neuropsychiatric syndrome such as bipolar illness and eventually go on to develop bvFTD or ALS. Some gene carriers also develop extrapyramidal findings such as dystonia in association with the FTD or ALS. Other unique features of this mutation are proneness for thalamic, occipital, and cerebellar disease (Sha et al. 2012).

VCP (CHROMOSOME 9), *ESCRT2* (CHROMOSOME 3), AND *EXT2*

Other mutations causing autosomal dominant forms of FTD have been found. Valosin,

produced by *VCP* on chromosome 9, is involved with protein processing and mitochondrial function, and its missense mutation can cause Paget's disease, an inclusion body myositis, or an FTD syndrome (30% of all cases) (Kimonis et al. 2008) We have reported on a patient with osteosarcomas, myopathy, and FTD associated with a mutation in *EXT2* (Narvid et al. 2009).

There is a large Danish family with a mutation in a protein involved with protein processing (ESCRT2). Additionally in 2012 Teepu Siddique found two new genes related to FTD and ALS, *Sequestosome 1* (*SQSTM1*) and *Ubiquilin-2* (*UBQLN2*) (Fecto & Siddique 2012). These genes are likely to explain small number of cases, but may prove valuable for understanding the two diseases at a mechanistic level (see Chapter 8: FTD Genes). Much less common than tau and progranulin, there is still little known about the clinical and molecular phenotype of these rare genetic causes for FTD (Figure 1–7).

OTHER FTD-ALS GENES

Just as the mutations in tau and progranulin proved strong links between the atypical parkinsonian syndromes PSP and CBD,

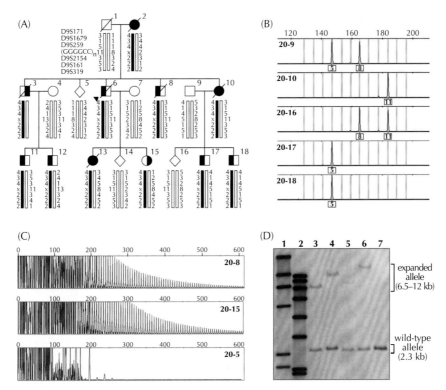

Figure 1–6. Expanded GGGGCC hexanucleotide repeat in *C9ORF72* causes FTD and ALS linked to chromosome 9p in family VSM-20. **(A)** Segregation of GGGGCC repeat in *C9ORF72* and flanking genetic markers in disguised linkage pedigree of family VSM-20. The arrowhead denotes the proband. For the GGGGCC repeat, numbers indicate hexanucleotide repeat units and the X denotes that the allele could not be detected. Black symbols represent patients affected with frontotemporal dementia (left side filled), amyotrophic lateral sclerosis (right side filled), or both. White symbols represent unaffected individuals or at-risk individuals with unknown phenotype. Haplotypes for individuals 20-1, 20-2, and 20-3 are inferred from genotype data of siblings and offspring. **(B)** Fluorescent fragment length analyses of a PCR fragment containing the GGGGCC repeat in *C9ORF72*. PCR products from the unaffected father (20-9), affected mother (2-10), and their offspring (20-16, 20-17, and 20-18) are shown illustrating the lack of transmission from the affected parent to affected offspring. Numbers under the peaks indicate number of GGGGCC hexanucleotide repeats. **(C)** PCR products of repeat-primed PCR reactions separated on an ABI3730 DNA Analyzer and visualized by GENEMAPPER software. Electropherograms are zoomed to 2,000 relative fluorescence units to show stutter amplification. Two expanded repeat carriers (20-8 and 20-15) and one noncarrier (20-5) from family VSM-20 are shown. **(D)** Southern blotting of four expanded repeat carriers and one noncarrier from family member of VSM-20 using genomic DNA extracted from lymphoblast cell lines. Lane 1 shows DIG-labeled DNA Molecular Weight Marker II (Roche) with fragments of 2,027; 2,322; 4,361; 6,557; 9,416; 23,130 bp. Lane 2 shows DIG-labeled DNA Molecular Weight Marker VII (Roche) with fragments of 1,882; 1,953; 2,799; 3,639; 4,899; 6,106; 7,427; and 8,576 bp. Patients with expanded repeats (lanes 3–6) show an additional allele from 6.5–12 kb, while a normal relative (lane 7) only shows the expected 2.3 kb wild-type allele.

there are a number of genes associated with both FTD and ALS. Families with these mutations show large variability in the age of onset and the clinical phenotype, with some individuals manifesting ALS and FTD, others developing only ALS or only FTD. The first known ALS mutation, superoxide dismutase (*SOD*), does not usually lead to FTD; and while mutations in dynactin and *TARDBP* typically cause ALS, FTD syndromes can emerge with these mutations. Fused in sarcoma (*FUS*) mutations cause familial forms of ALS, while FUS aggregates have been linked to a subtype of FTD that occurs in very young patients. More recently, intermediate repeats of *Ataxin-2* (*ATXN2*) were shown to predispose to both ALS and FTD (see Chapter 7: A Primer of FTLD Neuropathology; Chapter 8: FTD Genes).

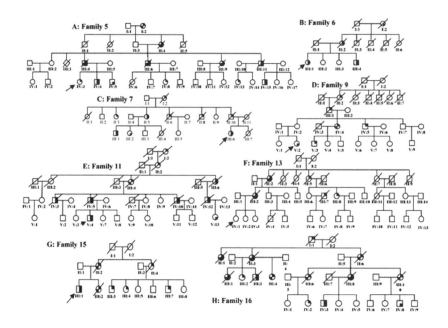

Figure 1–7. Pedigrees of IBMPFD families. The filled in top right corner of a symbol represents myopathy, the bottom right corner of a symbol represents Paget disease of the bone (PDB), and the bottom left corner of a symbol represents frontotemporal dementia (FTD). (Kimonis et al. 2008.)

Neuropathology

FROM PICK BODIES TO TAU

The neuropathological schemata of Pick, Alzheimer, Gans, Onari, and Spatz defined Pick's disease quite broadly to include a wide variety of patients with neurodegenerative disease. In the 1980s, Arne Brun began to subtype FTD. Dr. Brun clarified that the dominant form of FTD was not associated with Pick bodies and restricted the term "Pick's disease" to those FTD patients in whom the classical Pick bodies and Pick cells were present.

In the mid-1980s, it was discovered that the neuronal aggregates in PSP, CBD, Pick bodies, and the neurofibrillary tangles in AD all stained for tau. Ghetti, Delacourte, Kosik, Iqbal, Wisniewski, Binder, Ihara, Brion, Dickson, Lee, Trojanowski, and Selkoe all played an important role in delineating the important role of tau in neurodegeneration. It was soon discovered that many of the neuronal inclusions within neurons of patients dying with frontotemporal lobar degeneration (FTLD) neuropathology were not classical "Pick bodies" but were tau positive.

Suddenly a group of disorders with neuropathological inclusions with variable histological features were joined together by a specific molecule, tau. With the realization that tau mutations could cause FTD, staining with tau became a routine part of the neuropathological assessment of a dementia patient. Yet, FTD is not strictly a disorder of tau, and 50% of patients with FTD have inclusions that are ubiquitin-positive but tau-negative. One subtype of FTD in whom ubiquitin inclusions almost never stained positively for tau was the group of patients with FTD and ALS (Liscic et al. 2008).

It took more than 20 years to discover the major constituent of those tau-negative aggregates. In 2006 a hallmark study from Neumann and colleagues (Neumann et al. 2006) working in the laboratory of Virginia Lee, demonstrated that most of the ubiquitin-positive inclusions not staining for tau in FTD were positive for the RNA-binding protein TDP-43 (Figure 1–8). Not only were FTD cases positive for TDP-43, but the same was true for most of the inclusions in patients with sporadic (and familial ALS). Hence, FTD and ALS, already linked at a clinical level, were firmly associated molecularly as

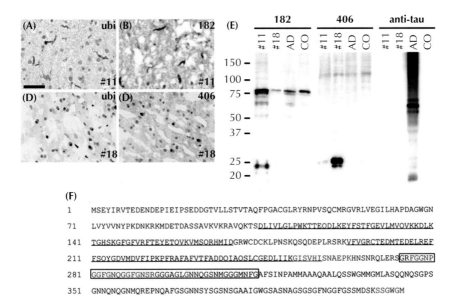

Figure 1–8. Identification of TDP-43 as the major disease protein in UBIs of FTLD-U. **(A to D)** mAb 182 specifically labeled neuritic UBIs in FTLD-U type 1 **(A and B)**, whereas mAb 406 immunostained UBIs in FTLD-U type 2 cases **(C and D)**. Scale bar in **(A)** corresponds to 25 µm for **(A)** to **(D)**. **(E)** mAbs 182 and 406 detected disease-specific bands ~24 kD and ~26 kD, respectively, in frontal gray matter urea fractions of FTLD-U type 1 and type 2 but not in those of AD or CO, whereas tau mAbs T14/46 detected only hyperphosphorylated AD tau. **(F)** Amino acid sequence of TDP-43 (accession no. NP_031401, Entrez Protein) depicting the two RNA-recognition motifs (underlined), glycine-rich sequence (boxed), and peptide sequences identified through LC-MS/MS analysis (red highlights). (Neumann et al. 2006.)

well. Ian Mackenzie and Manuela Neumann and colleagues completed the FTD-ALS story by showing that most of the patients in whom the ubiquitin inclusions were negative for TDP-43 had aggregates of the FUS protein, a protein that had recently been linked to ALS (Mackenzie et al. 2011).

ANATOMY AND PHYLOGENY: BRUN AND SEELEY

Paul Yakovlev's imaginative work on the ontogeny and phylogeny of the human brain (Yakovlev 1968) had a lasting influence on Arne Brun when the two worked together at Harvard. While studying FTD brains, Brun noticed that the most severe gliosis and neuronal loss in FTD were localized to the first three frontal layers. He went on to suggest that the late migration of neurons to the superficial frontal regions during embryogenesis might have made these brain regions particularly vulnerable to this neurodegenerative condition. Although this hypothesis remains unproven, it was one of the first attempts to explain a

neurodegenerative condition via an ontological theory (Brun 2007).

In 2006, Bill Seeley at UCSF (Seeley et al. 2006) made the remarkable discovery that long spindly neurons originally localized to the frontoinsular region by Konstantin von Economo were selectively vulnerable in patients with FTD. These von Economo neurons (VENs) became a source of great scientific fascination when John Allman and colleagues at California Institute of Technology discovered that VENs were phylogenetically new—present only in great apes and greatly expanded in humans. Seeley has pioneered exciting research into these neurons, attempting to understand why they are selectively vulnerable in FTD and how FTD spreads from this region (Seeley et al. 2011) (Figure 1–9).

FTD NOW: WHERE ARE WE?

FTD remains a fascinating, yet still relatively poorly understood, neurodegenerative

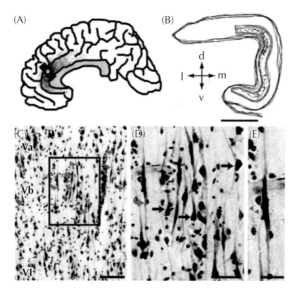

Figure 1–9. Anterior cingulate sampling site and von Economo neuron (VEN) characteristics in control subjects. **(A)** VENs are distributed throughout the mid- and anterior cingulate cortex. Dots, drawn schematically based on previous work, highlight the increasing posterior-to-anterior VEN gradient in the normal brain. For this study, tissue blocks were cut from the pregenual anterior cingulate cortex (ACC) (asterisk). **(B)** ACC VEN distribution in a representative nonneurological control subject. Overlaid contours of the ACC (outer) and Layer 5 (red, inner) were manually traced on 5 to 10 sections per subject. Dots represent VENs, which are concentrated in the crowns of the gyrus. **(C–E)** VENs (curved red arrows in **C**) are located in Layer 5b and are distinguished from neighboring neurons (e.g., straight black arrows in **D**) by their large size and bipolar dendritic architecture. VENs form vertically oriented clusters, often adjacent to small arterioles. Box in **(C)** is magnified in **(D)**. One of six VENs in **(D)** is highlighted (curved red arrow) and magnified in **(E)** to show the typical VEN morphology, including a large VEN axon (red arrowheads). Cresyl violet stain. Scale bars = 3mm **B**, 100μm **C**, 50μm **D**, and 25μm **E**. Photomicrographs are oriented with the pial surface at the top. d = dorsal; l = lateral, m = medial, v = ventral. (Seeley et al. 2006.)

condition that selectively attacks the frontal and anterior temporal regions. There are three major clinical presentations, all determined by the site of their regional onset. bvFTD is a right frontally predominant disorder that begins as a behavioral syndrome, the nonfluent/agrammatic variant is left frontoinsular predominant and the semantic variant begins in the anterior temporal regions. While FTD is classified based on its cortical onset, the basal ganglia including the substantia nigra, caudate, putamen, and nucleus accumbens are also involved early in the course of FTD. Similarly, a subtype of FTD is associated with selective vulnerability of motor neurons, a subtype associated with ALS.

Genetic and neuropathological approaches are beginning to clarify the etiology and pathogenesis of FTLD. Once considered a single biological etiology with a predilection for the front parts of the brain, FTLD is now understood to be a collection of disorders with distinctive genetics and neuropathology where the attack often goes beyond the frontotemporal regions.

Although approximately 60% of FTD does not appear to have a strongly familial component, the autosomal dominant forms of FTD, representing approximately 10% of all cases, have shed huge insights into FTD (Chow et al. 1999). Tau and progranulin represent the two major disease-causing mutations. Tau mutations lead to a toxic gain of function (Hong et al. 1998). By contrast, progranulin mutations cause a haploinsufficiency syndrome mediated by nonsense-mediated decay of progranulin (Ward & Miller 2011). Finally, the other major FTD-causing mutation, *C9ORF72*, causes neurodegeneration by generating long mRNA repeats that appear to poison nuclear function (DeJesus-Hernandez et al. 2011).

The careful phenotyping of FTD has led to interesting clinical pathological correlates. The bvFTD syndrome is associated with both tau and TDP-43 aggregates with approximately equal frequency; nearly all of the aggregates in svPPA are TDP-43 positive; the majority of nfvPPA cases show tau-positive pathology (CBD or PSP), and many other cases have TDP-43 as the major inclusion.

THE FUTURE

In many ways the study of FTD has lagged behind AD. With AD, the clinical and neuropathological diagnostic nomenclature systems are simple, and a clinical diagnosis is predicated on the assumption that the neuropathology consists of plaques and tangles. With FTD, the current nomenclature system is complex, and a clinical diagnosis does not easily translate into a definitive molecular or neuropathological entity. While the syndrome of svPPA usually predicts a nongenetic disorder with TDP type C inclusions, the patient with bvFTD can have mutations in tau, progranulin, TDP-43, valosin, or *C9ORF72* or be sporadic in etiology. Similarly, the pathology can be due to all of the major tau, TDP-43, or FUS subtypes.

Ultimately FTD will need a molecular classification system, as the different clinical subtypes will require different therapies. While most of the major mutations associated with FTD have been discovered and can be measured in clinical laboratories, susceptibility genes are still unknown. Similarly, molecular probes from the blood and spinal fluid or neuroimaging approaches are needed to help with a molecule-based prediction of neuropathology. Tau imaging is in its infancy but should be extremely helpful for defining tau-related cases of FTD whether the clinical presentation is bvFTD, PPA, PSP, or CBD.

Early diagnosis continues to be difficult, and many patients progress over many decades before they receive an accurate diagnosis. Subtle changes in personality lead to formal psychiatric diagnoses of bipolar illness or schizophrenia, and then functional impairment begins, finally becoming a case of bvFTD. Effective treatment will require early interventions and recognition of the molecular etiology in the prodromal, or possibly even preprodromal, phase. Functional connectivity mapping appears promising as an early marker, but more research will be needed to determine the most sensitive and specific pathways to early diagnosis of the FTD syndromes.

Finally, research into the pathogenesis and treatment of FTD is still in its infancy. Mouse models of the tau, progranulin, and TDP genetic forms of FTD have been created and appear to be the first step toward rational therapies. There are now neurons derived from skin cells (iPS), yeast, worm, fly, and mouse models of FTD (Kao et al. 2011). Tau-focused therapies for PSP are already underway, and progranulin-raising therapies are planned for patients with progranulin mutations (Cenik et al. 2011). The TDP-43, FUS, *C9ORF72*, and FTD-MND forms of FTLD appear to involve dysregulation of DNA and RNA and will be formidable to treat, although siRNA and other approaches to therapy are beginning. The day will come when susceptibility to FTD is determined at birth and prevented.

REFERENCES

Alzheimer A. Über eigenartige Krankheitsfälle des späteren Alters. Z Gesamte Neurol Psychiatr. 1911;4:356–85.

Alzheimer A. A contribution concerning the pathological anatomy of mental disturbances in old age, 1899. Alzheimer Dis Assoc Disord. 1991;5(2):69–70.

Baker M, Mackenzie IR, Pickering-Brown SM, Gass J, Rademakers R, Lindholm C, Snowden J, Adamson J, Sadovnick AD, Rollinson S, Cannon A, Dwosh E, Neary D, Melquist S, Richardson A, Dickson D, Berger Z, Eriksen J, Robinson T, Zehr C, Dickey CA, Crook R, McGowan E, Mann D, Boeve B, Feldman H, Hutton M. Mutations in progranulin cause tau-negative frontotemporal dementia linked to chromosome 17. Nature. 2006;442:916–9.

Brun A. Frontal lobe degeneration of non-Alzheimer type. I. Neuropathology. Arch Gerontol Geriatr. 1987;6(3):193–208.

Brun A. Identification and characterization of frontal lobe degeneration: historical perspective on the development of FTD. Alzheimer Dis Assoc Disord. 2007;21(4):S3–4.

Cenik B, Sephton CF, Dewey CM, Xian X, Wei S, Yu K, Niu W, Coppola G, Coughlin SE, Lee SE, Dries DR, Almeida S, Geschwind DH, Gao FB, Miller BL, Farese RV, Posner BA, Yu G, Herz J. Suberoylanilide hydroxamic acid (vorinostat) Cenik up-regulates progranulin transcription: rational therapeutic approach to frontotemporal dementia. J Biol Chem. 2011;286(18):16101–8.

Chow TW, Miller BL, Hayashi VN, Geschwind DH. Inheritance of frontotemporal dementia. Arch Neurol. 1999;56(7):817–22.

Constantinidis JJ, Richard J, Tissot R. Pick's disease: histological and clinical correlations. Eur Neurol. 1974;11(4):208–17.

Cruts M, Gijselinck I, van der Zee J, Engelborghs S, Wils H, Pirici D, Rademakers R, Vandenberghe R, Dermaut B, Martin JJ, van Duijn C, Peeters K,

Sciot R, Santens P, De Pooter T, Mattheijssens M, Van den Broeck M, Cuijt I, Vennekens K, De Deyn PP, Kumar-Singh S, Van Broeckhoven C. Null mutations in progranulin cause ubiquitin-positive frontotemporal dementia linked to chromosome 17q21. Nature. 2006;442(7105):920–4.

Cummings JL, Duchen LW. Kluver-Bucy syndrome in Pick disease: clinical and pathologic correlations. Neurology. 1981;31(11):1415–22.

DeJesus-Hernandez M, Mackenzie IR, Boeve BF, Boxer AL, Baker M, Rutherford NJ, Nicholson AM, Finch NA, Flynn H, Adamson J, Kouri N, Wojtas A, Sengdy P, Hsiung GY, Karydas A, Seeley WW, Josephs KA, Coppola G, Geschwind DH, Wszolek ZK, Feldman H, Knopman DS, Petersen RC, Miller BL, Dickson DW, Boylan KB, Graff-Radford NR, Rademakers R. Expanded GGGGCC hexanucleotide repeat in noncoding region of C9ORF72 causes chromosome 9p-linked FTD and ALS. Neuron. 2011;72(2):245–56.

Delay J, Brion S, Escourolle R. [Anatomo-clinical opposition between Pick's disease and Alzheimer's disease; diagnostic value of complementary examinations]. Presse Med. 1957;65:1515–8.

Dickson DW, Feany MB, Yen SH, Mattiace LA, Davies P. Cytoskeletal pathology in non-Alzheimer degenerative dementia: new lesions in diffuse Lewy body disease, Pick's disease, and corticobasal degeneration. J Neural Transm Suppl. 1996;47:31–46.

Fecto F, Siddique T. UBQLN2/P62 cellular recycling pathways in amyotrophic lateral sclerosis and frontotemporal dementia. Muscle Nerve. 2012;45:157–62.

Gans A. Betrachtungen über Art und Ausbreitung des krankhaften Prozesses in einem Fall von Pickscher Atrophie des Stirnhirns. Zeitschrift für die gesamte Neurologie und Psychiatrie. 1923;80:10–28.

Gibb WR, Luthert PJ, Marsden CD. Corticobasal degeneration. Brain. 1989;112:1171–92.

Gorno-Tempini ML, Dronkers NF, Rankin KP, Ogar JM, Phengrasamy L, Rosen HJ, Johnson JK, Weiner MW, Miller BL. Cognition and anatomy in three variants of primary progressive aphasia. Ann Neurol. 2004;55:335–46.

Gorno-Tempini ML, Hillis AE, Weintraub S, Kertesz A, Mendez M, Cappa SF, Ogar JM, Rohrer JD, Black S, Boeve BF, Manes F, Dronkers NF, Vandenberghe R, Rascovsky K, Patterson K, Miller BL, Knopman DS, Hodges JR, Mesulam MM, Grossman M. Classification of primary progressive aphasia and its variants. Neurology. 2011;76:1006–14.

Grover A, Houlden H, Baker M, Adamson J, Lewis J, Prihar G, Pickering-Brown S, Duff K, Hutton M. 5' splice site mutations in tau associated with the inherited dementia FTDP-17 affect a stem-loop structure that regulates alternative splicing of exon 10. J Biol Chem. 1999;274:15134–43.

Gustafson L, Hagberg B, Holley JW, Risberg J, Ingvar DH. Regional cerebral blood flow in organic dementia with early onset. Correlations with psychiatric symptoms and psychometric variables. Acta Neurol Scand. 1970;46:Suppl 43:74–5.

Harvey RJ, Rossor MN. Does early-onset Alzheimer disease constitute a distinct subtype? The contribution of molecular genetics. Alzheimer Dis Assoc Disord. 1995;9:S7–13.

Hodges JR, Patterson K, Oxbury S, Funnell E. Semantic dementia. Progressive fluent aphasia with temporal lobe atrophy. Brain. 1992;115:1783–806.

Hong M, Zhukareva V, Vogelsberg-Ragaglia V, Wszolek Z, Reed L, Miller B, Geschwind D, Bird T, McKeel D, Goate A, Morris J, Wilhelmsen K, Schellenberg GD, Trojanowski J, Lee V. Mutation-specific functional impairments in distinct tau isoforms of hereditary FTDP-17. Science. 1998;282(5395):1914–17.

Hosler BA, Siddique T, Sapp PC, Sailor W, Huang MC, Hossain A, Daube JR, Nance M, Fan C, Kaplan J, Hung WY, McKenna-Yasek D, Haines JL, Pericak-Vance MA, Horvitz HR, Brown RH Jr. Linkage of familial amyotrophic lateral sclerosis with frontotemporal dementia to chromosome 9q21-q22. JAMA. 2000;284:1664–9.

Hutton M, Lendon CL, Rizzu P, Baker M, Froelich S, Houlden H, Pickering-Brown S, Chakraverty S, Isaacs A, Grover A, Hackett J, Adamson J, Lincoln S, Dickson D, Davies P, Petersen RC, Stevens M, de Graaff E, Wauters E, van Baren J, Hillebrand M, Joosse M, Kwon JM, Nowotny P, Che LK, Norton J, Morris JC, Reed LA, Trojanowski J, Basun H, Lannfelt L, Neystat M, Fahn S, Dark F, Tannenberg T, Dodd PR, Hayward N, Kwok JB, Schofield PR, Andreadis A, Snowden J, Craufurd D, Neary D, Owen F, Oostra BA, Hardy J, Goate A, van Swieten J, Mann D, Lynch T, Heutink P. Association of missense and 5'-splice-site mutations in tau with the inherited dementia FTDP-17. Nature. 1998;393:702–5.

Ingvar D, Obrist W, Chivian E, Cronquist S, Risberg J, Gustafson L, Hägerdal M, Wittbom-Cigén G. General and regional abnormalities of cerebral blood flow in senile and "presenile" dementia. Scand J Clin Lab Invest Suppl. 1968;102:XII:B.

Jellinger KA. The enigma of vascular cognitive disorder and vascular dementia. Acta Neuropathologica. 2007; 113(4):349–88.

Josephs KA, Duffy JR, Strand EA, Whitwell JL, Layton KF, Parisi JE, Hauser MF, Witte RJ, Boeve BF, Knopman DS, Dickson DW, Jack CR Jr, Petersen RC. Clinicopathological and imaging correlates of progressive aphasia and apraxia of speech. Brain. 2006;129:1385–98.

Kao AW, Eisenhut RJ, Martens LH, Nakamura A, Huang A, Bagley JA, Zhou P, de Luis A, Neukomm LJ, Cabello J, Farese RV Jr, Kenyon C. A neurodegenerative disease mutation that accelerates the clearance of apoptotic cells. Proc Natl Acad Sc USA. 2011;108(11):4441–6.

Katzman R. Editorial: The prevalence and malignancy of Alzheimer disease. A major killer. Arch Neurol. 1976;33:217–8.

Kawamura M, Nakano I, Mizuno Y. Studies on Lewy bodies on their 100th year: a discussion. Brain Nerve. 2012;64(4):474–85.

Kimonis VE, Mehta SG, Fulchiero EC, Thomasova D, Pasquali M, Boycott K, Neilan EG, Kartashov A, Forman MS, Tucker S, Kimonis K, Mumm S, Whyte MP, Smith CD, Watts GD. Clinical studies in familial VCP myopathy associated with Paget disease of bone and frontotemporal dementia. Am J Med Genet. 2008;146A:745–57.

Knopman DS, Kramer JH, Boeve BF, Caselli RJ, Graff-Radford NR, Mendez MF, Miller BL, Mercaldo N. Development of methodology for conducting clinical trials in frontotemporal lobar degeneration. Brain. 2008;131(Pt 11):2957–68.

Liscic RM, Grinberg LT, Zidar J, Gitcho MA, Cairns NJ. ALS and FTLD: two faces of TDP-43 proteinopathy. Eur J Neurol. 2008;15:772–80.

Mackenzie IR, Munoz DG, Kusaka H, Yokota O, Ishihara K, Roeber S, Kretzschmar HA, Cairns NJ, Neumann M. Distinct pathological subtypes of FTLD-FUS. Acta Neuropathol. 2011;121(2):207–18.

Malamud N, Waggoner RW. Geneaologic and clinico-pathologic study of Pick's disease. Arch Neur Psych. 1943;50(3):288–303.

Mesulam MM. Slowly progressive aphasia without generalized dementia. Ann Neurol. 1982;11:592–8.

Miller BL, Cummings JL, Villanueva-Meyer J, Boone K, Mehringer CM, Lesser IM, Mena I. Frontal lobe degeneration: clinical, neuropsychological, and SPECT characteristics. Neurology. 1991;41(9):1374–82.

Narvid J, Gorno-Tempini ML, Slavotinek A, Dearmond SJ, Cha YH, Miller BL, Rankin K. Of brain and bone: the unusual case of Dr. A. Neurocase. 2009;15(3):190–205.

Neumann M, Sampathu DM, Kwong LK, Truax AC, Micsenyi MC, Chou TT, Bruce J, Schuck T, Grossman M, Clark CM, McCluskey LF, Miller BL, Masliah E, Mackenzie IR, Feldman H, Feiden W, Kretzschmar HA, Trojanowski JQ, Lee VM. Ubiquitinated TDP-43 in frontotemporal lobar degeneration and amyotrophic lateral sclerosis. Science. 2006;314:130–3.

Onari K, Spatz H. Anatomische Beitrage zur Lehre von der Pickschen umschriebenen Grosshirnrinden-Atrophie ("Picksche Krankheit"). Z Gesamte Neurol Psych. 1926;101:470–511.

Pick A. Über die Beziehungen der senilen Hirnatrophie zur Aphasie. Prag Med Wochenschr. 1892;17:165–7.

Pick A. Zur symptomatologie der linksseitigen Schlafenlappenatrophie. Monatsschr Psychiatr Neurologie. 1905;16:378–88.

Rebeiz JJ, Kolodny EH, Richardson EP Jr. Corticoden-tatonigral degeneration with neuronal achromasia: a progressive disorder of late adult life. Trans Am Neurol Assoc. 1967;92:23–6.

Riley DE, Lang AE, Lewis A, Resch L, Ashby P, Hornykiewicz O, Black S. Cortical-basal ganglionic degeneration. Neurology. 1990;40(8):1203–12.

Sammet K. Alfons Jakob (1884–1931). J Neurol. 2008;255(11):1852–3.

Seeley WW, Carlin DA, Allman JM, Macedo MN, Bush C, Miller BL, Dearmond SJ. Early frontotemporal dementia targets neurons unique to apes and humans. Ann Neurol. 2006;60:660–7.

Sha SJ, Takada LT, Rankin KP, Yokoyama JS, Rutherford NJ, Fong JC, Khan B, Karydas A, Baker MC, Dejesus-Hernandez M, Pribadi M, Coppola G, Geschwind DH, Rademakers R, Lee SE, Seeley W, Miller BL, Boxer AL. Frontotemporal dementia due to C9ORF72 mutations: Clinical and imaging features. Neurology. 2012;79:1002–11.

Sjogren H. Alzheimer disease-Pick's disease: a clinical analysis of 72 cases. Acta Psychiatr Neurol Scand Suppl. 1951;74:189–92.

Snowden JS, Neary D, Mann DM, Goulding PJ, Testa HJ. Progressive language disorder due to lobar atrophy. Ann Neurol. 1992;31:174–83.

Thibodeau MP, Miller BL. "Limits and current knowledge of Pick's disease: Its differential diagnosis" A translation of the 1957 Delay, Brion, Escourolle article. Neurocase. 2012 May 4. [Epub ahead of print]

Ward ME, Miller BL. Potential mechanisms of progranulin-deficient FTLD. J Mol Neurosci. 2011;45:574–82.

Wilhelmsen KC, Lynch T, Pavlou E, Higgins M, Nygaard TG. A localization of disinhibition-dementia-parkinsonism-amyotrophy complex to 17q21-22. Am J Hum Genet. 1994;55(6):1159–65.

Yakovlev PI. Telencephalon "impar," "semipar" and "totopar." (Morphogenetic, tectogenetic and architectonic definitions). Int J Neurol. 1968;6(3–4):245–65.

Chapter 2

The Clinical Syndrome of bvFTD

OVERVIEW

Behavioral variant frontotemporal dementia (bvFTD) is the most common clinical phenotype associated with frontotemporal lobar degeneration (FTLD) pathology, accounting for approximately 60% of FTD-spectrum cases (Johnson et al. 2005). The profound changes in personality and behavior that characterize bvFTD have a devastating effect on the patient and their loved ones. Additionally, bvFTD has proven to be a fascinating disorder with clinical overlap with many psychiatric disorders ranging from schizophrenia, bipolar illness, borderline personality disorder, obsessive-compulsive disorder, and addictive disorders.

Often, patients with bvFTD will present to a physician with midlife behavioral and personality changes. Yet, before these visits occur, there has been a profound disruption of the patient's social milieu. As the disease progresses, decreased language output and motor findings emerge. There is progressive atrophy, white matter degeneration and physiological dysfunction of the frontal cortex, anterior temporal lobes, and basal ganglia. In contrast to primary progressive aphasia (PPA), where atrophy is usually more severe in the left hemisphere, with bvFTD, the right hemisphere is usually more atrophic and dysfunctional. The disease course from the time of diagnosis to death typically takes somewhere between four to eight years. Because of the prominent behavioral and personality changes, many of these patients are misdiagnosed as suffering from a psychiatric syndrome before reaching a correct diagnosis (Woolley et al. 2011; Khan et al. 2012).

A careful history often reveals that the first symptoms of the illness occurred much earlier than the symptoms that brought the patient in for evaluation. Because this begins as a social disorder, many years prior to presentation there may have been changes that people close to the patient misconstrued as related to stress, midlife crisis, or normal aging. Of all the clinical subtypes of FTD, bvFTD is the most strongly genetic, particularly when it is associated with amyotrophic lateral sclerosis (ALS). Many such cases show mutations in *C9ORF72* (Sha et al. 2012).

CASE HISTORY

A 61-year-old male came for assessment of a progressive behavioral deterioration. Three years earlier this previously successful salesman began to have trouble meeting his sales quotas. For his 30th anniversary at age 59, he bought his wife a battery. He became distracted and remote and lost interest in sexual relations. On visits to a family counselor he resisted discussing his feelings. Whenever asked about whether he was depressed, he repetitively noted, "I couldn't feel better." His began to use words in a stereotyped manner and often repeated, "That's part of the puzzle." Drinking at work became common, and he was found intoxicated on the day of an important sales meeting. After counseling, he entered an alcohol rehabilitation facility.

The drinking stopped, but he began to smoke two packages of cigarettes daily and started to overeat, gaining 30 pounds. His wife complained, "that damn psychiatric facility replaced one addiction with two." After returning work he failed to return calls from clients and rarely left his office. Papers accumulated on his desk, and he kept a collection of cans in his closet. After counseling and a probation period, he was fired. He worked for less than one month delivering papers by bike

in his community, but delivery was erratic, and he lost this job as well.

Seeming undisturbed by his misfortune, he spent most of the time at home watching television. He drove through red lights and lost his license after he was arrested for driving 50 miles per hour in a school zone. He became more withdrawn from friends and family and began collecting cans from the garbage to sell. Although no longer interested in sexual activity with his wife, he brought pornographic magazines to the house, and he enjoyed showing them to his wife's friends when they visited. His eating dramatically increased, and he developed a craving for hamburgers, eating six every day.

There was no history of significant past illnesses, and family history was negative for dementia. Both of his parents were well and still living in their 80s.

On examination, the patient was restless and often left the room to pace or go to the bathroom. He was disinhibited—he commented on the female neuropsychologist's breasts and asked for a kiss. When asked about why he had come to the clinic he commented, "my memory's shot, Doc."

His Mini Mental Status Exam score was 26 with items missed for place, year, and two points lost for "world" spelled backward. His sentence on the MMSE said, "I love you," and he winked at the psychologist when she read it. He showed deficits in many, but not all aspects of frontal executive function. His digit span forward was 6 and backward was 5, both within normal limits. He generated a pathologically low three "d" words in one minute. On design fluency he generated one novel design, and there were 15 repetitions (Figure 2–1). By contrast, he named 15 animals, which was normal for his age. He was unable to complete a simplified alternating sequence task and made multiple errors and rule violations (Figure 2–2). Drawing, episodic memory, and naming were all within normal limits. Motor and sensory examinations were normal, and he had a normal EMG. An MRI showed prominent and severe atrophy in the frontal lobes and anterior temporal lobes (Figure 2–3).

At 62 years of age, he wandered away from home and was found two days later, dehydrated and confused, 15 miles away from home. At this point he was moved by his wife to a local nursing home, where he lived for 5 more years. Already overweight, he gained 70 more pounds over the next 2 years, often eating off of other patients' plates.

Top   Filled Dots

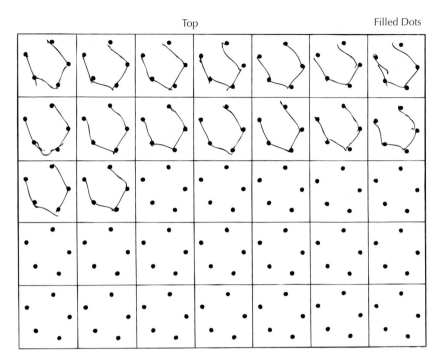

Figure 2–1. Patient's neuropsychological testing shows multiple perseverations on the design fluency task.

After 2 years he became mute but was still able to correctly copy complex drawings on paper.

At 65 years of age, he walked into the shower and turned on scalding hot water that gave him significant burns on his arms and body. By 66 years of age he began to show some motor slowing and subtle parkinsonian features. He had walked without major difficulty until his death and was able to eat a Thanksgiving dinner the day before he died. At 70 years of age, he attempted to swallow a small toy that became caught in his throat leading to a full respiratory and then cardiac arrest.

Neuropathology revealed massive atrophy in the orbital frontal, insular, and anterior temporal cortex. There was mild atrophy in the anterior parietal region, but the posterior parietal and occipital cortices were normal in size. There were round cytoplasmic inclusions within neurons that were positive with silver-staining (Pick bodies) and bloated silver-staining neurons (Pick cells). There were extensive 3R tau aggregates in the frontal and anterior temporal lobes within neurons

and glia. There were no amyloid plaques or Lewy bodies.

Comment. This is a fairly typical history for a patient with the behavioral variant of FTD (bvFTD) and is representative of the patients that we have seen who had underlying Pick's disease. Progression was slow and insidious, beginning with subtle changes in personality. He showed multiple addictive behaviors during the prodrome, and his poor work history was misconstrued as being secondary to alcohol abuse. Rather, orbital frontal, anterior insular, and ventral striatal degeneration led to a lowered threshold for addictions. As the disease spread, he became insensitive to pain, probably second to extensive bilateral degeneration of the insula. Like other bvFTD patients that we have seen, this patient suffered a serious injury secondary to a pain insensitivity.

Using the new international research criteria for bvFTD, the constellation of overeating, apathy, disinhibition, loss of empathy, repetitive motor behaviors, and loss of executive control meets possible bvFTD criteria. The presence of

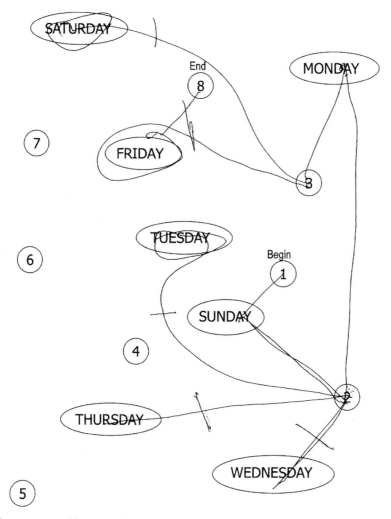

Figure 2–2. The patient is unable to complete a simplified alternating sequence task during neuropsychological testing.

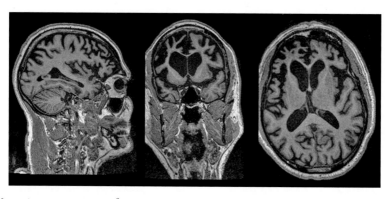

Figure 2–3. Magnetic resonance image of patient.

frontotemporal atrophy on MRI meets criteria for probable bvFTD (Rascovsky et al. 2011). The very slow progression, absence of motor findings, and lack of a family history is very typical of Pick's disease (Arne Brun, personal communication).

CLINICAL FEATURES AND ANATOMY

In the early stages of bvFTD, patients will typically show disinhibition, addictive behaviors, and abnormalities in the executive control system. These behavioral changes are varied and complex, driven by the specific anatomy of the patient's disease, premorbid brain wiring, and sociocultural factors. For example, men seem to be particularly prone to difficult behaviors in bvFTD, and certain families are able to shelter their loved ones from publicly embarrassing behaviors while for others protection from public disinhibition is not possible. In some patients there is a dramatic change in self-awareness, manifest by changes in well-established patterns of behavior suggesting a change in self-awareness and in loyalty to previous ideals and beliefs (Miller et al. 2001; Sturm et al. 2006).

Typical symptoms of bvFTD include:

- socially inappropriate behavior (loss of respect for interpersonal space, shoplifting, indecent exposure/touching, inappropriate familiarity with children or strangers, etc.);
- loss of social graces (use of crude language, telling off-color jokes, making offensive statements, rudeness, touching others, the absence of embarrassment etc.);
- loss of sympathy or empathy for others (inappropriate response to illness in a loved one, lack of interest in the problems of others, cruel comments to loved ones, children, or the elderly);
- misinterpretation of social cues provided by others such as continuing to talk while someone is trying to end the conversation, not taking turns in a conversation, or not understanding the emotional nuances of social interactions;
- apathy and social withdrawal with loss of interest in work, hobbies, and friends and diminished motor, verbal, or social activity;
- poor hygiene or grooming;

- repetitive motor behaviors such as collecting, counting, repetitive urination, or grooming;
- change in food habits with weight gain, overeating, preference for sweets, and poor table manners;
- bad decision making with impulsive, rash, or careless actions such as new-onset gambling, shoplifting, buying or selling property without regard for the future financial consequences, and not attending to safety risks of their children; and there is often poor planning in association with increased trust of strangers, even those who do not have the patient's best interest at heart;
- addictive behaviors including drinking, drug use, spitting, overeating, gambling, repetitive playing of computer games;
- personality change is often a first symptom with passivity, neuroticism, and anxiety as common prodromal findings.

The international research criteria for bvFTD capitalize on these features of the disease and require that patients show early in their illness at least of three of the following six features: disinhibition, apathy, loss of sympathy and empathy for others, hyperorality, repetitive motor behaviors, and frontal executive loss (Box 2.1).

These behaviors outlined in the international criteria develop insidiously but eventually cause devastating consequences for the patient and their loved ones. Unlike Alzheimer's disease (AD), where functional deficits parallel cognitive problems, traditional cognitive testing of patients with bvFTD may be relatively normal despite the patient's severe deficits in day-to-day function. Furthermore, by the time that a bvFTD patient presents to a neurologist, there has often been massive disruption of the family, legal problems for the patient, and financial losses (often bankruptcy).

Loss of insight into the illness is invariable (Rankin et al. 2005), and this contributes to the social chaos and functional decline associated with bvFTD (Rosen 2011). A striking mismatch between "knowing" and "doing" is typical of patients with frontal lobe disease, and the bvFTD patient may be able to say that shoplifting is wrong, but will still persist in shoplifting (Miller et al. 1997).

Another early sign of bvFTD is apathy or inertia. The apathy of bvFTD affects the motor, social, and cognitive domains. Motorically the patient moves less, moves more slowly, and is

Box 2.1 International Consensus Research Criteria for Behavioral Variant Frontotemporal Dementia (bvFTD) (Rascovsky et al. 2011)

I. Neurodegenerative disease

The following symptom must be present to meet criteria for bvFTD.
- I.A.   Shows progressive deterioration of behavior and/or cognition by observation or history (as provided by a knowledgeable informant)

II. Possible bvFTD

Three of the following behavioral/cognitive symptoms (II.A–II.F) must be present to meet criteria. Ascertainment requires that symptoms be persistent or recurrent, rather than single or rare events.
- II.A. Early* behavioral disinhibition
  [one of the following symptoms (II.A.1–II.A.3) must be present]:
  - II.A.1. Socially inappropriate behavior
  - II.A.2. Loss of manners or decorum
  - II.A.3. Impulsive, rash, or careless actions
- II.B. Early apathy or inertia
  [one of the following symptoms (II.B.1–II.B.2) must be present]:
  - II.B.1. Apathy
  - II.B.2. Inertia
- II.C. Early loss of sympathy or empathy
  [one of the following symptoms (II.C.1–II.C.2) must be present]:
  - II.C.1. Diminished response to other people's needs and feelings
  - II.C.2. Diminished social interest, interrelatedness, or personal warmth
- II.D. Early perseverative, stereotyped, or compulsive/ritualistic behavior
  [one of the following symptoms (II.D.1–II.D.3) must be present]:
  - II.D.1. Simple repetitive movements
  - II.D.2. Complex, compulsive, or ritualistic behaviors
  - II.D.3. Stereotypy of speech
- II.E. Hyperorality and dietary changes
  [one of the following symptoms (II.E.1–II.E.3) must be present]:
  - II.E.1. Altered food preferences
  - II.E.2. Binge eating, increased consumption of alcohol or cigarettes
  - II.E.3. Oral exploration or consumption of inedible objects
- II.F. Neuropsychological profile: executive/generation deficits with relative sparing of memory and visuospatial functions
  [all of the following symptoms (II.F.1–II.F.3) must be present]:
  - II.F.1. Deficits in executive tasks
  - II.F.2. Relative sparing of episodic memory
  - II.F.3. Relative sparing of visuospatial skills

III. Probable bvFTD

All of the following symptoms (III.A–III.C) must be present to meet criteria.
- III.A. Meets criteria for possible bvFTD

(continued)

> **Box 2.1 International Consensus Research Criteria for Behavioral Variant Frontotemporal Dementia (bvFTD) (Rascovsky et al. 2011) (cont.)**
>
> III.B. Exhibits significant functional decline (by caregiver report or as evidenced by Clinical Dementia Rating Scale or Functional Activities Questionnaire scores)
> III.C. Imaging results consistent with bvFTD
> *[one of the following (III.C.1–III.C.2) must be present]:*
> III.C.1. Frontal and/or anterior temporal atrophy on MRI or CT
> III.C.2. Frontal and/or anterior temporal hypoperfusion or hypometabolism on PET or SPECT
>
> ### IV. Behavioral Variant FTD with Definite FTLD Pathology
>
> Criterion IV.A and either criterion IV.B or IV.C must be present to meet criteria.
> IV.A. Meets criteria for possible or probable bvFTD
> IV.B. Histopathological evidence of FTLD on biopsy or at postmortem
> IV.C. Presence of a known pathogenic mutation
>
> ### V. Exclusionary Criteria for bvFTD
>
> Criteria V.A and V.B must be answered negatively for any bvFTD diagnosis. Criterion V.C can be positive for possible bvFTD but must be negative for probable bvFTD.
> V.A. Pattern of deficits is better accounted for by other nondegenerative nervous system or medical disorders
> V.B. Behavioral disturbance is better accounted for by a psychiatric diagnosis
> V.C. Biomarkers strongly indicative of Alzheimer's disease or other neurodegenerative process
>
> *As a general guideline, "early" refers to symptom presentation within the first three years.

less likely to engage in a motor solution to a problem (Chow et al. 2009; Merrilees et al. 2009). Socially, patients exhibit a lack of interest in their work, in previous hobbies, or in the concerns of others. Diminished interest in solving problems is evident. Activities that were previously engaging gradually extinguish, and the inability to initiate and sustain activities such as making a meal or maintaining a conversation appears. Many patients spend hours in front of the television or playing computer games. Commonly, this pattern of behavior is misinterpreted as depression, although when patients are queried they often deny any concerns related to mood (Merrilees et al. 2005).

For caregivers, one of the hardest symptoms to accept is the patient's loss of sympathy or empathy for others. The lack of understanding or indifference to other people's needs and feelings, along with the patient's decrease in social engagement and personal warmth, is common, and this withdrawal represents one of the factors that leads to the extreme caregiver burden associated with caring for a bvFTD patient. It is an important cause for the caregiver's feeling of loneliness and estrangement from the patient and is a factor in making the caregiving for FTD even more stressful than caregiving for AD (Merrilees et al. 2005).

Perseverative, stereotyped, or compulsive behaviors occur (Perry et al. 2012). These behaviors may be simple motor movements like tapping, standing up and down, clapping, rubbing, scratching, and so forth, or can be complex patterns of ritualized behavior or routines that the person feels compelled to complete (counting, collecting, walking particular routes, squishing ants, cleaning, singing, etc.). The same perseverative pattern may be seen in the speech, where words or phrases are repeated excessively.

In the prodromal period of bvFTD, addictive behaviors such as smoking, drinking, overeating, marijuana abuse, and excessive focus around exercise or shopping are commonly seen, sometimes years before the illness begins (Miller et al. 1995, Lebert & Pasquier 2008). Commonly, many caregivers, physicians, and neurologists tend to believe that the addictive behavior is the primary problem, even after cognitive symptoms emerge.

Many bvFTD patients gain weight due to changes in food preferences and habits (Miller et al. 1995, Ikeda et al. 2002). They crave foods (particularly sweets), keep eating when they are not hungry, or insist on eating specific foods or following ritualistic routines around food. Other oral behaviors like smoking, drinking, and chewing gum or tobacco may also increase. Table manners decay, and patients may try to take items off of other people's plates, stuff their mouth with food, or eat with their hands. In later stages of the illness, some patients will try to eat inedible objects (Woolley et al. 2007).

In the earliest stages of illness, patients show relatively normal executive function, but tests that tap reward or social cognition may be impaired (Rankin et al. 2003). Over time, the neuropsychological profile of bvFTD patients tends to show a decrease in executive function with relative sparing of visuospatial functions and language comprehension. This pattern reflects the frontal damage to planning and sequencing areas in the dorsolateral prefrontal cortex with preservation of more posterior parietal functions (Bozeat et al. 2000; Krueger et al. 2011).

Joel Kramer has led a national effort to develop neuropsychological tests that tap executive control and has a powerful battery called the EXAMINER. Examples of these tests are shown in Box 2.2. Table 2–1 shows the typical pattern of strength and weakness in the neuropsychological testing in a patient with bvFTD.

There are few things more valuable in the diagnosis of a patient with bvFTD than neuropsychological testing, but this cannot be performed without careful consideration of multiple factors. First, it is important to realize that modern neuropsychological testing must be anatomically oriented, and every task that is performed should focus on the brain structures being tested, while simultaneously understanding the cognitive process that is being tapped. Thinking anatomically is often helpful in understanding and interpreting neuropsychological testing. For example, tasks of working memory such as digits backward tap dorsolateral prefrontal cortex, but also require parietal lobe function. This probably explains why both AD and bvFTD patients fail this task. By contrast, letter fluency and the flanker and antisaccade tasks appear to be more specifically frontal (and subcortical), but not parietal. Hence, they are better at separating bvFTD from AD.

Second, the testing should tap the multiple cognitive domains that include working memory, verbal and visual episodic memory, fluency, comprehension, naming and repetition, visuoconstructive ability, letter, design and animal generation, alternating sequences, and abstraction. Screening tasks like the Mini Mental State Examination or the Montreal Cognitive Assessment are not sufficient for separating bvFTD from AD.

Additionally, while many neuropsychologists do not make observations about the patient's behavior, it is important to realize that many of the behaviors that are part of the international research criteria for bvFTD can be observed during testing. These behaviors may not always appear during testing but need to be systematically measured. Kate Rankin at the University of California, San Francisco (UCSF), has designed a social norms task and a behavioral checklist that is used during testing to capture the social deficits that characterized bvFTD including disinhibition, apathy, repetitive motor behaviors, coldness, and inattentiveness.

While previous data has emphasized the value of diminished executive control as a feature of bvFTD versus AD, our experience suggests that this is not always so simple. The tasks of executive control that are particularly sensitive to bvFTD versus AD include the antisaccade task, phonemic fluency, the behavioral checklist, and the social norms task.

Finally, it is important to remember that the frontal lobes have extensive connections with subcortical circuits, so many patients with subcortical diseases ranging from Huntington's disease, progressive supranuclear palsy, Parkinson's disease, and leukoencephalopathies can also show significant overlap on neuropsychological testing with bvFTD.

Imaging shows atrophy in frontal and/or anterior temporal regions on CT or MRI and

Box 2.2   Neuropsychological Tests Included in the EXAMINER Test Battery

Domain: Working Memory

- Dot counting

Domain: Inhibition

- Flanker
- Continuous performance test
- Antisaccades
- Dysexecutive errors

Domain: Set Shifting

- Set shifting

Domain: Fluency

- Phonemic fluency
- Category fluency

Domain: Planning

- Unstructured task

Domain: Insight

- Insight

Domain: Social Cognition and Behavior

- The social norms questionnaire
- Behavior rating scale

Table 2–1   Typical Pattern of Strength and Weakness in Neuropsychological Testing of a Patient with bvFTD

Syndrome	Behavior	Drive	Episodic Memory	Visuospatial function	Frontal Executive	Language
bvFTD	Disinhibition	Severe apathy	Variable, sometimes good	Good drawing, navigation	Impaired	Decreased output
AD	Normal	Mild apathy	Poor	Poor	Variable	Word-finding trouble

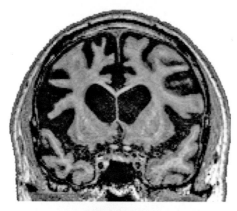

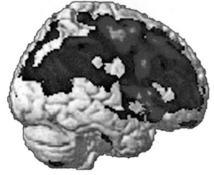

Figure 2–4. MRI showing typical atrophy pattern seen in bvFTD, and VBM group analysis of bvFTD versus healthy controls.

disproportionate frontal or frontotemporal hypometabolism or hypoperfusion on SPECT or PET (Miller et al. 1991) or fMRI (Figure 2–4). Application of newer imaging techniques is demonstrating widespread atrophy, hypoperfusion, and white matter changes in the frontoinsular networks, fairly early in the course of the illness (Tosun et al. 2012). These results reflect the underlying pathology disrupting the frontal and/or temporal networks and causing the signs and symptoms of bvFTD. The use of newer imaging techniques ranging from functional connectivity mapping to diffusion tensor mapping is discussed in the "Future Directions" segment of this chapter.

Unfortunately, radiologists (even neuro-radiologists) often ignore the atrophy that is evident on MRI in most bvFTD patients. In a study done at UCSF by Jomar Suárez, only four of 40 MRI reports from radiologists in patients with bvFTD reported the possibility of bvFTD (Suarez et al. 2009). Hence, the clinician needs to become expert at searching for the presence of frontotemporal and insular atrophy on the MRI scans of their patients (Table 2–2).

The startling array of behavioral disturbances seen with bvFTD is driven by the regional vulnerability of specific nondominant hemisphere frontoinsular and temporal circuits (Rosen et al. 2002). Disinhibition strongly correlates with the severity of atrophy in the right orbitofrontal region, apathy is associated with dysfunction in the right cingulate and medial frontal lobes, and repetitive motor behaviors are driven by the severity of atrophy in the right supplementary motor (Rosen et al. 2002, 2005). Additionally David Perry and colleagues suggest that loss in the bilateral globus pallidus, left putamen, and in the lateral temporal lobe, particularly the left middle and inferior temporal gyri, drive compulsions in bvFTD. Overeating correlates with hypothalamic and right ventral striatal and orbital insular tissue loss (Woolley et al. 2007, Piguet et al. 2011)

Table 2–2 **Radiologist Diagnostic Impressions in 40 Patients Clinically Diagnosed with Behavioral Variant Frontotemporal Dementia (bvFTD)**

Reported Diagnosis	Number (%)
Atrophy	20 (50)
White matter/ischemic	6 (15)
Unremarkable	5 (12.5)
Behavioral variant frontotemporal dementia	3 (7.5)
Normal pressure hydrocephalus/hydrocephalus	2 (5)
Alzheimer's disease vs. Pick's disease	1 (2.5)
Alzheimer's disease	1 (2.5)
Encephalomalacia	1 (2.5)
Mitochondrial/metabolic	1 (2.5)

(Suárez et al. 2009)

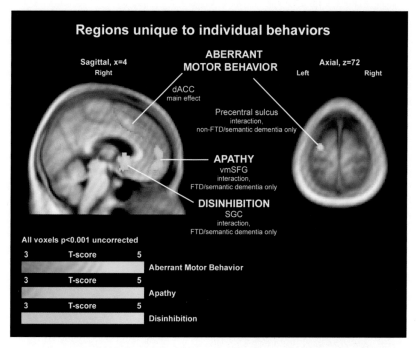

Figure 2–5. Regions where individual behaviors showed unique associations with focal regions of tissue loss. (Rosen et al. 2005.)

(Figures 2–5, 2–6). Diminished understanding of emotions on faces and diminished empathy for others strongly correlate with right anterior temporal and orbitoinsular cortex (Rosen et al. 2002; Rankin et al. 2006) (Figure 2–7).

Aspiration is a particularly troublesome problem for patients in the middle and later stages of the disease, as patients tend place large amounts of food in their mouth in the setting of progressively diminishing swallowing mechanisms. After years of FTD, patients may have trouble coordinating their muscles, swallowing, chewing, moving, and controlling their bladder and/or bowels. Death from FTD is usually caused by the consequences of these physical changes, most commonly infections in the lungs, skin, or urinary tract.

GENETIC AND PATHOLOGICAL CORRELATES

Motor deficits are common with bvFTD, and the timing and types of changes seen are clues to the molecular subtype responsible for the syndrome. The early presence of motor neuron disease usually means that the TDP-43 type B subtype is present, although more rarely FTD and ALS are due to fused in sarcoma protein (FUS) pathology. If a bvFTD syndrome is associated with prominent parkinsonism, particularly if the parkinsonism has marked axial rigidity and gaze disturbance, corticobasal degeneration (CBD) and progressive supranuclear palsy (PSP) should be considered. In Pick's disease and many of the FUS cases, motor findings occur only late in the course of the illness.

Definitive markers for bvFTD include pathogenic mutations in *C9ORF72*, *MAPT*, *PGRN*, *CHMP2B*, or *VCP* or the presence of histopathological evidence of FTLD on biopsy or at postmortem examination. Approximately one-half of all bvFTD cases show tau immunoreactive inclusions, the other cases show ubiquitin-positive TDP-43 aggregates. Other molecular varieties include FTLD with FUS immunoreactive inclusions, FTLD with ubiquitin or P62-only immunoreactive inclusions, FTLD with intermediate filament immunoreactive inclusions, and FTLD without immunoreactive inclusions (negative for all proteins). *C9ORF72* mutations are the most common genetic cause for bvFTD, while

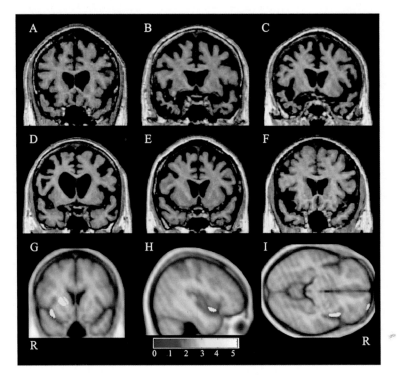

Figure 2–6. Structural MRI coronal sections of overeating patients and voxel-based morphometry (VBM). The overeating patients with frontotemporal dementia (FTD) have significantly more atrophy in the right ventral insula, striatum, and anterior orbitofrontal cortex (OFC). **(A–F)** Comparable structural MRI coronal sections obtained from the six overeating patients (Patients 1 through 6) are presented in native space. **(G–I)** VBM on high-resolution T1-weighted MR images was used to identify brain regions that showed significantly greater voxel-wise volume loss in the six overeating patients with FTD compared with 21 nonovereating patients with dementia and 47 control subjects. A priori region of interest included the insular, frontal, and temporal cortices as well as the basal ganglia bilaterally. The right inferior insula, striatum, and anterior OFC of overeating patients were significantly atrophied compared with controls and nonovereating patients ($p < 0.05$ corrected for multiple comparisons in the region of interest). Areas of significant atrophy are displayed on coronal **(G)**, sagittal **(H)**, and axial **(I)** sections of the mean of all subjects' brains and thresholded at $p < 0.05$ corrected for multiple comparisons (coordinates: $x = 41$, $y = 12$, $z = -13$). (Woolley et al. 2007.)

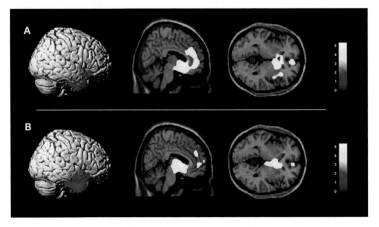

Figure 2–7. **(A)** Main effect of EC score, showing rendered sagittal ($x = 7$) and axial ($z = 0$) views of voxels significantly related to EC score at $p < 0.001$ uncorrected for multiple comparisons across the whole brain. Maps of significant correlation were superimposed on sections of a normal brain template image (SPM2: single_subj_T1.mnc). The design matrix for this analysis contained only EC score, with sex, age, and TIV included as nuisance covariates, and a t-test was used. **(B)** Main effect of PT score, showing voxels significantly related to PT score at $p < 0.001$ uncorrected. The design matrix for this analysis contained only PT score, with sex, age, and TIV included as nuisance covariates, and a t-test was used. (Rankin et al. 2006.)

a smaller percentage of familial cases are caused by tau or progranulin mutations (see Chapter 8: FTD Genes).

DIFFERENTIAL DIAGNOSIS

A comprehensive evaluation should include a detailed history (from the patient and an informant); neurological exam with a careful look for extrapyramidal, pyramidal, and lower motor neuron findings; neuropsychological testing with the inclusion of tasks of executive control; and observations regarding social behavior during the testing, imaging, and blood work. Together, these data will usually lead to a clear diagnosis.

Distinguishing FTD clinical syndromes from other neurological and psychiatric conditions can be challenging (Woolley et al. 2011, Manes 2012). bvFTD is often mistaken for depression, bipolar illness, personality disorder, drug or alcohol dependence, late-onset schizophrenia, AD, other FTD-spectrum disorders such as PSP or CBD, metabolic disorders, vascular dementia, structural brain disease, or less commonly with leukoencephalopathies (Box 2.3).

Alzheimer's Disease

There can be significant overlap between AD and FTD. In AD, symptoms such as disinhibition, overeating, loss of sympathy for others, and apathy are not usually prominent presenting features, but there are frontal variants of AD (Giovagnoli et al. 2008) and at least one example of an AD patient with frontal features in whom neuropathology exhibited frontally predominant neurofibrillary tangles (Johnson et al. 2004). While many patients with AD show deficits on some tasks of executive control, even at the time of first diagnosis, there are far fewer in whom the classical behavioral features of bvFTD are present early in the course of the illness.

We are often referred patients at the UCSF Memory and Aging Center with a diagnosis of bvFTD because there are deficits in executive control on neuropsychological testing. It is important to consider that many neurodegenerative conditions, including AD, may show this pattern.

In neuropsychological testing of someone with bvFTD, look for poor performance on executive control tests, better performance on verbal and visual recognition than recall, and normal calculation, drawing, and naming. Specifically, look for low performance on letter fluency and alternating tasks, but better performance on the verbal memory subscales, block design test, and drawing tests. Some patients with bvFTD exhibit a memory disturbance at presentation (Hornberger et al. 2010), although sparing of visuospatial function is very common.

On neuroimaging studies, most patients show marked orbitobasal, frontoinsular, and/or anterior temporal atrophy with relative sparing of the parietal and occipital lobes. With the advent of amyloid imaging there is now a strong biomarker to separate pure AD from FTD (Rabinovici et al. 2011), although patients with asymptomatic AD in the setting

---

Box 2.3 Differential Diagnosis of FTD

Alzheimer's disease
Psychiatric problems
Movement disorders
Chronic traumatic encephalopathy
Other FTD phenotypes
Vascular dementia
Metabolic disorders
Structural brain abnormalities (tumor, NPH, intracranial hypotension)

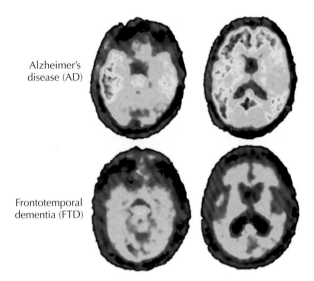

Alzheimer's
disease (AD)

Frontotemporal
dementia (FTD)

Figure 2–8. PIB-PET scans of a patient with Alzheimer's disease and a patient with FTD. Pittsburgh Compound B binds to beta-amyloid plaques in the cortex. (Image courtesy of Gil Rabinovici, MD.)

of FTD syndrome will not be distinguished with this approach (Figure 2–8). The presence of brain plaques in AD correlates very strongly with low levels of Aβ42 in the cerebrospinal fluid (CSF).

More typical of AD than FTD are the following:

- sparing of socially appropriate behavior,
- severe memory problems,
- difficulty with visuospatial tasks like navigation,
- a relatively normal neurological examination,
- generalized atrophy with marked parietal abnormalities, and
- a positive amyloid scan or a low CSF Aβ42.

Psychiatric Disorders

When it comes to psychiatric disorders, bvFTD is the great imitator, and many misdiagnoses of bvFTD fall into the psychiatric domain. The misdiagnoses work in both directions—there are patients with primary psychiatric disorders who are mistaken for bvFTD, and there are patients with true bvFTD who are initially considered to have a psychiatric condition. While the new international criteria for bvFTD usually facilitate the diagnosis of patients with true FTLD neuropathology, the complexity of

human behavior can complicate accurate diagnosis. For example, long-standing sociopathy or personality disorder can make a patient with AD appear to have bvFTD. Additionally, there are many caregivers who are poor historians, with some conjuring up behavioral disorders that do not exist, and still others are unaware of profound behavioral disorders in their loved ones. Similarly, not all bvFTD patients exhibit profound behavioral changes at the time of a medical visit, and if the disease is mild, neuropsychological testing can be normal.

The clinical syndrome of bvFTD is often initially misdiagnosed as psychiatric illness because of the profound changes in personality and behavior seen in the patient and because our society still tends to think of personality and behavior as falling into the psychiatric domain. In a systematic, retrospective, blinded chart review of 252 patients with a neurodegenerative disease diagnosis, 28% of patients received a prior psychiatric diagnosis (Woolley et al. 2011). Depression is the most common psychiatric diagnosis, but bvFTD patients are more likely to receive diagnoses of bipolar disorder or schizophrenia (Khan et al. 2012) than are patients with other neurodegenerative diseases.

Additionally, patients with schizophrenia or bipolar illness can develop cognitive impairment as they age, leading to overlap with bvFTD. Alcohol abuse can confound a diagnosis and needs to be stopped before bvFTD can be diagnosed with certainty. Finally, genetic forms of FTD can move very slowly, and some individuals with these mutations can adjust and even improve clinically over the course of several years. It is no surprise that schizophrenia and bipolar disorder can be mistaken for bvFTD as the atrophy patterns in these psychiatric disorders have significant overlap with what is seen in bvFTD with all of these conditions showing involvement of the anterior insular, orbitofrontal, and cingulate cortex (Bora et al. 2010, Sanders et al. 2012) (Figure 2–9).

Many FTD patients show symptoms of obsessive-compulsive disorder, and, in particular, repetitive compulsive behaviors are a core feature of FTD. Delusions and euphoria are also common with FTD, sometimes leading to the misdiagnosis of either schizophrenia or bipolar illness. Depression is not common

in FTD, but apathy and emotional withdrawal are, often leading to the misdiagnosis of depression. Even though FTD patients may appear to be depressed, when you ask them about their mood, they often offer that they feel happy (Rosen 2011).

The emotional volatility, aggressiveness, lack of empathy for others, and antisocial features of borderline personality and antisocial personality disorder have significant overlap with bvFTD. Some gene carriers are initially considered to suffer from these psychiatric conditions before the full-spectrum bvFTD syndrome emerges. The apathy and social withdrawal associated with bvFTD sometimes lead a patient to be described as a loner or schizoidal personality. The eccentric and sometimes mystical style of thinking overlaps with the schizotypal personality. Finally, addiction disorder is a common prodrome of bvFTD, while

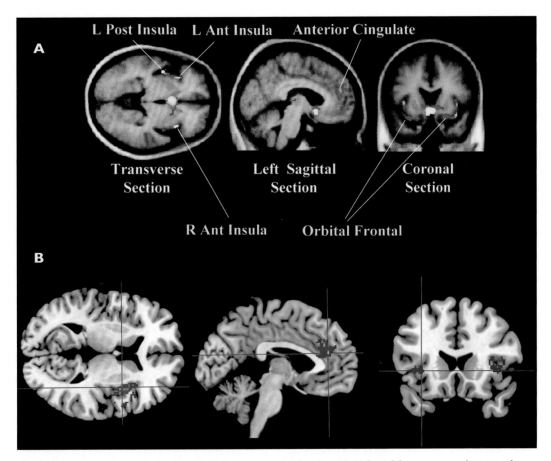

Figure 2–9. Similar atrophy patterns in FTD (**A**) and biopolar disorder (**B**). (Adapted from Rosen et al. 2002 and Bora et al. 2010.)

Box 2.4 Psychiatric Diagnoses Often Mistaken for bvFTD

- Major depressive disorder
- Bipolar affective disorder
- Schizophrenia
- Obsessive-compulsive disorder
- Borderline personality disorder
- Antisocial personality
- Schizoid personality
- Schizotypal personality
- Addiction disorder

there are many people in whom heavy alcohol abuse is mistaken for bvFTD (Box 2.4).

A small but significant percentage of patients diagnosed with bvFTD have what Kipps and Hodges have called the *FTD phenocopy* (Kipps et al. 2010). These patients show a normal MRI or only subtle atrophy patterns on imaging, progress very slowly or not at all, and tend to do relatively well on frontal-executive testing. In the few cases with neuropathology, no specific abnormality was seen, suggesting a nondegenerative etiology for many of these patients.

The documentation that there are patients who seem to meet the bvFTD phenotype in whom other etiologies might better account for the diagnosis has proven valuable for understanding the spectrum of disorders that present in an FTD clinic. In our experience, the FTD-phenocopy pattern tends to fall into four main subtypes:

1. FTD by proxy,
2. Self-diagnosed FTD,
3. A primary psychiatric disorder, and
4. Slow FTD.

In FTD by proxy, the caregiver becomes convinced that their loved one has bvFTD. Sometimes, this misconception is triggered by hearing a talk on the topic or by reading about FTD on the Internet. In other instances, intense conflicts within a marriage lead the spouse to believe that the person that he or she married has been changed by bvFTD. Despite a history strongly suggestive of bvFTD, when these patients are examined, they tend not to show the florid bvFTD syndrome that the history suggests, and imaging is nonspecific or normal. Often, there is significant turmoil in the relationship, and in many of these patients the marriage is relatively recent. The patient is often passive and defers to the observations of the partner. The etiology for patients with this presentation is variable. At least some suffer from a non-FTD dementia such as AD, but many others have a long-standing psychiatric disorder like mild Asperger syndrome. When the caregiver is told that their loved one does not suffer from bvFTD they are usually disappointed, or even angry, suggesting that there are profound psychological factors that bind them to this diagnosis.

There are many parallels in FTD by proxy and patients who self-diagnose as having bvFTD. Such patients become convinced that they have bvFTD, sometimes supported by the confirmation of a nonexpert, or even an expert, in the field. Because bvFTD attacks specific brain circuits that tend to lead to denial of illness and profound inability to self-reflect, it is unusual to see a patient who derives their own diagnosis. Like the FTD by proxy cases, such patients do not get satisfaction from hearing that they may not suffer from FTD and may get great joy from carrying a faux diagnosis.

As has been discussed, bipolar illness, schizophrenia, and obsessive-compulsive disorder can mimic bvFTD but typically start much earlier in life than bvFTD. Similarly, unlike bvFTD, patients with primary psychiatric disease typically fluctuate and often improve after treatment. Imaging tends not to show the severe atrophic changes of bvFTD with primary psychiatric disorders (Sanders et al. 2012).

Finally, there are patients who truly suffer from FTD in whom the progression is very slow. This is particularly true of patients with genetic variants of FTD. We have reported recently on two patients who were considered to have FTD phenocopy, one of whom who minimally changed over 11 years (Khan et al. 2012). Both had a C9 genetic mutation that explained their slow course. The bvFTD phenocopy syndrome emphasizes how difficult the evaluation of patients with suspected bvFTD can be (Kipps et al. 2010).

Movement Disorders

Many patients with FTD develop, or even present with, parkinsonian features. In classical Parkinson's disease (PD) a tremor is present, and the rigidity tends to involve the limbs, while in FTD a tremor is often absent, and the rigidity is usually axial. Falls at presentation or early in the disease course, poor response to levodopa, symmetry of motor signs, rapid progression, lack of tremor, and early dysautonomia are signs that identify patients with PSP or CBD as underlying pathology. The presence of PSP, CBD, or ALS shortens the life expectancy in patients with FTD (Roberson et al. 2005). Multiple system atrophy (MSA) patients can exhibit subtle frontal-executive difficulties, but the prominent dysautonomia and the presence of rapid eye movement (REM) behavior usually help to distinguish these patients from bvFTD.

Formal eye movement recordings may be useful to distinguish PD and other forms of parkinsonism from FTD. MRI and CT appear normal in PD, whereas the MRI of someone with FTD will typically show significant atrophy in the frontal and anterior temporal lobes. MRIs of patients with MSA may show abnormalities in the pons (the "hot-cross bun" sign) and lateral putamen with streaky linear densities outlining the lateral basal ganglia. PET may show low levels of dopaminergic activity in PD.

About 15% of all FTD patients develop ALS, while many patients with ALS go on to show FTD changes clinically or at postmortem examination (Lomen-Hoerth et al. 2002). Up to 50% of ALS patients also show loss of executive function, and up to 20% have full-blown signs and symptoms of FTD (Lomen-Hoerth et al. 2003). As a result, these ALS patients may lack the ability to fully understand the meaning of their illness, they may make poor decisions about their clinical care, or they may become agitated and difficult for caregivers who are trying to help them. They may have language problems that go beyond the expressive difficulties in ALS or show behavioral changes years before the ALS manifests. Extrapyramidal deficits are common, particularly as the disease progresses (Roberson et al. 2005). While the MRI in patients with FTD-ALS may lack the florid atrophy typical of typical bvFTD, both structural and functional imaging are helpful and typically show frontoinsular atrophy and dysfunction.

Chronic Traumatic Encephalopathy

Previously called *dementia pugilistica*, chronic traumatic encephalopathy (CTE) is used to describe a progressive degenerative dementia that follows traumatic brain disease (see Chapter 7: A Primer of FTLD Neuropathology). The typical syndrome occurs in a patient who has suffered multiple traumatic insults with initial partial, or complete, recovery. Subsequently, there is a prodrome with neuropsychiatric symptoms that include anxiety, depression, sleep disturbance, headache, and sometimes irritability or aggression. Many patients go on to develop a frontal or AD type dementia (Gavett et al. 2011). Parkinsonian features are common, and there may be increased susceptibility to ALS (McKee et al. 2010).

The neuropathological features of this syndrome include massive depositions of tau in the frontotemporal regions, with variable involvement of TDP-43, α-synuclein, or Aβ42. Research into this disorder is just beginning, and the factors that lead some individuals to develop dementia, while sparing many others, is largely unknown.

Other FTD Clinical Phenotypes

The other phenotypes of FTD, nonfluent/agrammatic variant primary progressive aphasia (nfvPPA) and the semantic variant of PPA (svPPA), can have significant clinical overlap with bvFTD. With nfvPPA, patients usually show relatively normal behavior until later in the course of the illness, but in some instances, a behavioral syndrome emerges soon after the aphasia. Similarly, svPPA, particularly when the right temporal lobe is involved, is associated with prominent behavioral problems (Edwards-Lee et al. 1997). Because the svPPA spreads into orbitofrontal cortex, many features of bvFTD soon emerge in most patients (Seeley et al. 2005).

Two tau-related diseases, often classified as motor disorders, CBD and PSP often begin as a frontal syndrome (Lee et al. 2011). Approximately one-third of patients with pathology-proven CBD exhibit a bvFTD syndrome, while many PSP patients begin with frontal-executive or behavioral disorders, prior to manifesting a motor syndrome (Yatabe et al. 2011). The emergence of axial rigidity or a supranuclear gaze palsy should make the clinician consider PSP.

Vascular Dementia

Commonly, patients with vascular dementia present with prominent apathy and disinhibition (Chin et al. 2012), although usually imaging shows infarctions or white matter disease that account for the clinical syndrome (Figure 2–10). An MRI is the best tool to look for vascular changes versus cortical atrophy. Blood tests and the history will also reveal any cerebrovascular risk factors.

Metabolic Causes

The physician should initially check to rule out any treatable causes of dementia symptoms.

- **Check medications and illicit drug use:** Some medications have side effects that mimic the symptoms of dementia. Chronic alcohol abuse can lead to a frontal disorder, although this usually disappears when the toxin is removed. Residual deficits in patients who discontinue alcohol abuse may be due to injuries sustained while drinking (i.e., head trauma). The same is true for cocaine or amphetamine abuse, but permanent frontal lobe syndromes can occur with these compounds due to their influence on cerebral blood vessels.
- **Check metabolic abnormalities:** Decreased thyroid function (hypothyroidism) can result in apathy or depression that mimics bvFTD. A single severe episode or repeated milder episodes of hypoglycemia can injure frontal systems. B12 deficiency or elevated homocysteine or methylmalonic acid have a predilection for frontal white matter and can lead to a frontal syndrome (Blundo et al. 2011). Similarly, heavy metal intoxication, albeit rare, can lead to symptoms that parallel bvFTD. Metachromatic dystrophy due to aryl-sulfatase deficiency (Skomer

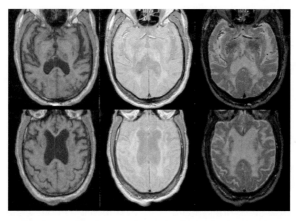

Figure 2–10. Magnetic resonance image of a patient with vascular dementia. (Image courtesy of Joel Kramer, PsyD.)

et al. 1983) can present as a frontal disorder, although usually patients show white matter disease that leads to the appropriate diagnose. Late-onset neuronal ceroid lipufuscinosis due to palmitoyl protein thioesterase mutations causes behavioral deficits, although myoclonic epilepsy and cerebellar changes usually are a tip-off to this diagnosis (Mole & Williams 2001). Late-onset Tay-Sachs disease (Neudorfer et al. 2005) can present with frontal syndromes, psychosis, primary lateral sclerosis, and even ALS. This usually occurs in Ashkenazi populations but has been seen in other ethnicities.

- **Nutritional deficiencies:** Vitamin B-1, B-3, and E deficiencies cause dementia, although there are no specific case reports suggesting that these syndromes overlap with FTD.
- **Infections:** Untreated syphilis or Lyme disease can cause chronic frontal lobe syndromes, and herpes simplex virus infection can leave patients with a frontotemporal syndrome.

Structural Brain Abnormalities

Brain tumors, subdural hematoma, and old developmental, traumatic, or vascular brain injuries can all mimic FTD and usually can be recognized with MRI. Normal pressure hydrocephalus presents with gait disturbance, urinary incontinence, and a dementia. Often, the dementia is characterized by apathy and sometimes disinhibition, overlapping with bvFTD.

Low intracranial pressure can lead to sagging of the frontotemporal regions onto the brainstem, causing a bvFTD syndrome with prominent apathy (Hong et al. 2002). Unlike typical bvFTD, these patients exhibit postural headache, and an MRI shows sagging frontal and temporal lobes.

TREATMENT

Treatment is discussed more extensively in Chapter 10. The management of bvFTD requires a comprehensive approach, and extensive guidance of the caregivers is particularly important (Jicha et al. 2011, Herrmann et al. 2012). Working to protect the family from the patient's poor insight is important, and decision making with bvFTD is almost always impaired (Hornberger et al. 2012, Strenziok et al. 2011). Companions can be helpful for protecting the patient from getting in trouble. Finding a supportive environment where the patient is not subject to danger is critical (Merrilees et al. 2010, Morhardt 2011).

Unfortunately a recent therapeutic trial with memantine was negative (Vercelletto et al. 2011, Boxer et al. 2013). Antidepressant medications including the selective serotonin reuptake inhibitors (SSRIs) and serotonin-norepinephrine reuptake inhibitors (SNRIs) have mild efficacy around symptoms related to the low serotonin associated with bvFTD including disinhibition, overeating, and repetitive motor behaviors (Swartz et al. 1997). Patients with bvFTD do not suffer from a significant cholinergic deficit, and cholinesterase inhibitors often make these patients worse (Vossel & Miller 2008). Medications that influence movement or swallowing such as antipsychotics should be avoided because patients often develop an extrapyramidal or ALS syndrome (Box 2.5).

bvFTD: CURRENT STATE AND RESEARCH ADVANCES

The understanding and diagnosis of bvFTD continues to improve. Less than one decade ago this disorder was rarely diagnosed, even in sophisticated memory clinics. Research and education have helped to make bvFTD widely recognized and increasingly more accessible to physicians and related health professionals, as well as caregivers. Across the world there are now experts in bvFTD, and there is increasing interest in the clinical manifestations of this condition. New international research criteria for bvFTD have simplified the diagnosis and are helping to establish standards for research databases and clinical trials.

Yet, bvFTD has not received widespread recognition, and the specialties where these patients may first present such as psychiatry, social work, psychology, and law enforcement do not have comprehensive efforts to diagnose or treat such patients. Indeed, the academic psychiatric journals rarely publish articles on bvFTD, despite the fact that these patients usually begin with psychiatric symptoms.

Box 2.5 Medications Used to Alleviate bvFTD Symptoms

Pharmacologic treatment in FTD is symptomatic and aimed at alleviating neurobehavioral symptoms.

- SSRIs have been used to treat compulsions, ritualistic behaviors, carbohydrate cravings, anxiety, and behavioral symptoms.

- Atypical antipsychotics such as quetiapine, olanzepine, or risperidone can be used for agitation, aggression, or psychotic behavior.

- NMDA-receptor antagonists such as memantine may provide some benefit.

- Valproic acid and derivatives may be useful for aggressive behavior and impulse control but can cause liver damage.

- Gabapentin may be helpful in managing behavioral problems.

Additionally, early diagnosis of bvFTD remains extremely difficult. The most promising area for research into early diagnosis is the study of genetic forms of bvFTD, where gene carriers can be recognized and followed through the early stages of their illness. Our preliminary work with this cohort of patients suggests that subtle neuropsychiatric syndromes range from addiction, depression, bipolar illness, and poor decision making to borderline and antisocial personality disorders (Khan et al. 2011). The study of these early behaviors in bvFTD will shed significant insights into the anatomic basis for psychiatric disorders.

While the diagnosis of bvFTD has dramatically improved, there are extensive efforts to determine the best biomarkers for both diagnosing and following the progression of this set of illnesses. While cerebrospinal fluid biomarkers have proven disappointing to date, there is still ongoing research into determining whether fragments of tau or other brain proteins will help to both improve diagnosis and follow the longitudinal progression of FTD (Grossman 2010).

Neuroimaging appears to show great promise for both of these goals. Howard Rosen at UCSF leads a longitudinal imaging study of FTD called Neuroimaging in Frontotemporal Dementia (NIFD) that includes sites at Mayo Clinic led by Brad Boeve and Dave Knopman and Harvard led by Brad Dickerson. Currently, diagnoses can be reliably obtained with simple structural imaging, but there have been ongoing efforts to determine the relative value of positron emission tomography (PET), perfusion, diffusion tensor, and connectivity mapping for the cross-sectional and longitudinal study of bvFTD. Cerebrospinal fluid is also collected.

The value of PET in the separation of AD from FTD has been explored since the early 1980s (Kamo et al. 1987). Fluorodeoxyglucose PET is now FDA approved for the differential diagnosis of FTD from AD and can precisely delineate a frontally predominant pattern of hypometabolism in FTD. Norman Foster has been the strongest advocate for the value of PET over MRI for early diagnosis of FTD (Foster et al. 2007). While his studies have been impressive, there are still some who believe that most of the abnormal signal associated with PET is volume averaging of atrophy. Howard Rosen's NIFD should answer this important question.

With diffusion tensor imaging it is clear that all of the subtypes of FTD are characterized by extensive white matter involvement (Borroni et al. 2007, Zhang et al. 2011). The UCSF group has described extensive white matter degeneration in FTD compared to AD (Zhang et al. 2009, Zhang et al. 2011), although the diagnostic value and pathologic underpinnings of this finding remain unknown. Additionally, Lillo and colleagues (Lillo et al. 2012) have suggested that FTD and FTD-ALS can be separated from ALS by the relative involvement of the corticospinal tract (ALS).

More recently, multimodal imaging has been explored to determine the best imaging technique for the diagnosis of FTD versus AD. In a study by Zhang and colleagues (Zhang et al. 2011), gray matter loss and white matter degeneration exceeded the reduced perfusion in FTD, whereas in AD, structural and functional damages were similar. Grossman and colleagues (McMillan et al. 2012) have also argued in multimodal imaging analyses that white matter degeneration adds diagnostic value.

Most exciting have been a series of studies on connectivity mapping led by Bill Seeley at UCSF. This technique allows the mapping of specific brain circuits by determining the brain regions that simultaneously activate together using the bold signal on fMRI. This technique was pioneered at Washington University by Randy Buckner and Marcus Raichle (Lustig et al. 2003) and was first applied to the study of AD by their group and by Michael Greicius at Stanford Medical School (Greicius et al. 2004). In AD they demonstrated decreased functional connectivity in a posterior network that includes precuneus, posterior cingulate, hippocampus, and a small region in the dorsal prefrontal cortex.

In an important study Seeley and colleagues (Seeley et al. 2009) demonstrated that AD, bvFTD, svPPA, nfvPPA, and CBS all had distinctive patterns of atrophy. Furthermore, they found that these diseases attacked, "five distinct, healthy, human intrinsic functional connectivity networks" and that there was a "direct link between intrinsic connectivity and gray matter structure" (Figure 2–11). The authors concluded that, "human neural networks can be defined by synchronous baseline activity, a unified corticotrophic fate, and selective vulnerability to neurodegenerative illness. Future studies may clarify how these complex systems are assembled during development and undermined by disease." This work set an important watermark for dementia research, defining the

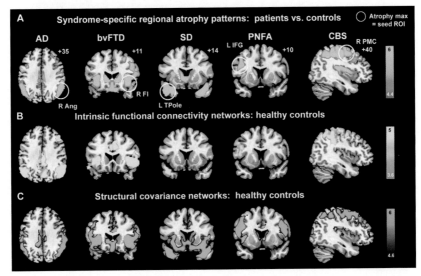

Figure 2–11. Convergent syndromic atrophy, healthy ICN, and healthy structural covariance patterns. (**A**) Five distinct clinical syndromes showed dissociable atrophy patterns, whose cortical maxima (circled) provided seed ROIs for ICN and structural covariance analyses. (**B**) ICN mapping experiments identified five distinct networks anchored by the five syndromic atrophy seeds. (**C**) Healthy subjects further showed gray matter volume covariance patterns that recapitulated results shown in (**A**) and (**B**). For visualization purposes, results are shown at p < 0.00001 uncorrected (**A and C**) and p < 0.001 corrected height and extent thresholds (**B**). In (**A–C**), results are displayed on representative sections of the MNI template brain. Color bars indicate t-scores. In coronal and axial images, the left side of the image corresponds to the left side of the brain. ANG, angular gyrus; FI, frontoinsula; IFGoper, inferior frontal gyrus, pars opercularis; PMC, premotor cortex; TPole, temporal pole. (Seeley et al. 2009.)

anatomic circuits associated with the major degenerative conditions, while offering hope that the longitudinal tracking of these circuits could be used to follow the illness.

In a fascinating follow-up study, Helen Zhou first-authored a paper from the Seeley group showing that in AD the posterior network (the default mode network) was diminished compared to healthy aged-matched controls, while the anterior network in the frontoinsular region (salience network) was actually increased in connectivity compared to controls. By contrast, the bvFTD group had decreased connectivity in the salience network but increased activity in the default mode network compared to the controls (Zhou et al. 2010) (Figure 2–12). Paradoxically, this study suggested that the loss of function in one of these reciprocal networks led to remodeling and enhancement of the other. This heightened connectivity in the network that was spared in AD and bvFTD improved separation from healthy controls and actually improved diagnostic accuracy.

Additionally, at a physiological and anatomical level this hints at why some patients with bvFTD develop visual creativity (increased posterior activity), or why some AD patients show normal or even enhanced social function (increased anterior activity).

Most recently, a third study published in the journal *Neuron* used connectivity mapping to predict longitudinal outcomes associated with distinctive degenerative disorders (Zhou et al. 2012). This paper demonstrated the major degenerative diseases all move predictably along specific circuits (Figure 2–13). Furthermore, the manner by which they traveled was best explained by a prion-like mechanism with steady movement from cell to cell. The authors suggested that similar findings from Raj and colleagues led to similar conclusions (Raj et al. 2012). These papers represent watershed findings because they suggest that functional connectivity mapping can be used for differential diagnosis, longitudinal tracking of disease, and understanding at a

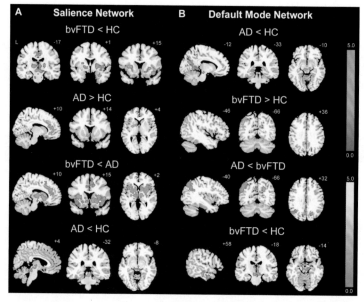

Figure 2–12. BvFTD and Alzheimer's disease feature divergent salience network and default mode network dynamics. Group difference maps illustrate clusters of significantly reduced or increased connectivity for each ICN. In the salience network **(A)**, patients with bvFTD showed distributed connectivity reductions compared to healthy controls (HC) and patients with Alzheimer's disease (AD), whereas patients with AD showed increased connectivity in anterior cingulate cortex and ventral striatum compared to healthy controls. In the DMN **(B)**, patients with AD showed several connectivity impairments compared to healthy controls and patients with bvFTD, whereas patients with bvFTD showed increased left angular gyrus connectivity. Patients with bvFTD and AD further showed focal brainstem connectivity disruptions within their "released" network (DMN for bvFTD, salience network for AD). Results are displayed at a joint height and extent probability threshold of P < 0.05, corrected at the whole brain level. Color bars represent t-scores, and statistical maps are superimposed on the Montreal Neurological Institute template brain. (Zhou et al. 2010.)

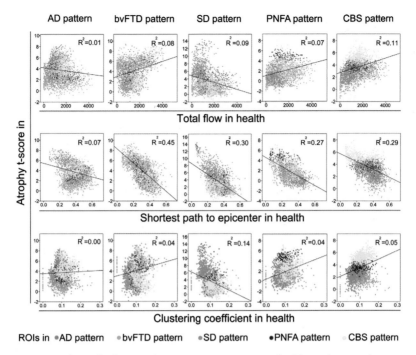

Figure 2–13. Transnetwork graph theoretical connectivity measures in health predict atrophy severity in disease. **Row 2:** ROIs showing greater disease-related atrophy were those featuring shorter functional paths, in the healthy brain, to the disease-associated epicenters (p < 0.05 familywise error corrected for multiple comparisons for AD, bvFTD, SD, PNFA, and CBS). **Rows 1 and 3:** Inconsistent weaker or nonsignificant relationships were observed between total flow or clustering coefficient and disease-related atrophy. (Zhou et al. 2012.)

mechanistic level how neurodegenerative diseases spread.

Drs. William Seeley, Christine Guo, and Suzee Lee at UCSF have applied this approach to early diagnosis with promising findings (Figure 2–14). As disease modifying and preventative therapies emerge, intervening during the earliest phase of the illness mandates better ways to know when the disease has started.

Another significant problem in bvFTD is determining the specific molecular subtype responsible for the clinical syndrome. While amyloid imaging is extremely valuable for separating patients with underlying AD, determining the molecular pathogenesis for bvFTD, whether neurodegenerative or psychiatric, remains difficult. Furthermore, unlike svPPA, nfvPPA, or PSP-syndrome, the diagnosis of bvFTD does not strongly help to narrow down the diagnosis to the molecular subtype—it can be caused by tau, TDP-43, or FUS.

Tau neuroimaging agents are under development, and a robust agent would become highly valuable for a variety of clinical syndromes including bvFTD, CTE, and PSP, and for neuropsychiatric patients with suspected FTD. Similarly, blood and CSF markers are needed. Finally, a better understanding of the risk factors for bvFTD, beyond genetics, needs to be determined.

As with AD, the future of bvFTD is early diagnosis and, ultimately, prevention. A time will come when individuals at risk for the different molecular forms of bvFTD will be recognized based on early life behavioral and imaging patterns as well as genetic background. Molecule and circuit-specific therapies will be initiated, and these devastating behavioral disorders will be eliminated. As will be described in the chapters on genetics and treatments, progranulin mutation carriers may be the first group of bvFTD patients for whom prevention may occur.

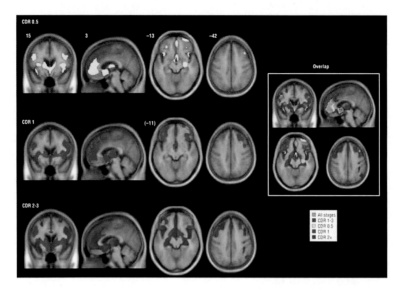

Figure 2–14. Stage-specific gray matter atrophy in behavioral variant frontotemporal dementia. Maps of significantly atrophied voxels (each group vs controls: P < 0.05, whole brain corrected) are overlaid on the study-specific brain template, using an inclusive gray matter mask for visualization purposes only. On the right, the same color scheme is overlaid on a single image to show overlap of stage-related atrophy patterns. The right side of the axial and coronal images corresponds to the right side of the brain. Numbers indicate the MNI (Montreal Neurological Institute) coordinate of the template brain magnetic resonance image shown. CDR indicates Clinical Dementia Rating; CDR 1–3, mild to severe; CDR 0.5, very mild; CDR 1, mild; and CDR 2+, moderate to severe. (Seeley et al. 2008.)

REFERENCES

Bora E, Fornito A, Yucel M, Pantelis C. Voxelwise meta-analysis of gray matter abnormalities in bipolar disorder. Biol Psychiatry. 2010;67:1097–105.

Borroni B, Brambati SM, Agosti C, Gipponi S, Bellelli G, Gasparotti R, Garibotto V, Di Luca M, Scifo P, Perani D, Padovani A. Evidence of white matter changes on diffusion tensor imaging in frontotemporal dementia. Arch Neurol. 2007;64(2):246–51.

Boxer AL, Knopman DS, Kaufer DI, Grossman M, Onyike C, Graf-Radford N, Mendez M, Kerwin D, Lerner A, Wu CK, Koestler M, Shapira J, Sullivan K, Klepac K, Lipowski K, Ullah J, Fields S, Kramer JH, Merrilees J, Neuhaus J, Mesulam MM, Miller BL. Memantine in patients with frontotemporal lobar degeneration: a multicentre, randomised, double-blind, placebo-controlled trial. Lancet Neurol. 2013;12:149–56.

Bozeat S, Gregory CA, Ralph MA, Hodges JR. Which neuropsychiatric and behavioural features distinguish frontal and temporal variants of frontotemporal dementia from Alzheimer's disease? J Neurol Neurosurg Psychiatry. 2000;69(2):178–86.

Blundo C, Marin D, Ricci M. Vitamin B12 deficiency associated with symptoms of frontotemporal dementia. Neurol Sci. 2011;32(1):101–5.

Chin J, Seo SW, Kim SH, Park A, Ahn HJ, Lee BH, Kang SJ, NA DL. Neurobehavioral dysfunction in patients with subcortical vascular mild cognitive impairment and subcortical vascular dementia. Clin Neuropsychol. 2012;26(2):224–38.

Chow TW, Binns MA, Cummings JL, Lam I, Black SE, Miller BL, Freedman M, Stuss DT, van Reekum R. Apathy symptom profile and behavioral associations in frontotemporal dementia vs. dementia of Alzheimer type. Arch Neurol. 2009; 66(7):888–93.

Edwards-Lee T, Miller BL, Benson DF, Cummings JL, Russell GL, Boone K, Mena I. The temporal variant of frontotemporal dementia. Brain. 1997;120(Pt 6): 1027–40.

Foster NL, Heidebrink JL, Clark CM, Jagust WJ, Arnold SE, Barbas NR, DeCarli CS, Turner RS, Koeppe RA, Higdon R, Minoshima S. FDG-PET improves accuracy in distinguishing frontotemporal dementia and Alzheimer's disease. Brain. 2007;130(Pt 10):2616–35.

Gavett BE, Cantu RC, Shenton M, Lin AP, Nowinski CJ, McKee AC, Stern RA. Clinical appraisal of chronic traumatic encephalopathy: current perspective and future direction. Current Opin Neurol. 2011;24(6):525–31.

Giovagnoli AR, Erbetta A, Reati F, Bugiani O. Differential neuropsychological patterns of frontal variant frontotemporal dementia and Alzheimer's disease in a study of diagnostic concordance. Neuropsychologia. 2008;46:1495–504.

Greicius MD, Srivastava G, Reiss AL, Menon V. Default-mode network activity distinguishes Alzheimer's disease from healthy aging: evidence from functional MRI. Proc Natl Acad Sci U S A. 2004;101(13):4637–42.

Grossman M. Biomarkers in frontotemporal lobar degeneration. Curr Opin Neurol. 2010;23(6):643–8.

Herrmann N, Black SE, Chow T, Cappell J, Tang-Wai DF, Lanctôt KL. Serotonergic function and treatment of behavioral and psychological symptoms of frontotemporal dementia. Am J Geriatr Psychiatry. 2012;20(9):789–97.

Hong M, Shah GV, Adams KM, Turner RS, Foster NL. Spontaneous intracranial hypotension causing reversible frontotemporal dementia. Neurology. 2002;58:1285–7.

Hornberger M, Piguet O, Graham AJ, Nestor PJ, Hodges JR. How preserved is episodic memory in behavioral variant frontotemporal dementia. Neurology. 2010;74(6):472–9.

Hornberger M, Yew B, Gilardoni S, Mioshi E, Gleichgerrcht E, Manes F, Hodges JR. Ventromedial-frontopolar prefrontal cortex atrophy correlates with insight loss in frontotemporal dementia and Alzheimer's disease. Hum Brain Mapp. 2012 Nov 5. [Epub ahead of print]

Ikeda M, Brown J, Holland AJ, Fukuhara R, Hodges JR. Changes in appetite, food preference, and eating habits in frontotemporal dementia and Alzheimer's disease. J Neurol Neurosurg Psychiatry. 2002;73(4):371–6.

Jicha GA, Nelson PT. Management of frontotemporal dementia: targeting symptom management in such a heterogeneous disease requires a wide range of therapeutic options. Neurodegener Dis Manag. 2011;1:141–56.

Johnson JK, Vogt BA, Kim R, Cotman CW, Head. Isolated executive impairment and associated frontal neuropathology. Dementi Geratr Cogn Disord. 2004;17(4):360–7.

Johnson JK, Diehl J, Mendez MF, Neuhaus J, Shapira JS, Forman M, Chute DJ, Roberson ED, Pace-Savitsky C, Neumann M, Chow TW, Rosen HJ, Forstl H, Kurz A, Miller BL. Frontotemporal lobar degeneration: demographic characteristics of 353 patients. Arch Neurol. 2005;62(6):925–30.

Kamo H, McGeer PL, Harrop R, McGeer EG, Calne DB, Martin WR, Pate BD. Positron emission tomography and histopathology in Pick's disease. Neurology. 1987;37(3):439–45.

Khan BK, Woolley JD, Chao S, See T, Karydas AM, Miller BL, Rankin KP. Schizophrenia or neurodegencrative disease prodrome? Outcome of a first psychotic episode in a 35-year-old woman. Psychosomatics. 2012;53(3):280–4.

Khan BK, Yokoyama JS, Takada LT, Sha SJ, Rutherford NJ, Fong JC, Karydas AM, Wu T, Ketelle RS, Baker MC, Hernandez MD, Coppola G, Geschwind DH, Rademakers R, Lee SE, Rosen HJ, Rabinovici GD, Seeley WW, Rankin KP, Boxer AL, Miller BL. Atypical, slowly progressive behavioural variant frontotemporal dementia associated with C9ORF72 hexanucleotide expansion. J Neurol Neurosurg Psychiatry. 2012;83:358–64.

Kipps CM, Hodges JR, Hornberger M. Nonprogressive behavioural frontotemporal dementia: recent developments and clinical implications of the "bvFTD phenocopy syndrome." Curr Opin Neurol. 2010;23:628–32.

Krueger CE, Laluz V, Rosen HJ, Neuhaus JM, Miller BL, Kramer JH. Double dissociation in the anatomy of socioemotional disinhibition and executive functioning in dementia. Neuropsychology. 2011;25(2):249–59.

Lebert F, Pasquier F. Frontotemporal dementia: behavioral story of a neurological disease. Psychol Neuropsychiatr Vieil. 2008;6(1):33–41.

Lee S, Wilson SM, Seeley W, Rankin K, Dearmond S, Huang EJ, Trojanowki JQ, Growdon M, Jang J, Sidhu M, See T, Karydas A, Jagust W, Weiner M, Gorno Tempini ML, Boxer A, Miller BL, Rabinovici GD. Correlates of Alzheimer's disease pathology in corticobasal syndrome. Annals of Neurology. 2011;70(2):327–40.

Lillo P, Mioshi E, Burrell JR, Kiernan MC, Hodges JR, Hornberger M. Grey and white matter changes across the amyotrophic lateral sclerosis-frontotemporal dementia continuum. PLoS One. 2012;7(8):e43993.

Lomen-Hoerth C, Anderson T, Miller B. The overlap of amyotrophic lateral sclerosis and frontotemporal dementia. Neurology. 2002;59(7):1077–9.

Lomen-Hoerth C, Murphy J, Langmore S, Kramer JH, Olney RK, Miller BL. Are amyotrophic lateral sclerosis patients cognitively normal? Neurology. 2003;60:1094–97.

Lustig C, Snyder AZ, Bhakta M, O'Brien KC, McAvoy M, Raichle ME, Morris JC, Buckner RL. Functional deactivations: change with age and dementia of the Alzheimer type. Proc Natl Acad Sci U S A. 2003;100(24):14504–9.

Manes F. Psychiatric conditions that can mimic early behavioral variant frontotemporal dementia: the importance of the new diagnostic criteria. Curr Psychiatry Rep. 2012;14:450–2.

McMillan CT, Brun C, Siddiqui S, Churgin M, Libon D, Yushkevich P, Zhang H, Boller A, Gee J, Grossman M. White matter imaging contributes to the multimodal diagnosis of frontotemporal lobar degeneration. Neurology. 2012;78(22):1761–8.

McKee AC, Gavett BE, Stern RA, Nowinski CJ, Cantu RC, Kowall NW, Perl DP, Hedley-Whyte ET, Price B, Sullivan C, Morin P, Lee HS, Kubilus CA, Daneshvar DH, Wulff M, Budson AE. TDP-43 proteinopathy and motor neuron disease in chronic traumatic encephalopathy. J Neuropathol Exp Neurol. 2010;69:918–29.

Merrilees J, Miller BL. Comparing Alzheimer's disease and frontotemporal lobar degeneration: implications for long-term care. Annals of Long-Term Care: Clinical Care and Aging. 2005;12:37–40.

Merrilees J, Hubbard E, Mastick J, Miller BL, Dowling GA. Rest-activity and behavioral disruption in a patient with frontotemporal dementia. Neurocase. 2009;15(6):515–26.

Merrilees J, Ketelle R. Advanced practice nursing: meeting the caregiving challenges for families of persons with frontotemporal dementia. Clin Nurse Spec. 2010;24(5):245–51.

Miller BL, Cummings JL, Villanueva-Meyer J, Boone K, Mehringer CM, Lesser IM, Mena I. Frontal lobe degeneration: clinical, neuropsychological, and SPECT characteristics. Neurology. 1991;41(9):1374–82.

Miller BL, Darby A, Benson DF, Cummings JL, Miller MH. Aggressive, socially disruptive and antisocial behavior in frontotemporal dementia. Brit J Psychiatry. 1997;170:150–56.

Miller BL, Darby AL, Swartz JR, Yener GG, Mena I. Dietary changes, compulsions and sexual behavior in frontotemporal degeneration. Dementia. 1995;6(4):195–9.

Miller BL, Mychack P, Seeley W, Rosen, H, Boone KB. Neuroanatomy of the self: evidence from patients with frontotemporal dementia. Neurology. 2001;57:817–21.

Mole SE, Williams RE. Neuronal ceroid-lipofuscinoses. In: Pagon RA, Bird TD, Dolan CR, Stephens K, Adam MP, editors. GeneReviews (Internet). Seattle (WA): University of Washington, Seattle; 1993–2001, updated 2010.

Morhardt D. Accessing community-based and long-term care services: challenges facing persons with frontotemporal dementia and their families. J Mol Neurosci. 2011;45(3):737–41.

Neudorfer O, Pastores GM, Zeng BJ, Gianutsos J, Zaroff CM, Kolodny EH. Late-onset Tay-Sachs disease: phenotypic characterization and genotypic correlations in 21 affected patients. Genet Med. 2005;7(2):119–23.

Perry DC, Whitwell JL, Boeve BF, Pankratz VS, Knopman DS, Petersen RC, Jack CR Jr, Josephs KA. Voxel-based morphometry in patients with obsessive-compulsive behaviors in behavioral variant frontotemporal dementia. Eur J Neurol. 2012;19(6):911–7.

Piguet O, Petersén A, Yin Ka Lam B, Gabery S, Murphy K, Hodges JR, Halliday GM. Eating and hypothalamus changes in behavioral-variant frontotemporal dementia. Ann Neurol. 2011;69:312–19.

Rabinovici GD, Rosen HJ, Alkalay A, Kornak J, Furst AJ, Agarwal N, Mormino EC, O'Neil JP, Janabi M, Karydas A, Growdon ME, Jang JY, Huang EJ, Dearmond SJ, Trojanowski JQ, Grinberg LT, Gorno-Tempini ML, Seeley WW, Miller BL, Jagust WJ. Amyloid vs FDG-PET in the differential diagnosis of AD and FTLD. Neurology. 2011;77:2034–42.

Raj A, Kuceyeski A, Weiner M. A network diffusion model of disease progression in dementia. Neuron. 2012;73:1204–15.

Rankin K, Kramer, JH, Mychack P, Miller BL. Double dissociation of social functioning in frontotemporal dementia. Neurology. 2003;60:266–71.

Rankin KP, Baldwin E, Pace-Savitsky C, Kramer JH, Miller BL. Self awareness and personality change in dementia. J Neurol Neurosurg Psychiatry. 2005;76(5):632–9.

Rankin KP, Gorno-Tempini ML, Allison SC, Stanley CM, Glenn S, Weiner MW, Miller BL. Structural anatomy of empathy in neurodegenerative disease. Brain. 2006;129:2945–56.

Rascovsky K, Hodges JR, Knopman D, Mendez MF, Kramer JH, Neuhaus J, van Swieten JC, Seelaar H, Dopper EG, Onyike CU, Hillis AE, Josephs KA, Boeve BF, Kertesz A, Seeley WW, Rankin KP, Johnson JK, Gorno-Tempini ML, Rosen H, Prioleau-Latham CE, Lee A, Kipps CM, Lillo P, Piguet O, Rohrer JD, Rossor MN, Warren JD, Fox NC, Galasko D, Salmon DP, Black SE, Mesulam M, Weintraub S, Dickerson BC, Diehl-Schmid J, Pasquier F, Deramecourt V, Lebert F, Pijnenburg Y, Chow TW, Manes F, Grafman J, Cappa SF, Freedman M, Grossman M, Miller BL. Sensitivity of revised diagnostic criteria for the behavioural variant of frontotemporal dementia. *Brain*. 2011;134:2456–77.

Roberson ED, Hesse JH, Rose KD, Slama H, Johnson JK, Yaffe K, Forman M, Miller C, Trojanowski JQ, Kramer JH, Miller BL. Frontotemporal dementia progresses to death faster than Alzheimer disease. Neurology. 2005;65:719–725.

Rosen HJ, Allison S, Schauer GF, Gorno-Tempini ML, Weiner MW, Miller BL. Neuroanatomical correlates of behavioral disorders in dementia. Brain. 2005;128:2612–25.

Rosen HJ, Gorno-Tempini ML, Goldman WP, Perry RJ, Schuff N, Weiner M, Feiwell R, Kramer JH, Miller BL. Patterns of brain atrophy in frontotemporal dementia and semantic dementia. Neurology. 2002;58:198–208.

Rosen HJ. Anosognosia in neurodegenerative disease. Neurocase. 2011;17:231–41.

Sanders F, Smeets-Hanssen MM, Meesters PD, van der Vlies AE, Kerssens CJ, Pinjnenburg YA. Frontotemporal dementia and schizophrenia in later life: a comparison of executive and general cognitive functions. Tijdschr Psychiatr. 2012;54:409–17.

Seeley WW, Bauer A, Miller BL, Gorno-Tempini ML, Kramer JH, Weiner M, Rosen HJ. The natural history of temporal variant frontotemporal dementia. Neurology. 2005;64:1384–90.

Seeley WW, Crawford R, Rascovsky K, Kramer JH, Weiner M, Miller BL, Gorno-Tempini ML. Frontal paralimbic network atrophy in very mild behavioral variant frontotemporal dementia. Arch Neurol. 2008;65:249–55.

Seeley WW, Crawford RK, Zhou J, Miller BL, Greicius MD. Neurodegenerative diseases target large-scale human brain networks. Neuron. 2009;62:42–52.

Sha SJ, Takada LT, Rankin KP, Yokoyama JS, Rutherford NJ, Fong JC, Khan B, Karydas A, Baker MC, Dejesus-Hernandez M, Pribadi M, Coppola G, Geschwind DH, Rademakers R, Lee SE, Seeley W, Miller BL, Boxer AL. Frontotemporal dementia due to *C9ORF72* mutations: Clinical and imaging features. Neurology. 2012;79:1002–11.

Skomer C, Stears J, Austin J. Metachromatic leukodystrophy (MLD. XV. Adult MLD with focal lesions by computer tomography. Arch Neurol. 1983;40(6):354–5.

Strenziok M, Pulaski S, Krueger F, Zamboni G, Clawson D, Grafman J. Regional brain atrophy and impaired decision making on the balloon analog risk task in behavioral variant frontotemporal dementia. Cogn Behav Neurol. 2011;24(2):59–67.

Sturm VE, Rosen HJ, Allison S, Miller BL, Levenson RW. Self conscious emotion deficits in frontotemporal lobar degeneration. Brain. 2006;129:2508–16.

Suárez J, Tartaglia MC, Vitali P, Erbetta A, Neuhaus J, Laluz V, Miller BL. Characterizing radiology reports in patients with frontotemporal dementia. Neurology. 2009;73:1073–4.

Swartz JR, Miller BL, Lesser IM, Darby AL. Frontotemporal dementia: treatment response to serotonin selective reuptake inhibitors. J Clin Psychiatry. 1997;58(5):212–6.

Tosun D, Rosen H, Miller BL, Weiner MW, Schuff N. MRI patterns of atrophy and hypoperfusion associations across brain regions in frontotemporal dementia. Neuroimage. 2012;59(3):2098–109.

Vercelletto M, Boutoleau-Bretonnière C, Volteau C, Puel M, Auriacombe S, Sarazin M, Michel BF, Couratier P, Thomas-Antérion C, Verpillat P, Gabelle A, Golfier V, Cerato E, Lacomblez L; French research network on Frontotemporal dementia. Memantine in behavioral variant frontotemporal dementia: negative results. J Alzheimers Dis. 2011;23(4):749–59.

Vossel KA, Miller BL. New approaches to the treatment of frontotemporal lobar degeneration. Curr Opin Neurol. 2008;21:708–16.

Woolley JD, Gorno-Tempini ML, Seeley WW, Rankin K, Lee SS, Matthews BR, Miller BL. Binge eating is associated with right orbitofrontal-insular-striatal atrophy in frontotemporal dementia. Neurology. 2007;69:1424–33.

Woolley JD, Khan BK, Murthy NK, Miller BL, Rankin KP. The diagnostic challenge of psychiatric symptoms in neurodegenerative disease: Rates of and risk factors for prior psychiatric diagnosis in patients with early neurodegenerative disease. J Clin Psychiatry. 2011;72:126–33.

Yatabe Y, Hashimoto M, Kaneda K, Honda K, Ogawa Y, Yuuki S, Matsuzaki S, Tuyuguchi A, Kashiwagi H, Ikeda M. Neuropsychiatric symptoms of progressive supranuclear palsy in a dementia clinic. Psychogeriatrics. 2011;11:54–9.

Zhang Y, Schuff N, Ching C, Tosun D, Zhan W, Nezamzadeh M, Rosen HJ, Kramer JH, Gorno-Tempini ML, Miller BL, Weiner MW. Joint assessment of structural, perfusion, and diffusion MRI in Alzheimer's disease and frontotemporal dementia. Int J Alzheimers Dis. 2011;2011:546871.

Zhang Y, Schuff N, Du AT, Rosen HJ, Kramer JH, Gorno-Tempini ML, Miller BL, Weiner MW. White matter damage in frontotemporal dementia and Alzheimer's disease measured by diffusion MRI. Brain. 2009;132(Pt 9):2579–92.

Zhou J, Greicius MD, Gennatas ED, Growdon ME, Jang JY, Rabinovici GD, Kramer JH, Weiner M, Miller BL, Seeley WW. Divergent network connectivity changes in behavioural variant frontotemporal dementia and Alzheimer's disease. Brain. 2010;133(Pt 5):1352–67.

Zhou J, Gennatas ED, Kramer JH, Miller BL, Seeley WW. Predicting regional neurodegeneration from the healthy brain functional connectome. Neuron. 2012;73(6):1216–27.

Chapter 3

The Clinical Syndrome of svPPA

OVERVIEW

The temporal variant of FTD is a fascinating disorder, and its study has offered unique insights into the functions of the amygdala and the anterior temporal neocortex. Tulving notes that, "Semantic memory (also called conceptual knowledge) is the aspect of human memory that corresponds to general knowledge of objects, word meanings, facts and people, without connection to any particular time or place" (Tulving 1987). In the semantic variant of primary progressive aphasia (svPPA; also called "semantic dementia"), selective degeneration of the left anterior temporal lobe leads to a disorder of semantic knowledge, slowly decimating the intricate classification and naming systems that we first develop as children to understand the world (Hodges et al. 1992; Patterson et al. 2007).

When the right anterior temporal lobe is the primary site of degeneration, profound deficits in empathy and recognition of other people's emotions or difficulty recognizing familiar faces are the first manifestations of the illness (Tyrrell et al. 1990, Perry et al. 2001, Rankin et al. 2006). When the degeneration of the temporal lobes progresses to the orbital frontal and anterior cingulate cortex, patients begin to exhibit many features suggestive of bvFTD (Seeley et al. 2005). Progression with both svPPA and the right temporal variant is slow, and there are patients who live as long as two decades with this form of FTD. Occasional patients develop ALS (and at autopsy show TDP-43 type B aggregates), but the vast majority shows TDP-43 type C pathology and never exhibit ALS (Mackenzie et al. 2011). Alzheimer's disease (AD) is an uncommon cause for svPPA.

CASE HISTORY

Mr. A, a 62-year-old male high school teacher began to notice difficulty finding words while speaking to colleagues and students. In his classroom when he came upon a word that he could not remember, he used the "Socratic method" to generate the word that he had lost from the class. "I am talking about that large park in the middle of San Francisco." The students would quickly respond, "Golden Gate Park?" "Yes," he would say, "Golden Gate Park." Eventually his principal asked him to retire, after receiving multiple complaints from the students regarding his inability to teach effectively. There was no family history of neurological disease, and the only other medical problem that the patient had was a recent diagnosis of Sjogren's syndrome with both dry eyes and dry mouth. He treated the dry eyes with artificial tears.

Neurological evaluation revealed a serious man with frequent word pauses. He had a 30/30 on the Mini Mental Status Exam (MMSE) but obtained only 7/15 on the abbreviated Boston Naming Test (BNT). He had particular trouble with the animals on the test including "octopus," which he called "fish," and "camel," which he called "cow." When the correct answers were read back to him, he said, "Octopus—what is an octopus?" There was evidence for surface dyslexia, and he read "yacht" as "yachet" and "knight" as "kuniyt," commenting

that he didn't know what either word meant. Verbal memory showed a flat learning curve (6 of 9 words on the fourth trial) and diminished recall (4 of 9 after 10 minutes). Like many patients with svPPA, he was not helped by category clues. Visual memory, working memory, and executive control were normal, and digit span backward was eight.

An MRI showed extensive left anterior temporal lobe atrophy, particularly severe in the middle and inferior temporal gyri. The left amygdala was small. There was mild atrophy of the right anterior temporal lobe and amygdala. A diagnosis of svPPA was made (Figure 3–1).

Upon retiring, he continued to oversee the family's finances while devoting himself to tennis, at which he improved steadily for two years. He played solitaire compulsively and began to paint, creating realistic copies of local animals, squirrels, chipmunks, cows, and horses. He became compulsive about taking vitamins and restricted his diet to low-fat frozen yogurt and chicken.

Within two years, the patient was restricted to the use of only 15 words, all verbs or vague descriptors. He called all animals "things." He continued to play tennis with a friend but transferred all financial matters to his wife. Solitaire began to take up four hours daily, and he began to compulsively collect cans from the trash. His dietary restrictions loosened, and he began to search his house for alcohol. His interest in painting ceased, although he helped with gardening and washing the dishes. His wife complained that he began to have trouble recognizing familiar faces and that he had become emotionally cold and indifferent to her feelings.

On examination Mr. A was cooperative. His MMSE had slipped to 14, and he missed all three points on following a sentence, two words on recall, and most of the orientation questions.

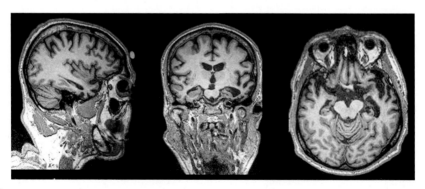

Figure 3–1. Typical atrophy of the right anterior temporal lobe and amygdala seen in this patient with svPPA.

He drew the pentagons and a more complex figure copy perfectly. All animals and tools were called "things," and he got 1/15 items on the BNT (bed). He could read phonetically but not when words were spelled in an irregular fashion. He failed on a task of emotion recognition, calling sad, surprised, and angry faces "happy" (Figure 3–2). When asked to draw an elephant, cow, fish, and bird, the animals had similar features, suggesting a prototypical animal that had come out of evolution (Figure 3–3). On the Neuropsychiatric Inventory (NPI), the family endorsed the items for disinhibition, eating disorder, repetitive motor behavior, apathy, and eating change. The basic neurological examination was normal.

Two years later, Mr. A required help with toileting and dressing, and his wife had to lock the door to prevent him from wandering away. He picked up items frequently and began to place them in his mouth. On one occasion, the police were called because Mr. A had touched a young child at a local store. When shopping, he had a tendency to place items into his pockets. Cognitive testing was hard to perform, but he obtained a 4 on the MMSE by repeating the three words and drawing correctly the intersecting pentagons. That year Mr. A was placed in a nursing home, where he began to show motor slowing and difficulty with

swallowing. Parkinsonism was evident. Within six months Mr. A aspirated on a piece of wood that he had found while walking.

Autopsy revealed extensive anterior temporal atrophy, left greater than right, with massive tissue loss in the amygdala. The orbital and medial frontal cortex were also atrophic, and there was mild atrophy in the dorsal-lateral convexity of the frontal lobe and in the caudate and putamen. Histologically there was extensive degeneration of white matter in the medial temporal lobe, frequent dendritic TDP-43, and sparse aggregates of cytoplasmic TDP-43 in the dentate region of the medial temporal lobe. This was diagnosed as a TDP-43 type C pattern (Mackenzie et al. 2011) (Figure 3–4).

Comment. This case illustrates the presentation and progression of svPPA. The disease begins with word-finding trouble, and it is often the patient who first notices the difficulty with words. The anomia of svPPA differs from what is seen with AD in that clues do not help the patient to find the word. Surface dyslexia and dysgraphia (the inability to read or write irregular words that do not follow the normal phonetic rules of the English language) occur early, while visuospatial abilities are often maintained late into the disease (Patterson & Hodges 1992; Brambati et al. 2006;

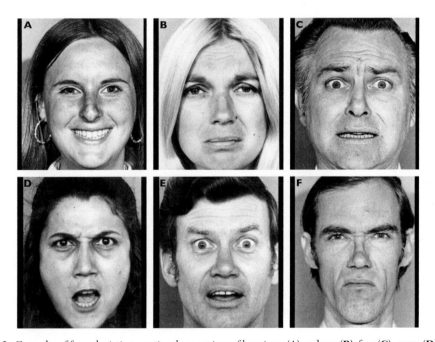

Figure 3–2. Examples of faces depicting emotional expressions of happiness (**A**), sadness (**B**), fear (**C**), anger (**D**), surprise (**E**), and disgust (**F**). (Ekman et al. 2002.)

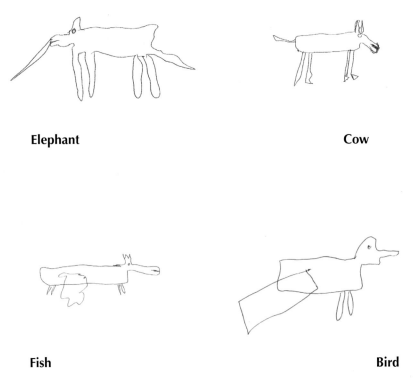

Elephant   **Cow**

Fish   **Bird**

Figure 3–3. Spontaneous animal drawings by patient.

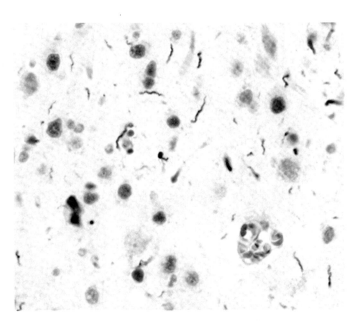

Figure 3–4. Patient histology showing a TDP43 type C pattern. (Image courtesy of Lea Grinberg, MD, PhD, and William Seeley, MD.)

Brambati et al. 2009). Compulsions are common, even in the early stages (Perry et al. 2012). As the disease moves to the right temporal lobe, patients lose the ability to recognize emotions in faces and forget the names of familiar people (Brambati et al. 2010). This can dramatically impair the ability to engage in social interactions. As was seen in Mr. A, svPPA is rarely genetic (Goldman et al. 2005) and nearly always shows TDP-43 type C pathology (Mackenzie et al. 2011).

CLINICAL FEATURES AND ANATOMY

Pick's case report in 1892 described a form of dementia associated with focal and progressive anterior temporal lobe atrophy that began clinically as a fluent, anomic aphasia. This temporally predominant form of FTD was largely neglected until 1982, when Mesulam coined the term "primary progressive aphasia" (PPA) to describe patients with at least two years of progressive language disorder with relative sparing of behavior and cognition and sparing of day-to-day function (Mesulam 1982). Patients with both fluent and nonfluent forms of aphasia were included under this PPA rubric.

In the 1990s John Hodges in Cambridge, England (Hodges et al. 1992), and Julie Snowden and David Neary in Manchester, England (Snowden et al. 1992), highlighted the language features of patients with selective degeneration of the left anterior temporal lobe, for which they applied the term "semantic dementia." Around the same time, patients with selective degeneration of the right anterior temporal lobe were described. Rossor and colleagues focused on the deficits in facial recognition associated with the right temporal lobe variant of FTD reporting on progressive prosopagnosia (Tyrrell et al. 1990), while my colleagues and I emphasized the odd and troubling social deficits of these patients (Miller et al. 1993).

New diagnostic criteria for PPA were published in 2011 with three major subtypes listed: nonfluent/agrammatic, logopenic, and semantic. Semantic variant primary progressive aphasia (svPPA) has both clinical and imaging-supported diagnostic components (Box 3.1) with the criteria requiring deficits in naming, single word comprehension, or knowledge about faces and people as the principal cause of impaired daily living. Also, they stipulate that the aphasia should be the most prominent deficit at symptom onset and during the initial phases of the

---

Box 3.1 International Consensus Research Criteria for Semantic Variant Primary Progressive Aphasia (svPPA) (Gorno-Tempini et al. 2011)

I. Primary progressive aphasia (PPA)

Inclusion: Criteria I.A.–I.C. must be answered positively.
- I.A. Most prominent clinical feature is difficulty with language
- I.B. These deficits are the principal cause of impaired daily living activities
- I.C. Aphasia should be the most prominent deficit at symptom onset and for the initial phases of the disease

Exclusion: Criteria I.D.–I.G. must be answered negatively for a PPA diagnosis.
- I.D. Pattern of deficits is better accounted for by other nondegenerative nervous system or medical disorders
- I.E. Cognitive disturbance is better accounted for by a psychiatric diagnosis
- I.F. Prominent initial episodic memory, visual memory, and visuoperceptual impairments
- I.G. Prominent, initial behavioral disturbance

(continued)

> ### Box 3.1 International Consensus Research Criteria for
> ###   Semantic Variant Primary Progressive Aphasia (svPPA)
> ###   (Gorno-Tempini et al. 2011) (cont.)
>
> ### II. Clinical diagnosis of semantic variant PPA
>
> Both of the following core features must be present:
> - II.A. Impaired confrontation naming
> - II.B. Impaired single-word comprehension
>
> At least 3 of the following other diagnostic features must be present:
> - II.C. Impaired object knowledge, particularly for low-frequency or low-familiarity items
> - II.D. Surface dyslexia or dysgraphia
> - II.E. Spared repetition
> - II.F. Spared speech production (grammar and motor speech)
>
> ### III. Imaging-supported semantic variant PPA diagnosis
>
> Both of the following criteria must be present:
> - III.A. Clinical diagnosis of semantic variant PPA
> - III.B. Imaging must show one or more of the following results: Predominant anterior temporal lobe atrophyPredominant anterior temporal hypoperfusion or hypometabolism on SPECT or PET
>
> ### IV. Semantic variant PPA with definite pathology
>
> Clinical diagnosis (criterion IV.A. below) and either criterion IV.B. or IV.C. must be present:
> - IV.A. Clinical diagnosis of semantic variant PPA
> - IV.B. Histopathologic evidence of a specific neurodegenerative pathology (e.g., FTLD-tau, FTLD-TDP, Alzheimer's disease, other)
> - IV.C. Presence of a known pathogenic mutation

disease. Additionally, imaging requires selective atrophy in the anterior temporal lobes (Gorno-Tempini et al. 2011) (Figure 3–5).

The language deficit associated with svPPA begins subtly. Initially patients exhibit occasional word-finding problems. Often it is nouns or names, not verbs or the grammatical components of language. While insight is variable with svPPA, many such patients are the first to notice their problem and become extremely self-critical about their word-finding disturbance, even hitting their heads in frustration when they fail to remember the word for which they were searching. When patients are tested in the early stages of the illness, they may show a subtle anomia without major semantic deficits. But, as the disease progresses, difficulty understanding the meaning of individual words becomes evident. The patient may repeat a word that has been spoken and ask what it

means, "Kite, what is a kite?" Eventually, so many words disappear that it becomes hard for the patient to communicate with others. Repetition is typically spared. The naming deficit is multimodal, and patients show poor knowledge of words and their meanings, whether the item is presented via the visual, auditory, or tactile modality (Ikeda et al. 2006).

Surface dyslexia and dysgraphia is the inability to read and write words that do not follow regular phonetic rules (Brambati et al. 2009). A low-frequency item like "gnat" is read, "gunat," and the patient does not realize that a gnat is an insect. In the early stages, names for people are lost, but the patient still recognizes faces. Over time, the disease spreads to the right temporal lobe, leading to profound deficits in knowledge about people, often disrupting social relationships.

To diagnose svPPA, neurodegenerative disease should be the best possible explanation for

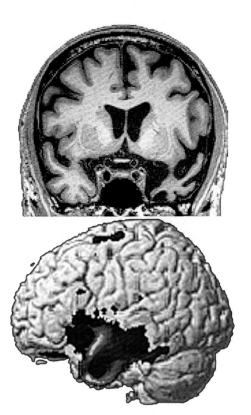

Figure 3–5. MRI showing typical atrophy pattern seen in svPPA, and VBM group analysis of svPPA versus healthy controls. (Image courtesy of Howard Rosen, MD.)

the symptoms. Medical and psychiatric disorders like neoplasms, cerebrovascular disease, hypothyroidism, depression, bipolar disease, schizophrenia, and personality disorder need to be ruled out as possible explanations. If the most prominent initial impairments are in episodic memory, visual memory, visuoperceptual skills, or behavior, then the patient most likely does not have svPPA, and another diagnosis like AD should be considered.

The two most basic symptoms of svPPA are poor confrontation naming of pictures or objects, particularly low familiarity or low frequency items, and impaired single-word comprehension. Both deficits must be present to make a diagnosis. Excellent grammar is evident in the patient's speech, which is structurally correct, and patients do remarkably well on tests of sentence comprehension as long as the nouns in the phrases are frequently used in the patient's vocabulary. Patients correctly comprehend even complex sentences such as "the boy is kissing the girl that the man with the hat

is hugging" because regions involved in grammatical processing in the left frontal and posterior left perisylvian regions are spared until the latest stages of this disorder.

svPPA is associated with anterior temporal lobe and ventromedial frontal gray matter atrophy, often with proportionate degeneration of anterior temporal white matter. Imaging should show predominant anterior temporal lobe atrophy on MRI or predominant anterior temporal hypoperfusion or hypometabolism on SPECT or PET. Diffusion tensor imaging typically shows microstructural damage to left hemisphere ventral white matter tracts. Activation fMRI during reading shows that the left midfusiform gyrus and superior temporal regions are less activated in patients with svPPA, probably due to damage of white matter tracts (i.e., inferior longitudinal fasciculus and arcuate) (Brambati et al. 2009). Conversely, svPPA patients show normal or increased activation of the left posterior inferior frontal gyrus and inferior parietal cortices when reading words that stress sublexical processes. Furthermore, these areas are not significantly atrophied and are connected by the spared frontoparietal superior longitudinal fasciculus (Figure 3–5).

One of the remarkable features of svPPA is the near complete sparing of syntax, despite profound deficits in semantic knowledge. Recent work from Wilson and colleagues (Wilson et al. 2011; Wilson et al. 2012) and Galantucci and colleagues (Galantucci et al. 2011) suggests that syntactic processing depends on well-functioning left frontal and posterior perisylvian regions and strong white matter connectivity between these two regions, areas that are largely spared until late in the course of svPPA. The anterior temporal lobe and its posterior connections play, at most, a minor role in syntax generation and comprehension. These fundamental insights surrounding grammar represent just one example of how the study of svPPA has enhanced our understanding of the anatomical substrates of language.

In the University of California, San Francisco (UCSF) neuropathology series, 22 of 23 svPPA patients demonstrated the TDP type C subtype. In the TDP type C subtype of svPPA, TDP-43 leaves the nucleus and accumulates in the cell bodies and dendritic processes of neurons (Mackenzie et al. 2011). Although the TDP-43 subtype is usually type C in svPPA, there is the occasional patient with comorbid amyotrophic lateral sclerosis who will show type B inclusions. More rarely, on autopsy, svPPA patients will show corticobasal degeneration, progressive supranuclear palsy, or AD neuropathology.

Right Temporal Lobe Syndrome

Degeneration of the right anterior temporal lobe leads to a fascinating syndrome with features of both svPPA and bvFTD. Often, the patients present with a long psychiatric prodrome, and we believe that many right temporal patients are never seen in a neurological setting.

Depression, hypochondriasis, compulsivity, and a tendency to seek social isolation are quite common (Miller et al. 1993; Edwards-Lee et al. 1997; Seeley et al. 2005). Additionally, many patients lose empathy for others in the early stages of the illness and profoundly alienate people around them (Rankin et al. 2006). Unlike patients with the classical left temporal lobe based svPPA who complain of their deficits and actively seek out medical consultation, the right-sided temporal patients often avoid social interactions and may refuse to be seen in medical environments. This may explain why we see approximately twice as many left temporal predominant as right temporal lobe predominant patients at UCSF; these patients with right temporal lobe disease refuse to be evaluated. Another intriguing, but in our opinion less likely, explanation for this disparity is that the left anterior temporal lobe is more vulnerable to neurodegeneration than is the right temporal lobe.

Many of these patients exhibit a lack of response to the emotions of others along with intensification of religious ideas and a new preoccupation for word games or writing in the early stages of the illness. At the time of diagnosis, patients can have features of svPPA or bvFTD, and some patients fall evenly between these clinical syndromes. An acquired disorder in understanding and recognizing faces (and people) and emotions emerges, and in many instances, the right temporal variant of FTD overlaps with Asperger syndrome due to this peculiar feature.

Howard Rosen has demonstrated that the severity of the deficit in emotional understanding correlates with the severity of atrophy in the right amygdala (Rosen et al. 2002) (Figure 3–6 and Figure 2–6). The loss of empathy is often the initial symptom in patients with this form of svPPA, and deficits in emotion recognition in the setting of dementia strongly correlate with atrophy in the right anterior temporal, orbital frontal, and ventral striatal regions.

Kate Rankin has found that personality profiles show a shift from warmth to coldness and agreeableness to disagreeableness (Rankin et al. 2003). Social pragmatics are profoundly altered, and these patients tend to speak in a long-winded, monotonous manner, interrupting others without allowing loved ones or caregivers either to interject or end the encounter. This trait has been called "viscosity" in the temporal lobe epilepsy literature (Geschwind 1983). We believe that one of the factors that lead these patients toward becoming viscous is that their ability to read emotions in others is altered, so that they are unable to understand irritation or their loved ones', strangers', and caregivers' desire to escape.

There is a rigid adherence to social rules, with lack of concern for the effects of this rigid adherence on the feelings of others. We had one patient who became fanatically religious and spent nearly every day in church. When a flood threatened his village, he became angered that the town's minister was out laying sandbags trying to prevent the flooding rather than preaching a Sunday sermon. Similarly, he suggested that his friends would suffer the wrath of God when they

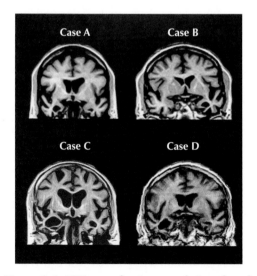

Figure 3–6. MRI scans showing coronal views through the anterior temporal lobe at the level of the amygdala.

bet small amounts of money on the Super Bowl. He listened to Christian music but ignored the melody and only cared about the religious words. These personality and behavioral changes are highly characteristic of right-temporal lobe patients and can be quantified using personality questionnaires asking a family to rate a patient's warmth and coldness using a series of adjectives (Rankin et al. 2003) (Figure 3–7).

Compulsive preoccupation with words may lead to hypergraphia. Some of these patients will write in journals, sometimes simply copying words from other books. They often play word games like "search and circle." This patient group also tends to exhibit hyperreligiosity and intensification of philosophical ideas (Edwards-Lee et al. 1997). The constellation of hypergraphia, religiosity, and viscosity (and sometimes hyposexuality) has features of the temporal lobe personality disorder originally described by Norman Geschwind and Henri Gastaut (Geschwind 1983a, 1983b).

In the early stages of right temporal lobe predominant neurodegeneration, patients have more trouble remembering the faces of friends and familiar people than the names of those faces. We have had many patients in the early stages of the illness who are unable to recognize

John Kennedy, Ronald Reagan, Martin Luther King, John Wayne, or Marilyn Monroe. Over time a profound prosopagnosia can develop. Eventually people with right-sided onset progress to the left side and then develop the classical language features of svPPA. Similarly, left-sided cases progress to involve the right temporal lobe, and then the person experiences difficulty recognizing faces, foods, animals, and emotions. Most patients eventually develop classical bvFTD behaviors including disinhibition, apathy, loss of empathy, and diminished insight (Seeley et al. 2005).

Additionally, there is some evidence that there are specific naming and recognition tasks that the right anterior temporal lobe is organized to perform. In a volume-based study of patients with dementia in 2006, Brambati and colleagues discovered that the ability to name living things correlated with the right anterior and medial temporal lobe volumes, while naming accuracy for "familiarity-matched nonliving items correlated with the volume of the left posterior middle temporal gyrus" (Brambati et al. 2006). This suggests some specificity for naming relating to animals versus tools in the right anterior temporal, and there are some patients where this disparity

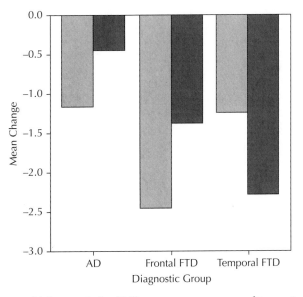

Figure 3–7. When Interpersonal Adjectives Scales (IAS) summary scores were used to examine overall personality style, patients with AD, frontal variant frontotemporal dementia (FLV), and temporal variant frontotemporal dementia (TLV) evidenced a significant interaction (p < 0.05). Patients with TLV showed a greater drop in affiliation (black bars) than in social dominance (gray bars), whereas patients with FLV showed the opposite pattern. Both frontotemporal dementia subtypes showed a greater overall degree of change than did AD. (Rankin et al. 2003.)

in naming living things versus nonliving items is evident.

Because many of the patients with the right temporal variant present with such disordered, and often unpleasant behavioral constellations, they are often diagnosed clinically as bvFTD. Yet, the MRI does not show frontal atrophy, and the disorder initially involves only the temporal. There are other patients with right-sided disease, particularly those with significant left temporal dysfunction, who have enough language disturbance that they are classified clinically as svPPA.

As with the left-predominant svPPA syndrome, patients with right temporal predominant disease tend to show TDP type C neuropathology, although a scattering of patients have been reported in whom TDP type B or tau pathology was found.

Neuropsychological testing is invaluable in the diagnosis of svPPA and right-temporally predominant versions of svPPA, but it is important for the patients to be evaluated using tasks that tap into knowledge of words, faces, and emotions (Kramer et al. 2003). Because the only task of semantics on the Mini Mental State Examination is naming of two very high frequency words, "pencil" and "watch," this task is insensitive to svPPA. The animals on the Montreal Cognitive Assessment, "rhinoceros" and "camel" are more difficult, so this task can hint at a semantic problem. The Boston Naming Task captures the anomia of svPPA unless the disease is very early. Unlike patients with other nontemporal forms of anomia, the svPPA patients are not usually helped by clues, or even multiple choices. Commonly, the patients repeat the word when it is spoken and repeat back the word, without understanding its meaning. Sentence comprehension may be normal because the patients maintain syntactic knowledge, although comprehension on a task like the Peabody Picture Vocabulary Test will show deficits in single-word comprehension. Fluency, repetition, and verbal agility are all normal. Reading tasks that use both regular and irregular words will capture a patient's surface dyslexia. Semantic generation tasks such as listing "animals" are more impaired than tasks of phonemic fluency such as generating "d" words.

If the patient has more right temporal atrophy they may do reasonably well on tests that tap verbal semantic knowledge. Many of these individuals will have difficulty recognizing familiar faces from their past such as Elvis Presley, Marilyn Monroe, John Wayne, John Kennedy, or Margaret Thatcher. In the early stages of the disease before left temporal regions are too severely devastated, they may even make comments like, "Elvis Presley, oh yes, he sang songs," but still not be able to recognize the face. Another early deficit is the recognition of emotions on faces. In the early stages of the disease, patients mistake complex facial emotions such as disgust, or pride, while still maintaining the ability to recognize emotions like happiness. Eventually the loss of recognition of all emotions is evident. It is important to have the family provide some formal documentation of the patient's previous level of empathy and to determine how much this has changed from the premorbid personality.

As important as are the patient's deficits on neuropsychological testing are the pattern of strengths. Visuoconstructive abilities such as copying remain normal, even late in the illness. Unlike patients with bvFTD, many svPPA patients show excellent working memory and may perform well on tasks like the "N back" (Waltz et al. 1999) and design generation. Additionally, tasks of calculations, syntax comprehension, and motor speed remain normal.

Creativity

Some individuals with svPPA develop new artistic skills in the context of their illness. While most of the patients have with this pattern have had classical svPPA, some have had right temporal atrophy and a more mixed anatomical picture. Visual activities such as drawing, painting, or sculpting appear as the patient is losing their capability for communicating verbally. In the setting of svPPA, we have seen the emergence of creativity in visual art, music, gardening, and mechanical design (Miller et al. 1996, Miller et al. 1998, Miller et al. 2000, Liu et al. 2009).

The artwork of people with svPPA tends to be literal versus abstract, and the use of color is striking. We have seen compelling use of purple, yellow, and green colors. Pictures of animals are common, while the details of faces are often neglected. We have had svPPA patients who made beautiful colored paper flowers, sculptures, and crafted spectacular gardens (Miller & Hou 2004). As the illness encroaches on the right anterior temporal lobe, faces becomes distorted, bizarre, and even alien, reflecting their specific deficits in recognizing faces, emotions, and their meaning (Figure 3–8). Hence, the paintings developed by the patient reflect his or her understanding and perceptions of the external visual world.

As the disease progresses, the images become more vague and eccentric. The items in the picture show no contextual meaning or relationships to other elements and are reduced to reflecting the pure perception of the visual properties. While the composition may not represent a planned, coherent creative expression of an idea, the arrangement and representation of the fundamental pieces,

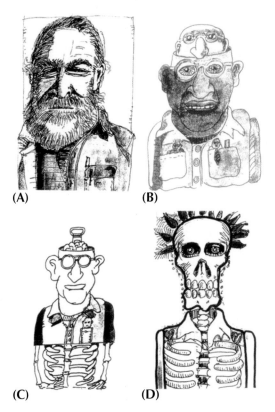

(A)   (B)

(C)   (D)

Figure 3–8. Caricatures made by patient. The patient's facial drawings became bizarre, with portraits of people emerging out of the heads or bellies of other people and eventual skeletal depictions, as if seeing through to their bones. Fig. (**A**) was made many years before his illness. Figs. (**B**) and (**C**) were made in the first two years of his dementia, and Fig. (**D**) at least three years into his disease. (Mendez & Perryman 2003.)

shapes, patterns, colors, and lines can be highly original. Generally, the paintings are realistic or surrealistic without a significant symbolic or abstract component. The work is approached compulsively, and a painting may be repeated over and over until a new theme is explored (Figure 3–9).

We worked with a remarkable man with an svPPA syndrome who showed bitemporal but right greater than left atrophy. Previously a lawyer, he began to paint as he lost words. In his life he had become socially isolated and attempted to connect to another human being by ordering a mail order bride. This relationship lasted less than one month. Markedly impaired in his ability to comprehend emotions in faces, he focused on painting couples whose faces showed distorted patterns of emotion. This curious distortion gave the pictures a beautiful but haunting quality and reflected the problems that this patient had with understanding emotion in others (Liu et al. 2009) (Figure 3–10).

Additionally, Indre Viskontas, in collaboration with Adam Boxer and me, (Viskontas et al. 2011) showed that svPPA patients view the world differently than do healthy controls and other patients with dementia. Using sophisticated eye-tracking systems in Dr. Boxer's laboratory, the authors were able to demonstrate that, in contrast to healthy and dementia controls, svPPA patients looked at complex pictures without spending extra time on semantically meaningful items. For example, while looking at a complex picture of penguins on ice floats, the patients were equally likely to look at water as penguins, and tended to look more thoroughly at the whole picture, without targeting any particular item. This tracking distinction may allow these individuals to capture an image of the world that is more unique than what they might see with an ordinary visual tracking strategy.

Recently we have seen a few patients with the right temporal variant of FTD in whom verbal creativity emerged shortly prior to the onset of their illness. Several wrote books, while another wrote poetry. Neither had shown a verbal proclivity or preoccupation prior to the onset of the right-sided temporal lobe neurodegeneration. This release of verbal creativity seemed to parallel the visual creativity found in patients with the svPPA suggesting that the anterior temporal lobes have a role in human

Figure 3–9. Painting of "Pi" by Anne Adams, who had a diagnosis of nfvPPA. (Gouache, 1998.)

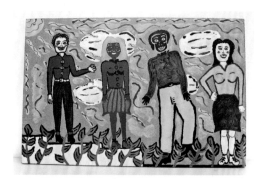

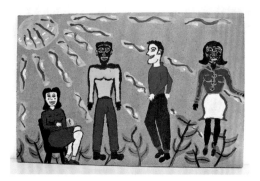

Figure 3–10. The artwork of a man with an svPPA syndrome that shows the problems that this patient had with understanding emotion.

preferences for words. All of these patients with verbal creativity showed sparing of left lateral temporal cortex, and preservation of this brain region may have contributed to their ability to think about and play with words.

GENETIC AND PATHOLOGICAL CORRELATES

svPPA is the least genetic of all the FTD subtypes, and in one study from our group led by Jill Goldman, less than 5% of all patients with svPPA had a family history of FTD (Goldman et al. 2005). While there may be multiple genes that contribute to svPPA, rarely is there an autosomal dominant gene that is responsible for svPPA. Additionally, at least a subset of svPPA patients seem to be prone to autoimmune disorders suggesting another nongenetic etiology (see "svPPA: Current State and Research Advances" below).

Other research suggests that the seeds of svPPA may be sown fairly early in life, possibly even *in utero* in some individuals. In a large international study on occupation and FTD in 588 patients, occupation information showed a relationship to the quadrant of tissue that was involved. Patients with right-sided atrophy had professions more dependent on verbal abilities than those with left-sided or symmetrical atrophy. Most of this lateralization effect was localized to the temporal lobes, and the patients with verbal and mathematical professions had preserved left temporal relative to right temporal volumes. All of the artists had left-sided disease (Spreng et al. 2010).

In at least some patients with nfvPPA or svPPA, unusual constellations of cognitive abilities and deficits suggest that subtle features of svPPA were already present early in life. Mesulam and colleagues were the first to demonstrate that at least some patients with svPPA show dyslexia early in life or show a family history of learning disabilities (Rogalski et al. 2008). Similarly, he and colleagues (Alberca et al. 2004) found left hemicranial skull anomalies or left temporal lobe cysts in two patients with PPA.

In interpreting the data found in the study from Spreng and colleagues (Spreng et al. 2010), perhaps early visual deficits may have influenced the interest and choice of verbal occupations for the cohorts with right hemisphere atrophy. Conversely, subtle left hemisphere abnormalities may have led their subjects to a right hemisphere–dominant skill, painting. In svPPA there is often, but not always, a hint of language dysfunction, or atypical cortical wiring from very early in life. In the UCSF and Mayo Clinic cohorts, left-handedness is overrepresented. Therefore, with this form of FTD, perhaps very early brain asymmetry or dysfunction is a marker for the predisposition to svPPA.

DIFFERENTIAL DIAGNOSIS

The differential diagnosis of svPPA is usually fairly straightforward, although approximately 20% of our patient's symptoms are initially considered psychiatric in origin. The subtle anomia seen in the early stages of svPPA can be somewhat nonspecific and is easily mistaken for the anomia of AD, although the imaging features of left temporal atrophy usually point to a non-AD diagnosis. As the disease progresses, the profound anomia associated with semantic deficits, loss of word meaning, makes the diagnosis more apparent. Profound naming deficits that are not improved with clues and loss

of knowledge about the world are common. In contrast, there is relatively good day-to-day memory (Patterson et al. 1992; Gorno-Tempini et al. 2011).

By contrast, the right temporal variant is far more difficult to diagnose, and any disease that begins with a loss of empathy for others, emotional coldness, or depression will initially be referred to social workers, marriage counselors, family physicians, or psychiatrists (Edwards-Lee et al. 1997; Seeley et al. 2005). Yet, decreased empathy is not typical of the psychiatric profile associated with aging and should always trigger a search for FTD. Deficits in the recognition of emotions on faces or familiar faces and the presence of temporal atrophy on MRI make the diagnosis of FTD (Brambati et al. 2010). The temporal lobes are prone to trauma, and the loss of tissue in the anterior temporal lobes can be misinterpreted as encephalomalacia. Conversely, there are patients in whom tissue loss that was secondary to old trauma can lead to the mistaken diagnosis of svPPA or the right temporal variant of FTD.

The right temporal variant of FTD sometimes presents as bvFTD, while at other times the semantic deficits are sufficiently severe so that the patient is diagnosed with svPPA. The atrophy in the temporal lobes confirms the diagnosis and helps with the prediction of a TDP-43 C neuropathology.

TREATMENT

Treatment of svPPA is difficult. In the early stages of the illness, patients are extremely motivated to participate in speech and language therapy. While the results of this approach are somewhat limited, it is possible to teach patients to remember words used frequently in their environment that are key for their ability to communicate effectively. The repetitive compulsive behaviors seen with both the left- and right-sided temporal variants of FTD seem to respond to a limited degree to SSRI- and SNRI-type compounds (Swartz et al. 1997).

The compulsive behaviors with svPPA can lead patients to exceptional creativity in the visual or, less commonly, the musical or athletic domain. Encouraging patients to participate in visual activities, capitalizing on skills that may be enhanced such as painting or music can be uplifting for the patient and for their caregivers. As svPPA progresses, the full-blown behavioral syndrome seen with bvFTD often emerges, causing huge stress for the caregivers, often leading to institutionalization of the patient. It is particularly important to explain to family members that the patient's lack of concerns for others is a natural part of the disease process and does not represent a failure of either the patient or of them.

svPPA: CURRENT STATE AND RESEARCH ADVANCES

Semantic Knowledge and the Anterior Temporal Lobes

svPPA has proven to be a powerful model for understanding how the brain processes and stores semantic knowledge. The anterior temporal regions are rarely infarcted due to stroke, and therefore severe semantic deficits are uncommon in the setting of ischemic brain injury. Similarly, subtle, but not profound, verbal learning and sometimes semantic deficits occur with anterior temporal lobectomy, temporal brain tumors, or traumatic brain injury (Viskontas et al. 2000, Schwarz & Pauli 2009). In fact, full-blown semantic deficits occur in only three major clinical settings: svPPA, herpes simplex viral infection (Lambon Ralph et al. 2007), or paraneoplastic limbic encephalitis (Vernino et al. 2007). Extensive bilateral anterior temporal lobe dysfunction seems to be necessary to generate profound semantic deficits. Such lesions occur with svPPA, herpes encephalitis, and autoimmune encephalitis, but not with temporal lobectomy, trauma, or stroke.

Additionally, even functional imaging has failed to delineate a precise anatomy for semantics because the anterior temporal lobar regions where semantics appear to be localized are so prone to artifact. Therefore, while previous efforts to understand the anatomical underpinnings of semantic knowledge in the brain were impeded by the lack of an anatomical model, svPPA has become a valuable syndrome from which semantic knowledge can become better understood.

Karalyn Patterson and Matthew Lambon Ralph have studied the unique linguistic features of svPPA, leading them to interesting

hypotheses regarding how the brain stores semantic knowledge. Dr. Patterson notes, "Only a few decades ago, one respectable position held that semantic memory might arise from 'universal connectivity' in the brain, and hence have no corresponding stable neural architecture" (Patterson et al. 2007). Yet, the selective disruption of semantic or conceptual knowledge with focal anterior temporal lobe lesions has made this idea untenable.

While previous hypotheses suggested that semantic knowledge was associated with the multiple visual, auditory, tactile, olfactory, and motor associations, this concept cannot explain the complex ways in which individuals compute semantic associations. For example, the determination of what features of an animal make a human categorize it as a cat cannot be explained by this multiple associations theory. Dr. Patterson explains that while there are many similarities visually across all cats, there are small dogs that have the long tail and pointy ears seen with most cats, and there are cats like the Chinese hairless cat that have long ears and no fur, making visual recognition alone impossible (Patterson et al. 2007). svPPA patients tend to be drawn by the featural lures—so that a small dog with pointy ears likely to be called a cat. These mistakes in naming are better explained by theories that hypothesize a system in the anterior temporal lobes that is needed for centrally classifying words (Figure 3–11).

From the work of Patterson and Lambon Ralph, it is clear that svPPA patients make specific types of errors that fall into the categories of "undergeneralization" and "overgeneralization." Hence, cats like a lion or Chinese hairless are no longer recognized as cats by the patient with svPPA because they lack prototypical visual features (undergeneralization). By the same token, there are dogs like the shiba inu and chihuahua that are misidentified as cats because they have some visual features that are seen in cats (overgeneralization).

The phenomenology of these findings has led them to propose a "hub and spoke" hypothesis. They suggest, "No single feature defines them as a single group but instead they form a group through partial, overlapping features. In computational terms, this problem cannot be solved by a single layer of feature-coding units (a single-layer perceptron), because the representations are not linearly separable. They can, however, be grouped properly if an

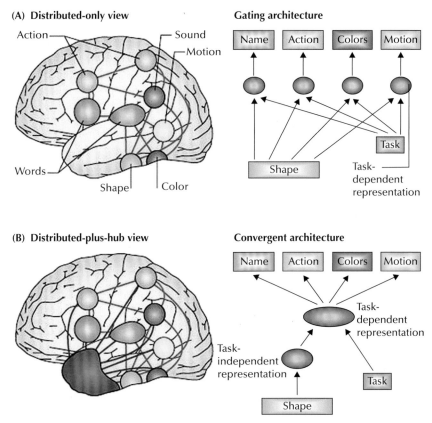

Figure 3–11. Both positions hold, in agreement with most investigators, that the network is widely distributed and partly organized to conform to the neuroanatomy of sensory, motor, and linguistic systems. **(A)** The distributed-only view suggests that these widely distributed regions, along with the diverse connections between them (shown as green lines), constitute the whole semantic network. The flow of activation through this network can be "gated" by a representation of the current task (right-hand panel): for instance, if the task is to name a line drawing of a familiar object, activation will flow from a representation of object's shape to a representation of its name. Associations between different pairs of attributes are encoded along different neuroanatomical pathways. **(B)** By contrast, the distributed-plus-hub view posits that, in addition to these modality-specific regions and connections, the various different surface representations (such as shape) connect to (shown as red lines), and communicate through, a shared, amodal "hub" (shown as a red area) in the anterior temporal lobes. At the hub stage, therefore, associations between different pairs of attributes (such as shape and name, shape and action, or shape and color) are all processed by a common set of neurons and synapses, regardless of the task. The right-hand panel (labeled "convergent architecture") illustrates the model equivalent of the distributed-plus-hub view. (Patterson et al. 2007.)

additional (hidden) layer is added because this allows re-representation of the feature input." (Lambon Ralph et al. 2010).

More recently Christine Guo and William Seeley at UCSF have studied the changes in brain connectivity in patients with svPPA and are supporting the concept of a central anterior temporal hub with connections to the various association cortices that allows the modality-specific categorization of items. While svPPA leaves these association cortices intact, it is the central hub that degenerates first and

prevents the patient from making the proper associations with specific items.

While these studies (Lambon Ralph et al. 2010; Visser et al. 2011) are beginning to delineate the functional role of the anterior temporal regions in understanding and separating semantic features of items, they do not explain the mechanism for the difference between the function of the right versus the left semantic deficits that differ between the left and right anterior temporal lobes. More research is needed to determine the mechanism for why right anterior degeneration leads to deficits in visual knowledge about people and diminished empathy for others, while the left anterior temporal degeneration limits verbal semantic knowledge. The connections that are critical for these differences also remain unknown, although they are being actively investigated at UCSF and elsewhere.

Additionally, there have been only limited efforts to rehabilitate patients with these deficits, and placebo-controlled studies of clinic trials for svPPA are greatly needed. Such studies have been started by Maya Henry and Marilu Gorno-Tempini at UCSF, and Peaghie Beeson at the University of Arizona, but large placebo-controlled studies are still needed.

Autoimmunity, Left-Handedness, Head Trauma, and svPPA

In the 1960s Norman Geschwind hypothesized a relationship between left-handedness, autoimmunity, and dyslexia (Geschwind & Behan 1982). Zachary Miller has shown in the UCSF cohort that svPPA patients show a greater than expected frequency of left-handedness while the lvPPA cohort showed a greater than expected frequency of dyslexia, and this paper is currently under review at *Brain* (Zac Miller, personal communication). Additionally, recent collaborations between UCSF, Mayo Clinic, and Stanford and reports from other groups all suggest that svPPA patients also have alterations in their peripheral immune system. Previously, a Swedish study found that FTD was associated with changes in inflammatory markers including TNFα (Sjögren et al. 2004), while several cases reports from Mesulam and colleagues and Heilman and colleagues have hypothesized autoimmune mechanisms in PPA and bvFTD (Weintraub et al. 2006, Decker & Heilman 2008). In the study by Weintraub and colleagues vasectomy may have triggered an autoimmune process that led to progressive aphasia. Hence, the old hypotheses generated by Norman Geschwind more than 40 years ago about immunity and handedness may have very modern relevance to the understanding of svPPA.

Paralleling the Weintraub and colleagues study, research on paraneoplastic syndromes suggests that the anterior temporal lobes can be the site of autoimmune attacks against tumor antigens. Remote tumors in the testes, ovaries, or lungs can lead to subacute or rapid behavioral and semantic changes with an anatomy that is parallel to svPPA (Rosenbloom et al. 2009). In some individuals, the generation of these antibodies (and other immune-based molecules) seems to occur spontaneously without a precipitating tumor antigen.

While paraneoplastic mechanisms do not explain the slowly evolving dementia of svPPA, there is new data suggesting that these patients may be prone to autoimmune conditions such as rheumatoid arthritis, lupus, sarcoid, inflammatory bowel disease (chronic lymphocytic colitis), and Sjögren's syndrome, and this work is in press at *Journal of Neurology, Neurosurgery & Psychiatry* (Zac Miller, personal communication). Many of these conditions show an altered innate immunity profile and are associated with activation of cytokines including TNF, interleukins, and complement pathways.

Proteomic studies performed at UCSF by Zac Miller and at Stanford by Trisha Stan and Tony Wyss-Coray have found that there is an inflammatory phenotype with high levels of tumor necrosis factor alpha (TNFα), interleukin 12, interleukin 27, and nuclear factor kappa-light-chain-enhancer of activated B cells (NF-κB) (Tony Wyss-Coray, personal communication). Additionally, lymphocytes from these individuals are overrepresented by the presence of CD8+ C27+ and CD8+ CD85j+ helper T cell subtypes (Tony Wyss-Coray, personal communication). Remarkably, a very similar proteomic pattern is seen in patients with progranulin mutations, and it is well accepted that progranulin plays a role in the body's and brain's inflammatory response. Progranulin seems to have an anti-inflammatory effect by turning down TNFα, while its deficiency leads to a hyperactivated innate immune response. It appears that the whole progranulin model protects the body and the brain from inflammation, while TNFα and other cytokines participate in the inflammatory process. Additionally in the setting of brain trauma some have suggested that lowered progranulin may play a role in the pathogenesis of FTD later in life (Jawaid et al. 2009).

Whether or not the findings in svPPA and patients with progranulin mutations represent an overactive immune profile still remains to be determined, but if true, this line of investigation holds the potential to offer inroads into new and exciting therapeutic approaches for these disorders. Similarly, the specificity of these changes to svPPA versus other forms of FTD remains unknown, although AD patients do not show this pattern in our preliminary proteomic studies.

Finally, because the anterior temporal lobes sit adjacent to bone and are particularly vulnerable to trauma, the possibility that early trauma might play a role in svPPA needs further exploration. As better research on brain trauma and neurodegeneration emerges, it will be important to think about the role of trauma in the pathogenesis of svPPA.

SUMMARY

svPPA is a fascinating disorder associated with focal degeneration of left and right anterior temporal circuits involved with semantic knowledge about words and people. The semantic losses related to words offer fundamental insights into the way that words contribute to the way that we understand the world, while the surprising deficits in emotion comprehension and empathy associated with the right temporal variant of svPPA point to the important role that the right anterior temporal lobe and amygdala play in emotion perception and emotion regulation. The deficits seen in the svPPA patients have parallels with what is seen in schizophrenia, autism, and sometimes bipolar illness. Similarly, there are parallels between the diminished empathy of right temporal lobe patients and antisocial, borderline, and schizoidal personality disorders (Rankin et al. 2003; Rankin et al. 2006).

Because this is the least genetic of the FTD variants, our group has sought out other potential mechanisms for svPPA. Some evidence suggests that svPPA individuals have abnormal temporal lobe development, and early in life have visual (left temporal variant) or verbal (right temporal variant) preferences that influence choice of occupation (Spreng et al. 2010). Additionally, they show a higher prevalence of left-handedness than do our healthy controls and all of our dementia cohorts. Because left-handedness is set early in life, this is further evidence for a development component to svPPA.

Finally, there is an emerging literature pointing to an abnormal inflammatory profile in peripheral blood. Whether or not these inflammatory markers will eventually become targets for therapies that diminish their levels remains unknown, although it is clear that this clinical and pathological variant of FTD is distinctive from the other FTD subtypes and will require distinctive approaches toward early recognition and therapies.

REFERENCES

Alberca R, Montes E, Russell E, Gil-Néciga E, Mesulam M. Left hemicranial hypoplasia in 2 patients with primary progressive aphasia. Arch Neurol. 2004;61(2):265–8.

Brambati SM, Benoit S, Monetta L, Belleville S, Joubert S. The role of the left anterior temporal lobe in the semantic processing of famous faces. Neuroimage. 2010;53:674–81.

Brambati SM, Myers D, Wilson A, Rankin KP, Allison SC, Rosen HJ, Miller BL, Gorno-Tempini ML. The anatomy of category-specific object naming in neurodegenerative disease. J Cogn Neurosci. 2006;18:1644–53.

Brambati SM, Ogar J, Neuhaus J, Miller BL, Gorno-Tempini ML. Reading disorders in primary progressive aphasia: a behavioral and neuroimaging study. Neuropsychologia. 2009;47(8–9):1893–900.

Decker DA, Heilman KM. Steroid treatment of primary progressive aphasia. Arch Neurol. 2008;65:1533–5.

Ekman P, Friesen WV, Hager JC. Facial action coding system: the manual network. Salt Lake City [UT]: Information Research Corporation; 2002.

Edwards-Lee T, Miller BL, Benson DF, Cummings JL, Russell GL, Boone K, Mena I. The temporal variant of frontotemporal dementia. Brain. 1997;120 (Pt 6):1027–40.

Galantucci S, Tartaglia MC, Wilson SM, Henry ML, Filippi M, Agosta F, Dronkers NF, Henry RG, Ogar JM, Miller BL, Gorno-Tempini ML. White matter damage in primary progressive aphasias: a diffusion tensor tractography study. Brain. 2011;134:3011–29.

Geschwind N, Behan P. Left-handedness: association with immune disease, migraine, and developmental learning disorder. Proc Natl Acad Sci U S A. 1982;79 (16):5097–100.

Geschwind N. Interictal behavioral changes in epilepsy. Epilepsia. 1983;24 Suppl 1:S23–30.

Geschwind N. Pathogenesis of behavior change in temporal lobe epilepsy. Res Publ Assoc Res Nerv Ment Dis. 1983;61:355–70.

Goldman JS, Farmer JM, Wood EM, Johnson JK, Boxer A, Neuhaus J, Lomen-Hoerth C, Wilhelmsen KC, Lee VM, Grossman M, Miller BL. Comparison of family histories in FTLD subtypes and related tauopathies. Neurology. 2005;65(11):1817–9.

Gorno-Tempini ML, Hillis AE, Weintraub S, Kertesz A, Mendez M, Cappa SF, Ogar JM, Rohrer JD, Black S, Boeve BF, Manes F, Dronkers NF, Vandenberghe R, Rascovsky K, Patterson K, Miller BL, Knopman DS, Hodges JR, Mesulam MM, Grossman M. Classification of primary progressive aphasia and its variants. Neurology. 2011;76:1006–14.

Hodges JR, Patterson K, Oxbury S, Funnell E. Semantic dementia. Progressive fluent aphasia with temporal lobe atrophy. Brain. 1992;115:1783–806.

Ikeda M, Patterson K, Graham KS, Ralph MA, Hodges JR. A horse of a different colour: Do patients with semantic dementia recognize different versions of the same object as the same? Neuropsychologia. 2006;44:566–75.

Jawaid A, Rademakers R, Kass JS, Kalkonde Y, Schulz PE. Traumatic brain injury may increase the risk for frontotemporal dementia through reduced progranulin. Neurodegener Dis. 2009;6:219–20.

Kramer JH, Jurik J, Sha SJ, Rankin KP, Rosen HJ, Johnson JK, Miller BL. Distinctive neuropsychological patterns in frontotemporal dementia, semantic dementia, and Alzheimer disease. Cogn Behav Neurol. 2003;16(4):211–8.

Lambon Ralph MA, Lowe C, Rogers TT. Neural basis of category-specific semantic deficits for living things: evidence from semantic dementia, HSVE and a neural network model. Brain. 2007;130:1127–37.

Lambon Ralph MA, Sage K, Jones RW, Mayberry EJ. Coherent concepts are computed in the anterior temporal lobes. Proc Natl Acad Sci USA. 2010;107;2717–22.

Liu A, Rankin K, Werner K, Roy S, Morgan-Kane U, Miller BL. A case study of an emerging visual artist with frontotemporal lobar degeneration and amyotrophic lateral sclerosis. Neurocase. 2009;15:235–47.

Mackenzie IR, Neumann M, Baborie A, Sampathu DM, Du Plessis D, Jaros E, Perry RH, Trojanowski JQ, Mann DM, Lee VM. A harmonized classification system for FTLD-TDP pathology. Acta Neuropathol. 2011;122(1):111–3.

Mendez MF, Perryman KM. Disrupted facial empathy in drawings from artists with frontotemporal dementia. Neurocase. 2003;9:44–50.

Mesulam MM. Slowly progressive aphasia without generalized dementia. Ann Neurol. 1982;11:592–8.

Miller BL, Boone K, Cummings JL, Read SL, Mishkin F. Functional correlates of musical and visual ability in frontotemporal dementia. Br J Psychiatry. 2000;176:458–63.

Miller BL, Chang L, Mena I, Boone K, Lesser IM. Progressive right frontotemporal degeneration: clinical, neuropsychological and SPECT characteristics. Dementia. 1993;4(3–4):204–13.

Miller BL, Cummings J, Mishkin F, Boone K, Prince F, Ponton M, Cotman C. Emergence of artistic talent in frontotemporal dementia. Neurology. 1998;51(4):978–82.

Miller BL, Hou CE. Portraits of artists: emergence of visual creativity in dementia. Arch Neurol. 2004;61:842–4.

Miller BL, Ponton M, Benson DF, Cummings JL, Mena I. Enhanced artistic creativity with temporal lobe degeneration. Lancet. 1996;348:1744–5.

Patterson K, Hodges J. Deterioration of word meaning: implications for reading. Neuropsychologia. 1992;30(12):1025–40.

Patterson K, Nestor PJ, Rogers TT. Where do you know what you know? The representation of semantic knowledge in the human brain. Nature Rev Neurosci. 2007;8:976–87.

Perry DC, Whitwell JL, Boeve BF, Pankratz VS, Knopman DS, Petersen RC, Jack CR Jr, Josephs KA. Voxel-based morphometry in patients with obsessive-compulsive behaviors in behavioral variant frontotemporal dementia. Eur J Neurol. 2012;19(6):911–7.

Perry RJ, Rosen HR, Kramer JH, Beer JS, Levenson RL, Miller BL. Hemispheric dominance for emotions, empathy and social behaviour: evidence from right and left handers with frontotemporal dementia. Neurocase. 2001;7:145–60.

Rankin KP, Gorno-Tempini ML, Allison SC, Stanley CM, Glenn S, Weiner MW, Miller BL. Structural anatomy of empathy in neurodegenerative disease. Brain. 2006;129:2945–56.

Rankin KP, Kramer JH, Mychack P, Miller BL. Double dissociation of social functioning in frontotemporal dementia. Neurology. 2003;60:266–71.

Rogalski E, Johnson N, Weintraub S, Mesulam M. Increased frequency of learning disability in patients with primary progressive aphasia and their first-degree relatives. Arch Neurol. 2008;65(2):244–8.

Rosen HJ, Perry RJ, Murphy J, Kramer JH, Mychack P, Schuff N, Weiner M, Levenson RW, Miller BL. Emotion comprehension in the temporal variant of frontotemporal dementia. Brain. 2002;125(Pt 10):2286–95.

Rosenbloom MH, Smith S, Akdal G, Geschwind MD. Immunologically mediated dementias. Curr Neurol Neurosci Rep. 2009;9(5):359–67.

Schwarz M, Pauli E. Postoperative speech processing in temporal lobe epilepsy: functional relationship between object naming, semantics and phonology. Epilepsy Behav. 2009;16(4):629–33.

Seeley WS, Bauer A, Miller BL, Gorno-Tempini ML, Kramer JH, Weiner M, Rosen HJ. The natural history of temporal variant frontotemporal dementia. Neurology. 2005;64:1384–90.

Sjögren M, Folkesson S, Blennow K, Tarkowski E. Increased intrathecal inflammatory activity in frontotemporal dementia: Pathophysiological implications. J Neurol Neurosurg Psychiatry. 2004;75:1107–11.

Snowden JS, Neary D, Mann DM, Goulding PJ, Testa HJ. Progressive language disorder due to lobar atrophy. Ann Neurol. 1992;31:174–83.

Spreng RN, Rosen HJ, Strother S, Chow TW, Diehl-Schmid J, Freedman M, Graff-Radford NR, Hodges JR, Lipton AM, Mendez MF, Morelli SA, Black SE, Miller BL, Levine B. Occupation attributes relate to location of atrophy in frontotemporal lobar degeneration. Neuropsychologia. 2010;48:3634–41.

Swartz JR, Miller BL, Lesser IM, Darby AL. Frontotemporal dementia: treatment response to serotonin selective reuptake inhibitors. J Clin Psychiatry. 1997;58(5):212–6.

Tulving E. Multiple memory systems and consciousness. Hum Neurobiol. 1987;6:67–80.

Tyrrell PJ, Warrington EK, Frackowiak RS, Rossor MN. Progressive degeneration of the right temporal lobe studied with positron emission tomography. J Neurol Neurosurg Psychiatry. 1990;53(12):1046–50.

Vernino S, Geschwind M, Boeve B. Autoimmune encephalopathies. Neurologist. 2007;13(3):140–7.

Viskontas IV, Boxer AL, Fesenko J, Matlin A, Heuer HW, Mirsky J, Miller BL. Visual search patterns in semantic dementia show paradoxical facilitation of binding processes. Neuropsychologia. 2011;49(3):468–78.

Viskontas IV, McAndrews MP, Moscovitch M. Remote episodic memory deficits in patients with unilateral temporal lobe epilepsy and excisions. J Neurosci. 2000;20(15):5853–7.

Visser M, Lambon Ralph MA. Differential contributions of bilateral ventral anterior temporal lobe and left anterior superior temporal gyrus to semantic processes. J Cogn Neurosci. 2011;23:3121–31.

Waltz J, Knowlton B, Holyoak K, Boone KB, Mishkin FS, Santos M, Thomas CR, Miller BL. A system for relational reasoning in human prefrontal cortex. Psychol Sci. 1999;10:119–125.

Weintraub S, Fahey C, Johnson N, Mesulam MM, Gitelman DR, Weitner BB, et al. Vasectomy in men with primary progressive aphasia. Cogn Behav Neurol. 2006;19:190.

Wilson SM, Galantucci S, Tartaglia MC, Gorno-Tempini ML. The neural basis of syntactic deficits in primary progressive aphasia. Brain Language. 2012; 122:190–8.

Wilson SM, Galantucci S, Tartaglia MC, Rising K, Patterson DK, Henry ML, Ogar JM, Deleon J, Miller BL, Gorno-Tempini ML. Syntactic processing depends on dorsal language tracts. Neuron. 2011;72:397–403.

Chapter 4

The Clinical Syndrome of nfvPPA

OVERVIEW

CLINICAL FEATURES AND ANATOMY

GENETIC AND PATHOLOGICAL CORRELATES

DIFFERENTIAL DIAGNOSIS

TREATMENT

nfvPPA: CURRENT STATE AND RESEARCH ADVANCES
Diagnosis from Clinical Syndrome to Molecular Diagnosis
Neurolinguistic and Neuroplasticity Discoveries

REFERENCES

OVERVIEW

The nonfluent/agrammatic variant of primary progressive aphasia (nfvPPA) is the third major clinical disorder that is considered under the rubric of FTD. Until recently the logopenic variant of PPA (lvPPA) was often included under the nfvPPA category, leading to a misleadingly high number of these patients with a diagnosis of Alzheimer's disease (AD) (Knibb et al. 2006). With refinement of the clinical phenomenology that truly defines nfvPPA, the likelihood that this syndrome will be associated with FTLD neuropathology has dramatically increased (Gorno-Tempini et al. 2004; Rogalski et al. 2011). In a recent look at the neuropathology of patients with nfvPPA, one-half had tau-related changes, the other half had TDP-43, and none had AD as the primary cause for the syndrome.

This language-predominant syndrome (PPA) is characterized by progressive difficulty with language output and word finding with relative preservation of behavior, day-to-day function and memory (Gorno-Tempini et al. 2011). Subtle word-finding problems evolve into a full-blown nonfluent aphasia syndrome with effortful speech, decreased phrase length, decreased number of words, and dysprosody of speech. Often, this is associated with apraxia of speech (Ogar et al. 2006; Ogar et al. 2007).

At an anatomical level, nfvPPA often begins with very focal degeneration in the left fronto-opercular region (Josephs et al. 2006). When the disease eventually spreads to the right frontal lobe, patients usually go on to exhibit findings suggestive of a frontal disorder with apathy, disinhibition, and widespread loss of executive control. Additionally, involvement of the basal ganglia and midbrain leads to atypical parkinsonian syndromes with axial rigidity, falls, and often abnormalities of extraocular motility. These extrapyramidal features can guide the clinician to the diagnosis of either progressive supranuclear palsy (PSP) or corticobasal degeneration (CBD). When the disease goes very slowly and parkinsonian features do not emerge later in the illness, we tend to consider Pick's disease or TDP-43 type A (see below).

At a pathological level, nfvPPA is commonly associated with abnormal aggregates of tau, leading to confirmation of a diagnosis of CBD, PSP, or Pick's disease (Knibb et al. 2006; Josephs et al. 2006). While most tau-related cases of nfvPPA are sporadic, there are case reports regarding patients with nfvPPA who suffered from tau mutations.

Additionally, *GRN* mutations can lead to an nfvPPA syndrome with TDP-43 type A neuropathology. More puzzling are the patients with nfvPPA who show TDP-43 type A aggregates at autopsy, in whom there is no known genetic syndrome.

CASE HISTORY

This case history is an amalgam of several cases of nfvPPA that we have seen, including some features of a patient previously reported in the journal *Neurocase* (Gorno-Tempini et al. 2004).

At 62 years of age, Mrs. B began to notice that she was having trouble finding the correct words in her work as an architect. A year later, her son noticed the problem and told his mother, "Spit it out mom. You sound tongue-tied." The patient was seen by a neurologist who performed an abbreviated cognitive assessment, along with a neurological examination, and an MRI scan. He suggested that her problem was psychological in origin and that her MRI was normal.

In the next six months Mrs. B started to exhibit noticeable stuttering, and her clients began to complain. Her word output diminished, and she began to notice trouble reading. Despite these problems, she continued to manage well at work and looked after a large family.

There was no other history of medical problems. An aunt on the maternal side of the family had died with a diagnosis of AD in her late 80s.

On examination Mrs. B was bright and cooperative but quiet and reserved. She admitted to

frustration and mild depression related to her symptoms. She scored highly on the Geriatric Depression Scale. Her MMSE was 30/30. Her speech output was diminished, and her speech had an effortful, halting, and stuttering quality. There were occasional paraphasic errors where she replaced one consonant with another. On one occasion she mispronounced the word "flower," saying "plower" instead. Repetition was difficult, and she had an apraxic pattern of output. When asked to repeat multisyllabic words like "catastrophe" she said, "capasprosee," "no cakastofe," "no caramoti," before finally saying the word correctly. She scored 15/15 on the Boston Naming Task. Verbal memory and visual memory were both above average, and on tasks of executive control she did reasonably well, except for mild slowing on Trails B. She generated only nine words beginning with the letter "d" but was able to generate the names of 16 novel animals. Neurological examination revealed mild but subtle incoordination in the right hand. A diagnosis of nfvPPA was made, and the patient was started on a serotonin-boosting antidepressant. A vigorous exercise program and speech therapy were recommended, and both offered some symptomatic relief.

During the next year she began to exhibit more problems with language. For a period of 6 months, she was able to communicate better with handwriting than speaking, although written output was effortful and agrammatical. She found that working with a speech pathologist was valuable and helped her to articulate more slowly and precisely. She retired due to her inability to communicate with clients but continued to help around the house with cooking and cleaning. Subtle behavioral problems emerged—she tended to sweep dishes off the table before people were finished, and she was easily distractible.

Three years after initial presentation, speech output was down to a few strangled words, although the patient's understanding remained normal. Her drive began to diminish, and she spent much of the day in the house walking aimlessly or sitting on the couch. Her family noticed that she grabbed items inadvertently and had trouble letting go of them. Her memory remained normal, and she took long walks around the neighborhood without getting lost.

On examination the patient was alert, and she responded to questions by nodding her head "yes" or "no." Comprehension was normal for short questions that did not require remembering long sequences of words. She could not name items on request but pointed appropriately to pictures of the words when she was given multiple choices. Verbal memory was untestable, but she copied and remembered well a complex figure. Oral-buccal apraxia was evident, and she couldn't lick her lips, whistle, or cough on command.

There was a grasping and groping dominant (right) hand, and the patient grabbed objects placed in front of her and had difficulty releasing them. Also, there was a prominent grasp reflex of the right hand. Basic neurological examination showed difficulty moving the eyes horizontally on gaze and a subtle right facial droop. Mrs. B's right arm and leg showed subtle cogwheel rigidity. Her right hand had a dystonic posture at rest, and she held her fingers in a clenched fashion. Gait was characterized by mild axial rigidity, decreased arm swing, and posturing of her right hand when she was asked to walk on her toes.

Initially treatment with Sinemet (carbidopa-levodopa) helped with the rigidity of the right side with maximum effect at 500 mg. Unfortunately, over the following six months a painful right hand dystonia emerged that improved with botulinum toxin injections. Swallowing difficulty emerged, and 4 1/2 years after her initial symptoms, the patient died from aspiration pneumonia. Figure 4–1 shows the voxel-based morphometry patterns of atrophy from the patient over the course of the illness. Neuropathology showed massive left fronto-opercular and basal ganglia atrophy

with milder right frontal atrophy. Histologically there was mild frontal gliosis with abundant gliala astrocytic plaques that stained positively for 4R tau. Coiled neurofibrillary tangles were present within the left and right frontal region. A neuropathological diagnosis of corticobasal degeneration was made (Figure 4–2).

Comment. This patient is a typical example of nfvPPA. She began with subtle word-finding problems that were considered psychiatric in origin. Word-finding difficulty is a very common symptom and is not always diagnostic for a neurodegenerative condition, as many healthy individuals can complain of this problem. Yet, her symptoms persisted and worsened prior to her evaluation, and by the time she sought neurological assistance, the word-finding difficulty was already evident to both the patient and to her children. While her first MRI appeared normal, a statistical analysis using voxel-based-morphometry suggested statistically that there was significant atrophy in the left frontoinsular and in the left caudate regions.

As the disease progressed, the classical findings of nonfluent aphasia became obvious: effortful speech, decreased phrase length, decreased number of words per minute, apraxia of speech, and agrammatism. Furthermore, bilateral frontal findings became problematic, and she demonstrated disinhibition and distractibility, although a full-blown bvFTD syndrome never emerged. In the later stages of the illness, she exhibited

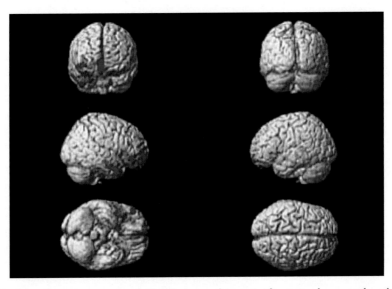

Figure 4–1. Voxel-based morphometry reveals that the areas of most significant atrophy are in the orbital and medial frontal and right greater than left orbitofrontal regions. The insula was involved as well. (Narvid et al. 2009.)

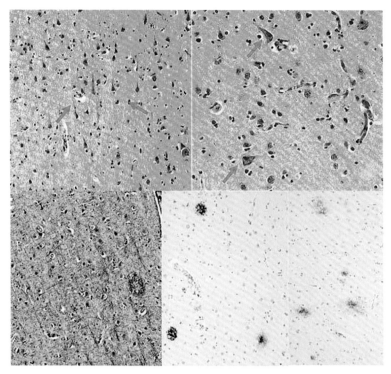

Figure 4–2. Multiple foci of neuronal degeneration are shown in H&E staining above (shown by blue arrows). Neuritic plaques in the frontal lobe shown below (middle) with rare NF tangles (right). (Narvid et al. 2009.)

motor findings, demonstrating that the disease had spread into the basal ganglia. As she approached death, motor symptoms predominated, and a focal dystonia of the right hand became painful and disabling (Gorno-Tempini et al. 2004).

Alien hand is a type of disconnection syndrome described by Norman Geschwind in the 1960s (Geschwind 1965). A classical alien dominant hand emerged, and she grabbed items in her environment without voluntary intent. This symptom complex correlated with progression of the atrophy in her left supplementary motor regions. CBD leads to severe degeneration of the dorsal and medial prefrontal and premotor cortex as well as the corpus callosum. We have seen some patients with end-stage CBD in whom a groping dominant alien hand is present due to left medial frontal degeneration and a nondominant hand that competes with the dominant side is present due to degeneration of the anterior corpus callosum and right medial prefrontal and supplementary motor cortex.

Based on the clinical pattern, CBS neuropathology was strongly suspected and eventually confirmed (Sanchez-Valle et al. 2006). While PSP can cause nfvPPA, the absence of dysarthria and the lack of a vertical gaze disturbance made this diagnosis unlikely. Pick's disease, another tauopathy, can cause nfvPPA, although often the course is slower and, typically, motor findings occur very late.

While no treatment is known to slow the progression of nfvPPA, this patient's mood improved with an antidepressant, and her parkinsonism was partially responsive to the Sinemet. Additionally, a painful dystonia responded to botulinum toxin injections. Patients with CBD can develop profoundly self-deprecatory depression and this can be highly resistant to treatment, although antidepressants somewhat ameliorate these symptoms. Additionally, even though CBD was initially thought to be a movement disorder, the majority of patients present with a bvFTD or nfvPPA syndrome.

A *MAPT*, *GRN*, or *C9ORF72* mutation were all unlikely due to the lack of a significant family history of dementia, but TDP-43 type A (typically associated with *GRN* mutations) can attack a very similar network, even when mutations in *GRN* are absent.

CLINICAL FEATURES AND ANATOMY

The diagnostic criteria for nfvPPA, also known as progressive nonfluent aphasia (PNFA) or as agrammatic PPA, have two components. The first is based on the clinical features, while the diagnosis is secondarily supported by imaging findings (Box 4.1).

To meet an nfvPPA diagnosis, the most prominent clinical feature should be difficulty in the area of language associated with word-finding deficits, paraphasias, effortful speech, and agrammatism in spoken and written language. Many patients exhibit subtle difficulty with comprehension of grammatically difficult sentences. These deficits should be the principal cause of impaired daily living activities, and the aphasia should be the most prominent deficit at symptom onset and the most prominent abnormality for the initial phases of the disease.

There are characteristic features on neuropsychological testing that include nonfluent speech with decreased numbers of words and shortened phrase length in spoken and written speech. Additionally, there may be errors in tense and word order. If an anomia is present the words are usually quickly retrieved with small clues like the first letter of the word. Repetition is much like spontaneous speech

---

Box 4.1 International Consensus Research Criteria for Nonfluent/Agrammatic Variant Primary Progressive Aphasia (nfvPPA) Are Listed Below (Gorno-Tempini et al. 2011)

I. Primary progressive aphasia (PPA)

Inclusion: Criteria I.A.–I.C. must be answered positively.
   I.A. Most prominent clinical feature is difficulty with language
   I.B. These deficits are the principal cause of impaired daily living activities
   I.C. Aphasia should be the most prominent deficit at symptom onset and for the initial phases of the disease
Exclusion: Criteria I.D.–I.G. must be answered negatively for a PPA diagnosis.
   I.D. Pattern of deficits is better accounted for by other nondegenerative nervous system or medical disorders
   I.E. Cognitive disturbance is better accounted for by a psychiatric diagnosis
   I.F. Prominent initial episodic memory, visual memory, and visuoperceptual impairments
   I.G. Prominent, initial behavioral disturbance

II. Clinical diagnosis of nonfluent/agrammatic variant PPA

Both of the following core features must be present:
   II.A. Agrammatism in language production
   II.B. Effortful, halting speech with inconsistent speech sound errors and distortions (apraxia of speech)
At least 2 of 3 of the following other features must be present:
   II.C. Impaired comprehension of syntactically complex sentences
   II.D. Spared single-word comprehension
   II.E. Spared object knowledge

(continued)

Box 4.1 International Consensus Research Criteria for Nonfluent/Agrammatic Variant Primary Progressive Aphasia (nfvPPA) Are Listed Below (Gorno-Tempini et al. 2011) (cont.)

III. Imaging-supported nonfluent/agrammatic variant PPA diagnosis

Both of the following criteria must be present:
   III.A. Clinical diagnosis of nonfluent/agrammatic variant PPA
   III.B. Imaging must show one or more of the following results:
       III.B.1. Predominant left posterior frontoinsular atrophy on MRI or
       III.B.2. Predominant left posterior frontoinsular hypoperfusion or hypometabolism on SPECT or PET

IV. Nonfluent/agrammatic variant PPA with definite pathology

Clinical diagnosis (criterion IV.A. below) and either criterion IV.B. or IV.C. must be present:
   IV.A. Clinical diagnosis of nonfluent/agrammatic variant PPA
   IV.B. Histopathologic evidence of a specific neurodegenerative pathology (e.g., FTLD-tau, FTLD-TDP, Alzheimer's disease, other)
   IV.C. Presence of a known pathogenic mutation

and comprehension, except for grammatically complex phrases, is normal. Executive functions may be perfectly normal except for decreases in verbal working memory and phonemic fluency. Visuospatial functions are remarkably spared.

The pattern of deficits should be not be better accounted for by other nondegenerative nervous system or medical disorders, psychiatric diagnosis, or include prominent initial episodic memory, visual memory, and visuoperceptual impairments or behavioral disturbance.

On examination of a patient with nfvPPA, effortful speech is the most obvious finding at the bedside. Speech tends to be slow and halting with labored speech production, inconsistent distortions, deletions, substitutions, insertions, or transpositions of speech sounds. These deficits can be particularly evident when the patient attempts to speak or repeat polysyllabic words such as "catastrophe" or "Methodist Episcopal." When attempting to speak, some patients exhibit stuttering (even though they never stuttered as a child), gesticulation with the hands and effortful movements of the face. As with other types of nonfluent aphasia, effortful speech is part of a constellation of findings that include shortened phrase length (often several words) and fewer spoken words

per minute, agrammatism in speech and writing, dysprosody (Benson & Ardila 1996), and often apraxia of speech.

In the early stages of the illness, some patients may exhibit relatively better written than spoken output (aphemia), but eventually written output becomes impaired as well. Argye Hillis has emphasized that patients with nfvPPA have more trouble with verbs, while those with svPPA have greater deficits with nouns (Hillis et al. 2004).

Muteness can occur relatively early in the course of the illness. The anatomic correlate of muteness is a large perisylvian and insular lesion that involves the operculum, insula, and portions of the inferior and middle frontal gyrus (Gorno-Tempini et al. 2006) (Figure 4–3).

Many, but not all, patients exhibit difficulty with the production and comprehension of grammar in the early stages of the illness. Agrammatism is characterized by shortened, simple phrases of speech associated with grammatical errors. The grammatical simplification and deficits in both word sequence and tense (morphosyntactic errors) is typical of nfvPPA. Longer phrases such as "I live in a big house" become "I lived house, big." The tense (lived) is wrong and the word sequence is altered.

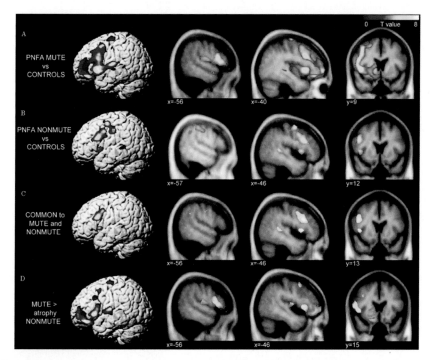

Figure 4–3. Areas of atrophy in mute patients versus control subjects (**A**) and nonmute patients versus control subjects (**B**) (simple main effects). Area of common atrophy in mute and nonmute patients versus control subjects (**C**) and areas of greater atrophy in mute versus nonmute patients and control subjects (**D**). Atrophy maps are displayed on the three-dimensional rendering of the Montreal Neurologic Institute standard brain and on sections of the customized template image used for normalization. Results are displayed at p < 0.001 uncorrected for multiple comparisons. (Gorno-Tempini et al. 2006.)

This inability to put together groups of phonemes (syllables) is called "apraxia of speech" and is present in many nfvPPA patients (Josephs et al. 2006). One characteristic feature of apraxia of speech is that patients have marked trouble with repetition, often making multiple different mistakes each time they attempt to repeat a word. For example, "episcopal" might be pronounced sequentially "pepiscopal," "metiscopal," "episcosal," and so forth (Ogar et al. 2006; Ogar et al. 2007).

While it is widely accepted that apraxia of speech is due to injury in anterior dominant hemisphere structures, Argye Hillis at Johns Hopkins has argued that left fronto-opercular injury is the critical lesion (Jordan & Hillis 2006) while Nina Dronkers at UC Davis and her colleagues (Ogar et al. 2006) have pointed to the critical role of the left anterior insula in apraxia of speech (Figure 4–4).

Agrammatism and motor speech errors begin in a subtle fashion, and often it is the patient who is the first to notice these changes. When patients present to physicians at this early stage of disease, it may be difficult to detect their abnormalities in speech or language with routine clinical bedside measures. Lower performance on tasks of word generation from a letter ("D," "F," "A," or "S") is often evident by the time a patient reaches a neurologist. Similarly, deficits on motor speech evaluations that require multiple repetitions of multisyllabic words are evident. Impaired comprehension of syntactically complex sentences, spared single word comprehension, and spared object knowledge are typical of nfvPPA.

The language deficits in the understanding and production of grammar, apraxia of speech, and dysarthria are followed by asymmetric right-hand and -leg parkinsonism with dystonia and alien hand. The motor problems can be extrapyramidal due to involvement of the basal ganglia or pyramidal due to motor strip degeneration.

Of all the clinical variants of FTD, nfvPPA is the most focal, often restricted to the left frontal regions on the initial neuroimaging studies (Gorno-Tempini et al. 2004; Seeley et al. 2009). In many cases the atrophy is so minimal that

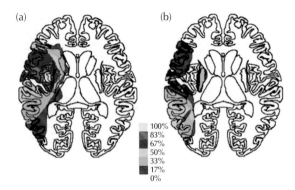

Figure 4–4. Comparison of computerized lesion overlapping in patients with and without apraxia of speech (AOS). **(A)** Overlapping the lesions of 18 patients with AOS lesions shows a common area of infarction (in bright yellow). **(B)** Overlapping the lesions of 8 patients without AOS lesions shows damage to much of the left hemisphere, but not the superior precentral gyrus of the insula (SPGI). (Ogar et al. 2006.)

the MRI is called normal, although statistical analyses of the atrophy pattern in these patients usually shows mild frontoinsular changes (Gorno-Tempini et al. 2004). nfvPPA is associated with focal degeneration of circuits in the left frontal, basal ganglia, and insular region. Structural imaging of these patients typically shows predominant left posterior frontoinsular atrophy on MRI or predominant left posterior frontoinsular hypoperfusion or hypometabolism on SPECT or PET. These structural or functional deficits involve circuits that are critical for the understanding and production of language, executive control, and movement in the left inferior frontal gyrus, insula, premotor, and supplementary motor areas (see Figure 4–5).

GENETIC AND PATHOLOGICAL CORRELATES

Most nfvPPA patients show FTLD-tau or FTLD-TDP-43 type A pathologic changes. Patients with tau pathology usually have PSP or CBD pathology at autopsy. The presence of a vertical gaze disturbance or dysarthria should bring PSP to consideration, and an asymmetric motor syndrome suggests CBD. While motor asymmetry was once considered pathognomonic for CBD, it is now realized that PSP, Pick's disease, AD, and dementia with Lewy bodies can all show asymmetric motor findings.

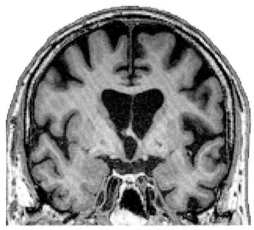

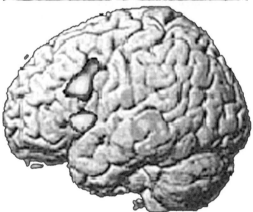

Figure 4–5. MRI showing typical atrophy pattern seen in nfvPPA, and VBM group analysis of nfavPPA versus healthy controls. (Image courtesy of Howard Rosen, MD.)

If nfvPPA develops in the setting of a strong family history, *GRN* is the most likely etiology, and this mutation often leads to an asymmetric cognitive, behavior, and motor syndrome (Behrens et al. 2007; Caso et al. 2012). nfvPPA with CBD motor features has been seen in patients with selective left frontoinsular and medial prefrontal cortical degeneration. *GRN* mutations are associated with spread of atrophy to the parietal and sometimes even occipital regions, so when nfvPPA is associated with posterior involvement *GRN* should be considered. nfvPPA does occur with *MAPT*, although this syndrome appears to be less common in the setting of *C9ORF72* mutations, as these genes tend to cause more symmetrical neurodegeneration.

DIFFERENTIAL DIAGNOSIS

The diagnosis of nfvPPA is usually straightforward, and the effortful speech, diminished language output, and relative sparing of other cognitive domains are easily recognized as a distinctive entity. Often, oculomotor or motor deficits are present at the time of diagnosis or emerge soon afterward, although we have seen patients with nfvPPA in whom the syndrome stays isolated for many years (Lee et al. 2011; Caso et al. 2012). This overlap between language and motor syndromes in a single patient can cause diagnostic dilemmas. Whether to call a patient nfvPPA or PSP or CBD is often a difficult decision that depends on the presenting features and relative severity of the language or motor findings. Yet, the guidelines around diagnosis are still somewhat vague. So for example, when a patient with nfvPPA for several years develops classical eye movement findings of PSP, is the initial diagnosis changed, or does the presenting syndrome preempt the new syndrome, even though PSP (the second diagnosis) is more highly predictive of the patient's underlying neuropathology than was the first diagnosis, nfvPPA?

At the University of California, San Francisco (UCSF), we have tended to make two diagnoses, one that captures the clinical syndrome and another that emphasizes predicted pathology. Hence the patient described above would be nfvPPA with predicted PSP pathology. Even this layered approach is fraught with problems, and one dilemma is whether to change the underlying clinical diagnosis when a new diagnosis comes along. Ultimately, as our precision for predicting the underlying molecule responsible for the clinical syndrome improves, molecular diagnosis is likely to be emphasized over clinical syndromes.

Another major differential diagnostic problem in the patient with nfvPPA is the separation of this syndrome from lvPPA. Some of the diagnostic uncertainty relates to similarities in the way that both disorders present. Both nfvPPA and lvPPA are subtypes of PPA that begin with slowly progressive word-finding problems that spare other aspects of cognition and behavior. Additionally, there are problems with the understanding of grammar in both lvPPA and nfvPPA. Another similar feature of both forms of PPA is that unlike other AD subtypes, many lvPPA patients do not exhibit significant memory difficulties.

While lvPPA does not truly cause a classical nonfluent aphasia, as phrase length and words per minute are often perfectly normal when the patient is relaxed and comfortable, however when the lvPPA patient searches for words, the speech output may begin to sound choppy. Similarly, as the patient loses confidence in her ability to speak without errors, this leads to a cautious word output that has nonfluent features.

Yet, there are significant differences between these patients that help to differentiate them from each other. While true nfvPPA patients rarely produce normal output, the lvPPA patient is often fluent unless stumped by generating a specific word. While both nfvPPA and lvPPA patients have deficits with working memory, only lvPPA patients have problems with echoic memory, so their ability to list numbers forward or repeat long sentences is markedly impaired in contrast to the patient with nfvPPA. Finally, the lvPPA patient often has subtle hippocampal and posterior biparietal and bitemporal abnormalities. Hence, these patients can have more significant memory, drawing, navigational, and calculation problems than the patient with nfvPPA. The addition of amyloid imaging is greatly improving separation of these two conditions, and a positive amyloid scan greatly increases the likelihood that the aphasia is lvPPA with AD neuropathology.

Patients with Creutzfeldt-Jakob disease can present with nfvPPA, although cortical ribboning is usually evident on MRI in these cases leading to the easy diagnosis of prion disease.

Rarely, we have seen patients with psychiatric conditions that mimic nfvPPA. The lack of progression over time, the marked fluctuation of symptoms—sometimes from day to day—and the atypical (nonphysiological) features of the aphasia usually help to separate out these psychologically mediated cases from true nfvPPA.

TREATMENT

Taking care of patients with nfvPPA can be heartbreaking, as their insight often remains intact, and depressive symptoms are very common. There is almost no medical evidence to support any specific therapy for nfvPPA. With that said, the early patient often benefits from speech therapy and may eventually find some solace using a computer or board to help with communication. Some groups have tried music-based therapies, although the literature on this approach is still scant. Exercise can help hold off motor symptoms for a while, and SSRIs often help with the mood disturbance that these patients exhibit. Parkinsonian symptoms may improve for a short while with Sinemet (carbidopa-levodopa), and in the later stages of nfvPPA injections of botulinum toxin can alleviate painful dystonias.

nfvPPA: CURRENT STATE AND RESEARCH ADVANCES

Diagnosis from Clinical Syndrome to Molecular Diagnosis

As is described in this chapter, the recognition of nfvPPA is relatively recent, noted first by Marsel Mesulam in the 1980s (Mesulam 1982). The new research criteria for nfvPPA that were formalized by Marilu Gorno-Tempini and international colleagues in 2011, with generous advice and collaboration from Marsel Mesulam, have allowed harmonized diagnosis of this syndrome across the world (Gorno-Tempini et al. 2011).

The early issue, separating nfvPPA patients from those with AD has been largely solved, but the current challenge of nfvPPA is molecular diagnosis. With the advent of amyloid imaging, it is now possible to reliably separate AD from FTLD-spectrum causes. This technique is particularly valuable in patients who are under

70 years of age, because amyloid aggregation can occur without causing symptoms. We have reported on one such patient with nfvPPA who had a positive amyloid scan in whom neuropathology confirmed Pick's disease and incidental cortical amyloid (Caso et al. 2012).

The percentage of patients that suffer from tau- versus TDP-43-related disease varies from center to center, but the vast majority of nfvPPA patients show CBD, PSP, Pick's disease, or TDP-43 type A neuropathology (Josephs et al. 2006). As has been described previously in this chapter, other features of the illness can be diagnostic. PSP patients almost always develop a supranuclear vertical gaze palsy, CBD patients go on to have grasping and groping alien hand (or foot), Pick's disease patients have a long clinical course, show massive orbitofrontal and anterior temporal atrophy, and tend to exhibit motor symptoms only late in the illness, and patients with *GRN* or tau mutations have a family history of FTD. Still, greater precision is needed. Tau imaging may further help to separate tau cases from TDP-43, greatly improving molecular separation of these disorders. There are current efforts in tau imaging directed at neurofibrillary tangles (Jensen et al. 2011; Watanabe et al. 2012) but *in vivo* imaging efforts to define the tau subtypes associated with PSP, CBD, and Pick's disease and to follow longitudinally these biomarkers are still greatly needed.

Still poorly understood is the relationship between the nfvPPA cases with *GRN* mutations and TDP-43 type A neuropathology versus those without a mutation. If the pathogenesis of the *GRN* mutation negative cases is similar to *GRN* positive nfvPPA, *GRN*-boosting approaches might work for both groups of patients, expanding the therapeutic opportunities for these patients while increasing the need to recognize this nfvPPA subtype during life, not only at autopsy.

Neurolinguistic and Neuroplasticity Discoveries

Through the study of patients with slow degeneration of the left frontoinsular degeneration, new insights into the brain's organization of language have been made possible. nfvPPA has allowed investigators to compare the linguistic features of this left frontoinsular degenerative condition to those of a disorder of the left anterior temporal lobe, svPPA. The distinctive word outputs of patients with these conditions helps to understand the way that differing anatomical regions handle various components of language. Even simple analyses of verb output (worse in nfvPPA) versus noun output (worse in svPPA) point to the use of different circuitry to communicate.

Several groups, including those led by Murray Grossman and colleagues at the University of Pennsylvania (Gunawardena et al. 2010) and Steven Wilson (University of Arizona) and Marilu Gorno-Tempini and colleagues at UCSF have correlated language functions that are either lost or spared to the specific white matter circuits that are lost or still function (Galantucci et al. 2011; Grossman 2012; Wilson et al. 2012). The dorsal white matter tracts, including the superior longitudinal fasciculus and arcuate fasciculus, seem to play a critical role in syntactic processing. Diffusion tensor imaging suggests that damage to left hemisphere dorsal tracts strongly correlates with abnormalities in the understanding and production of syntax (Wilson et al. 2011; Wilson et al. 2012) (Figure 4–6). Hence, nfvPPA patients have devastating deficits in syntax, while patients with svPPA do not.

Finally, there is a small but tantalizing set of findings to suggest that the slow progression of this disorder can be associated with remodeling of posterior cerebral cortex, generating visual creativity in a small subset of patients (Seeley et al. 2008). All of the visual artists in an international study on occupation in FTD had a form of progressive aphasia (Spreng et al. 2010) suggesting the possibility that subtle early

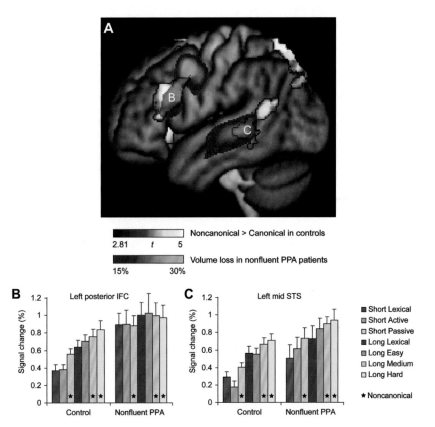

Figure 4–6. Functional abnormalities for syntactic processing in nonfluent PPA. **(A)** In age-matched controls, frontal and temporal regions were modulated by syntactic complexity (hot colors, p < 0.05, corrected for multiple comparisons), and these regions overlapped regions that were atrophic in nonfluent PPA patients (blue–green). **(B)** Inferior frontal cortex was modulated by syntactic complexity in controls, but not in nonfluent PPA patients. **(C)** Left superior temporal cortex showed normal modulation by syntactic complexity in patients, despite atrophy in this region. (Reprinted, with modifications, from Wilson et al. 2010a). (Wilson et al. 2012.)

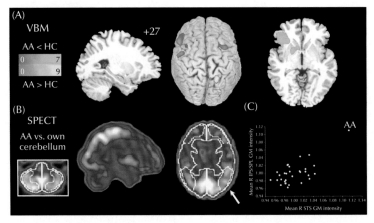

Figure 4–7. Neuroimaging results. **(A)** Gray matter reductions in AA versus controls (blue colorscale) were accompanied by focal areas of increased gray matter intensity in right posterior neocortex (orange colorscale). Bars indicate t-scores. Displayed voxels are significant at P < 0.001 (whole brain, uncorrected). **(B)** AA showed increased cerebral perfusion in only one ROI examined, the right parietal cortex (arrow, 112% of cerebellar baseline). **(C)** Mean gray matter intensities from right IPS/SPL and right STS ROIs (arbitrary units), plotted against each other for each subject, show the degree to which AA's values exceeded those of controls. For axial images, the left side of the image corresponds to the left side of the brain. Sagittal images are from right hemisphere. VBM data are superimposed on slice and surface-rendered images of the Montreal Neurological Institute template brain. HC = healthy controls. (Seeley et al. 2008.)

changes in language areas led to reorganization and strengthening of posterior brain circuits involved with visual processing.

In a comprehensive study of an artist with nfvPPA due to CBD, we described a patient in whom neuroimaging was performed prior to the onset of aphasia. Her brain showed extensive atrophy of the left frontoinsular brain circuit that ultimately was the site generating her symptoms of aphasia and greater volume in the right posterior parietal lobe than 30 age-matched control subjects (Figure 4–7).

There are multiple possible explanations for this distinctive atrophy pattern, including the possibility that this pattern happened by chance. We suspect that as the language circuit degenerated there was functional release of right parietal circuits involved with visual processing. Another possible mechanism for the enlarged right parietal lobe is that her increased interest in art led to increased use of this brain region that in turn led to parietal lobe remodeling. Finally, it is possible that she always had brain structural changes that were exhibited at the time of her first image. Whatever the mechanism, these patients offer a unique opportunity to explore the capability of posterior brain structures to remodel in the setting of an anterior neurodegenerative disorder.

REFERENCES

Behrens MI, Mukherjee O, Tu PH, Liscic RM, Grinberg LT, Carter D, Paulsmeyer K, Taylor-Reinwald L, Gitcho M, Norton JB, Chakraverty S, Goate AM, Morris JC, Cairns NJ. Neuropathological heterogeneity in HDD1: a familial frontotemporal lobar degeneration with ubiquitin-positive inclusions and progranulin mutation. Alz Dis Assoc Disord. 2007;21:1–7.

Benson DF, Ardila A. Aphasia: A Clinical Perspective. Oxford, England: Oxford University Press; 1996.

Caso F, Gesierich B, Henry M, Sidhu M, Lamarre A, Babiak M, Miller BL, Rabinovici GD, Huang EJ, Seeley WW, Gorno-Tempini ML. Nonfluent/agrammatic PPA with in-vivo cortical amyloidosis and Pick's disease. Behav Neurol. 2013;26:95–106.

Caso F, Villa C, Fenoglio C, Santangelo R, Agosta F, Coppi E, Falautano M, Comi G, Filippi M, Scarpini E, Magnani G, Galimberti D. The progranulin (GRN) Cys157LysfsX97 mutation is associated with nonfluent variant of primary progressive aphasia clinical phenotype. J Alzheimers Dis. 2012;28:759–63.

Galantucci S, Tartaglia MC, Wilson SM, Henry ML, Filippi M, Agosta F, Dronkers NF, Henry RG, Ogar JM, Miller BL, Gorno-Tempini ML. White matter damage in primary progressive aphasias: a diffusion tensor tractography study. Brain. 2011;134:3011–29.

Geschwind N. Disconnexion syndromes in animals and man. II. Brain. 1965;88:585–644.

Gorno-Tempini ML, Dronkers NF, Rankin KP, Ogar JM, Phengrasamy L, Rosen HJ, Johnson JK, Weiner MW, Miller BL. Cognition and anatomy in three variants of primary progressive aphasia. Ann Neurol. 2004;55:335–46.

Gorno-Tempini ML, Hillis AE, Weintraub S, Kertesz A, Mendez M, Cappa SF, Ogar JM, Rohrer JD, Black S, Boeve BF, Manes F, Dronkers NF, Vandenberghe R, Rascovsky K, Patterson K, Miller BL, Knopman DS, Hodges JR, Mesulam MM, Grossman M. Classification of primary progressive aphasia and its variants. Neurology. 2011;76:1006–14.

Gorno-Tempini ML, Murray RC, Rankin KP, Weiner MW, Miller BL. Clinical, cognitive and anatomical evolution from nonfluent progressive aphasia to corticobasal syndrome: a case report. Neurocase. 2004;10(6):426–36.

Gorno-Tempini ML, Ogar JM, Brambati SM, Wang P, Jeong JH, Rankin KP, Dronkers NF, Miller BL. Anatomical correlates of early mutism in progressive nonfluent aphasia. Neurology. 2006;67:1849–51.

Grossman M. The non-fluent/agrammatic variant of primary progressive aphasia. Lancet Neurol. 2012;11(6):545–55.

Gunawardena D, Ash S, McMillan C, Avants B, Gee J, Grossman M. Why are patients with progressive nonfluent aphasia nonfluent? Neurology. 2010;75:588–94.

Hillis AE, Oh S, Ken L. Deterioration of naming nouns versus verbs in primary progressive aphasia. Ann Neurol. 2004;55:268–75.

Jensen JR, Cisek K, Funk KE, Naphade S, Schafer KN, Kuret J. Research towards tau imaging. J Alzheimers Dis. 2011;26 Suppl 3:147–57.

Jordan LC, Hillis AE. Disorders of speech and language: aphasia, apraxia and dysarthria. Curr Opin Neurol. 2006;19(6):580–5.

Josephs KA, Duffy JR, Strand EA, Whitwell JL, Layton KF, Parisi JE, Hauser MF, Witte RJ, Boeve BF, Knopman DS, Dickson DW, Jack CR Jr, Petersen RC. Clinicopathological and imaging correlates of progressive aphasia and apraxia of speech. Brain. 2006;129:1385–98.

Knibb JA, Xuereb JH, Patterson K, Hodges JR. Clinical and pathological characterization of progressive aphasia. Ann Neurol. 2006;59:156–65.

Lee S, Wilson SM, Seeley W, Rankin K, Dearmond S, Huang EJ, Trojanowki JQ, Growdon M, Jang J, Sidhu M, See T, Karydas A, Jagust W, Weiner M, Gorno Tempini ML, Boxer A, Miller BL, Rabinovici GD. Correlates of Alzheimer's disease pathology in corticobasal syndrome. Annals of Neurology. 2011;70(2):327–40.

Mesulam MM. Slowly progressive aphasia without generalized dementia. Ann Neurol. 1982;11:592–8.

Narvid J, Gorno-Tempini ML, Slavotinek A, Dearmond SJ, Cha YH, Miller BL, Rankin K. Of brain and bone: the unusual case of Dr. A. Neurocase. 2009;15:190–205.

Ogar J, Willock S, Baldo J, Wilkins D, Ludy C, Dronkers N. Clinical and anatomical correlates of apraxia of speech. Brain Lang. 2006;97:343–50.

Ogar JM, Dronkers NF, Brambati SM, Miller BL, Gorno-Tempini ML. Progressive nonfluent aphasia and its characteristic motor speech deficits. Alzheimer Dis Assoc Disord. 2007;21:S23–30.

Rogalski E, Cobia D, Harrison TM, Wieneke C, Weintraub S, Mesulam MM. Progression of language decline and cortical atrophy in subtypes of primary progressive aphasia. Neurology. 2011;76:1804–10.

Sánchez-Valle R, Forman MS, Miller BL, Gorno-Tempini ML. From progressive nonfluent aphasia to corticobasal syndrome: a case report of corticobasal degeneration. Neurocase. 2006;12(6):355–9.

Seeley WW, Crawford RK, Zhou J, Miller BL, Greicius MD. Neurodegenerative diseases target large-scale human brain networks. Neuron. 2009;62(1):42–52.

Seeley WW, Matthews BR, Crawford RK, Gorno-Tempini ML, Foti D, Mackenzie IR, Miller BL. Unravelling Boléro: progressive aphasia, transmodal creativity and the right posterior neocortex. Brain. 2008;131:39–49.

Spreng RN, Rosen HJ, Strother S, Chow TW, Diehl-Schmid J, Freedman M, Graff-Radford NR, Hodges JR, Lipton AM, Mendez MF, Morelli SA, Black SE, Miller BL, Levine B. Occupation attributes relate to location of atrophy in frontotemporal lobar degeneration. Neuropsychologia. 2010;48:3634–41.

Watanabe H, Ono M, Kimura H, Matsumura K, Yoshimura M, Okamoto Y, Ihara M, Takahashi R, Saji H. Synthesis and biological evaluation of novel oxindole derivatives for imaging neurofibrillary tangles in Alzheimer's disease. Bioorg Med Chem Lett. 2012;22(17):5700–3.

Wilson SM, Galantucci S, Tartaglia MC, Gorno-Tempini ML. The neural basis of syntactic deficits in primary progressive aphasia. Brain Lang. 2012;122(3):190–8. doi: 10.1016/j.bandl.2012.04.005. Epub 2012 Apr 29.

Wilson SM, Galantucci S, Tartaglia MC, Rising K, Patterson DK, Henry ML, Ogar JM, DeLeon J, Miller BL, Gorno-Tempini ML. Syntactic processing depends on dorsal language tracts. Neuron. 2011;72:397–403.

Chapter 5

Related Disorders: FTD-ALS

OVERVIEW

The cortically predominant syndromes of the behavioral variant of frontotemporal dementia (bvFTD), semantic variant of primary progressive aphasia (svPPA), and the nonfluent variant of PPA (nfvPPA) are strongly linked to disorders of movement, including amyotrophic lateral sclerosis (ALS), corticobasal degeneration (CBD), and progressive supranuclear palsy (PSP). In some individuals, neurodegeneration begins in brain regions that control movement, and only later does the disease move to cortical regions, while in others, disease begins cortically and later spreads to the basal ganglia or motor neurons.

Yet, from an etiological and treatment perspective, there are only minor differences between a CBD or PSP patient who starts with a movement abnormality and one who begins as a disorder of executive control, behavior, or language (Huey et al. 2012). Similarly, many patients begin with ALS only later to evolve into bvFTD, while for others the behavioral or personality changes herald the disease, yet the underlying neuropathology is often identical for both patients (Rademakers et al. 2012). Even when ALS is caused by a specific genetic mutation like *C9ORF72*, one family member may begin with ALS, another with bvFTD, a third with a mixture of both ALS and bvFTD, and still another with a parkinsonian syndrome with dystonia (Boxer et al. 2011; Takada et al. 2012). Similarly, FTD-associated with *GRN* or *MAPT* mutations can begin with either parkinsonian features or an FTD syndrome.

For nearly every FTD syndrome, whether genetic or sporadic, the clinical heterogeneity is extensive. In one individual the disease may start as a change in movement, yet in another the disease begins as an aphasia or behavioral disorder. For these reasons, I discuss neurodegenerative disorders of movement whose cognitive features are often overlooked, ALS, PSP, and CBD, and I outline their links to FTD. In this chapter I describe links between ALS and FTD; in Chapter 6 I focus on the links between PSP, CBD, and FTD.

AMYOTROPHIC LATERAL SCLEROSIS

ALS, also called Lou Gehrig's disease, is a progressive, fatal disease that attacks the pyramidal system and lower motor neurons. Some ALS patients who exhibit deficits in higher cortical function or behavior at the time of their first evaluation or soon after presentation go on to develop symptoms of bvFTD (Lomen-Hoerth et al. 2003; Lillo et al. 2011). Although the coassociation between bvFTD and ALS varies from study to study, in a 2002 University of California, San Francisco/Los Angeles (UCSF/UCLA), series, approximately 15% of FTD patients developed findings suggestive of ALS (Lomen-Hoerth et al. 2002), and up to 50% of ALS patients exhibited frontal-executive changes on neuropsychological testing (Lomen-Hoerth et al. 2003).

Full-blown bvFTD, svPPA, or nfvPPA will often emerge in a sizable minority of patients who were first diagnosed with ALS. Furthermore, even patients in whom no features of bvFTD are seen show more atrophy in the frontal regions than do age-matched controls, suggesting that these patients might be in the early preclinical stage of bvFTD but have not yet reached a clinical threshold for the diagnosis.

CASE HISTORY

A 55-year-old male was accused of sexual harassment at work. Although eight different women in the office complained of grossly offensive language and inappropriate touching over the previous 18 months, the patient denied these accusations.

At the same time, it was learned that the patient had illegally taken money from the office kitty. His wife described that he had mild withdrawal from his children and hobbies and a loss of interest in sexual intimacy. He began to compete aggressively with his children and called his 4-year-old daughter a "loser" when he beat her in a game of checkers. He was fired from his work as an office manager and briefly obtained work as a car salesman but lost his job within 1 week.

At home, he developed a compulsive interest in buying clothes from the Internet and was swindled out of $150,000 in a deal buying land in the Caribbean. Apathy grew profound, and the patient lay on his couch watching television throughout the day. When awake he searched the house for food and gained 15 pounds. His manners deteriorated, he stuffed food in his mouth and licked his plate clean. When forced to watch his teenage son's football game, he spent most of the time at the food stand eating hot dogs.

Finally, his wife insisted that he obtain a neurological evaluation. The patient's father had died in a mental institution, and his father's brother was diagnosed with ALS in his sixth decade.

On examination, Mr. C was inappropriately familiar with the female staff and asked the receptionist for a date in front of his wife. He stared without blinking and giggled at many questions. When asked if anything was wrong he responded, "No, it is my wife who is crazy."

Neuropsychological testing revealed an MMSE of 25 with points missed for incorrectly identifying what floor he was on and that he was in a hospital, one word on recall and two points on spelling "world" backward. He generated three "d" words, and he repeated, "dumb, damn, dog" 10 times. He made multiple perseverative errors on the trails and flanker task and repeated seven digits forward and three backward. On the Boston Naming Test he correctly named 13/15 words, and he did well on verbal and visual memory and drawing. His results on the NPI scored high for apathy, disinhibition, repetitive motor, and euphoria. His neurological examination was normal. His MRI showed mild frontal and subtle occipital atrophy.

The patient was placed in a daycare center but was quickly expelled due to inappropriate touching of female staff and a tendency to spit while indoors. His wife found a male companion for him who accompanied him for hours around his neighborhood where he looked for cans to bring home. SSRIs mildly decreased his repetitive behaviors.

The patient deteriorated behaviorally and cognitively over the next year. He broke into his neighbor's house to find liquor. He paced up and down the stairs in his house and worried that strangers were trying to enter. At meals he began to choke on food, and his wife noticed that his voice was becoming softer. At night, his muscles rippled intensely and his muscle bulk diminished. He began to have trouble climbing the stairway, and his wife noticed that he was gasping for air at night.

Examination revealed an apathetic man who stared at the examiners. His MMSE was 22 with losses on items of orientation, spelling "world" backward, and writing a complete sentence. Speech was slurred and suggested a combination of pyramidal and lower motor neuron involvement. Gag was diminished, and there was tongue atrophy. Muscle bulk diminished in the arms and hands, and fasciculations were evident. The reflexes were diffusely increased, including the jaw jerk, and toes were upgoing. An MRI showed worsening of the frontal atrophy. FTD-ALS was diagnosed. Within three months, the patient aspirated and died in a nursing home.

Autopsy showed mild frontal, occipital, and cerebellar atrophy. Histology revealed neuron loss in the hypoglossal nucleus, extensive lower motor neuron loss in the cervical spinal cord, and TDP-43 positive inclusions in the frontal lobes and motor neurons. FTD-ALS with TDP-43 type B was diagnosed. Later he was discovered to have a *C9ORF72* mutation.

Comment. This patient had a typical bvFTD presentation and had all six of the items in the international research criteria (Box 3.1), early disinhibition, apathy, loss of sympathy and empathy, repetitive motor behavior, overeating, and deficits in executive control with sparing of spatial skills. Insight into the behavioral syndrome from which the patient suffers is almost never evident, and it is usually family members or coworkers that observe disturbing changes in behavior. This led the patient to facilely suggest that it was his wife, not he, who suffered from a mental illness and that the multitude of women at work who accused him of sexual harassment were the ones at fault, not him. Treatment with SSRIs showed mild efficacy, but hiring a companion was particularly valuable.

Like many patients with bvFTD, he went on to develop an ALS syndrome. Management of his behavior was difficult, and his FTD-ALS was proven be due to a mutation in *C9ORF72* (deJesus-Hernandez et al. 2011). This subtype of FTD can show occipital, thalamic, and cerebellar atrophy with milder frontal atrophy than other subtypes (Sha et al. 2012). The presence of this mutation has profound implications for the patient's children, who are at a 50% risk for developing either FTD, ALS, or both. The *C9ORF72* mutation can now be measured in Clinical Laboratory Improvement Amendments (CLIA) approved laboratories, although genetic counseling is strongly suggested for anyone, whether presymptomatic or symptomatic, before performing this test. Few of our asymptomatic subjects choose to know the results of their genetic status. When effective therapies for *C9ORF72* emerge this will certainly change.

CLINICAL FEATURES AND ANATOMY

ALS is associated with a combination of upper and lower motor neuron findings, and the diagnosis of FTD should trigger a systematic search for evidence of ALS. Upper motor neuron findings suggestive of ALS include slow, strangled speech; spasticity in the upper and lower extremities; hyperactive gag and jaw jerks; brisk limb reflexes; and a Hoffman or Babinski's sign. Lower motor neuron findings include a weak, dysarthric voice; diminished gag; atrophy of the facial, tongue, arm, or leg muscles; fasciculations; weakness; and hyporeflexia. Most patients with FTD-ALS exhibit a combination of upper and lower motor neuron findings, although a small minority will show either pure upper motor findings (called progressive lateral sclerosis) or pure lower motor neuron findings (called motor neuron disease). Geser and colleagues have shown that pure motor neuron disease is a TDP-43 proteinopathy similar to that in patients with both upper and lower motor neuron disease (Geser et al. 2011).

While all clinical variants have been reported in association with ALS, far and away the most common FTD variant is bvFTD (Sha et al. 2012). In a patient with well-established ALS, bvFTD can manifest with subtle behavioral changes such as apathy, anxiety, disinhibition, or paranoia. There are sometimes subtle differences in the clinical features of the bvFTD patient with ALS and, unlike typical bvFTD, FTD-ALS patients show prominent anxiety and weight loss. In fact, in a patient with bvFTD, weight loss should lead to the suspicion of the new onset of ALS. As was demonstrated by Rick Olney at UCSF, the presence of ALS in a patient with FTD or FTD in an ALS patient is associated with a greatly shortened life span compared to the patient with either pure FTD or pure ALS (Olney et al. 2005). ALS-FTD is strongly familial, and in the UCSF cohort of patients with both disorders the majority of the familial cases are explained by mutations in the *C9ORF72* gene (Sha et al. 2012).

El Escorial Criteria

The diagnosis of ALS is based primarily on clinical presentation, with supportive data from electrodiagnostic, imaging, and laboratory studies. In 1994 the World Federation of Neurology published the El Escorial criteria for the diagnosis of ALS (Brooks, 1994). They defined three categories of certainty based on clinical signs:

- **Clinically Definite ALS:** Upper and lower motor neuron signs in three or more regions. Regions are defined as bulbar, cervical, thoracic, or lumbar.
- **Clinically Probable ALS:** Upper and lower motor neuron findings in two regions or upper motor neuron findings anatomically rostral to (above) lower motor neuron findings. (Therefore increased reflexes in the arms with wasting and fasciculations in the legs would qualify, but not the other way around.)
- **Clinically Possible ALS:** Upper and lower motor neuron findings in one region or lower motor neuron findings anatomically above upper motor neuron findings.

In addition to the motor neuron signs as defined above, the diagnosis is supported by the spread of signs and symptoms from one region to another with a linear increase in severity. The diagnosis of ALS should be questioned if sensory, cerebellar, oculomotor, or bowel or bladder symptoms are present. The laboratory studies below are helpful in confirming the diagnosis and ruling out other possible diagnoses.

- **Blood tests**: Creatine phosphokinase (CPK) may be normal or moderately elevated (2–3 times normal) in ALS. CPK may be ordered to rule out muscle disease, which in some cases can cause a high elevation of CPK.

Other studies that should be considered to rule out diseases that can mimic FTD-ALS include B12, Lyme titers or western blot, Anti-GM1 antibody titers, and serum protein electrophoresis.

- **Electromyography (EMG)**: The presence of fibrillations and positive waves (together referred to as spontaneous activity) and decreased recruitment in a muscle qualify as lower motor neuron findings and can be used to upgrade the probability of the diagnosis based on the El Escorial criteria outlined above.
- **MRI of the spine:** Multifocal spinal cord disease can mimic the findings of ALS and therefore should be ruled out with an anatomical study.
- **Muscle biopsy:** Not routinely performed, but muscle biopsy is done in selected cases where the diagnosis is problematic. In ALS, a muscle biopsy will show a neurogenic pattern.

GENETIC AND PATHOLOGICAL CORRELATES

Most familial FTD-ALS cases are caused by mutations in *C9ORF72*. Rarely, mutations in *TARDBP* or *FUS* can lead to familial ALS with FTD, but most of these mutations have been described in association with ALS alone. Even more rarely, a mutation in valosin (Koppers et al. 2012), dynactin, tau, or an expansion in ataxin-2 will lead to an FTD-ALS syndrome (Swarup & Julien 2011). A *SOD* mutation is a common cause for ALS but rarely causes FTD and does not lead to TDP-43 aggregates. A recent review discusses the different molecules linked to familial ALS (Siddique & Ajroud-Driss 2011).

FTD-ALS is the most strongly genetic of the major clinical phenotypes of FTD, and Jill Goldman and colleagues found that approximately 30% of FTD-ALS cases were familial and suggested a dominant form of inheritance (Goldman et al. 2005). DNA testing should be considered after consultation with a genetic counselor in any patient with the combination of FTD and ALS.

Michael Strong and colleagues have proposed research criteria for FTD-ALS (Strong et al. 2009). In this effort they note, "The recommendations arising from this research workshop address the requirement for a concise clinical diagnosis of the underlying motor neuron disease (Axis I), defining the cognitive and behavioural dysfunction (Axis II), describing additional non-motor manifestations (Axis III) and identifying the presence of disease modifiers (Axis IV)." This international effort emphasizes the strong links between the two disorders.

Neuropathology

In FTD-ALS, ubiquitin-positive, tau negative aggregates are found in the medial temporal lobe, frontal lobe, and motor neurons. In 2006, Manuela Neumann in collaboration with Virginia Lee and colleagues demonstrated that most of these inclusions contained the transactive response (TAR)-DNA-binding protein 43 (TDP-43) (Neumann et al. 2006). This finding transformed the approach to ALS and led to a new emphasis on the links between FTD and ALS.

In the typical FTD-ALS case, TDP-43 leaves the nucleus and forms aggregates within the cytoplasm. It is still unknown whether the loss of DNA and RNA regulation within the nucleus or cytotoxic damage from TDP-43 aggregates within the cytoplasm is responsible for the FTD or for the ALS. Although both processes are likely important, there is increasing evidence that the translocation of TDP-43 plays a critical role in the neurodegenerative process and leads to dysregulation of RNA, DNA, and protein synthesis. Within the spinal cord in ALS the cytoplasmic aggregates are relatively sparse and diffusely spread but they are not associated with disease spread. This is evidence against the concept that the TDP-43 aggregates are the only toxic mechanism for FTD-ALS (Bodansky et al. 2010)

In 2009, Neumann and Mackenzie found that another DNA- and RNA-binding protein, fused in sarcoma (FUS), was present in the small minority of cases where TDP-43 was lacking (Neumann et al. 2009). Mutations in *FUS* cause familial ALS (Kwiatkowski et al. 2009), but FTD appears to be less common as a phenotype in these patients. While FUS aggregates are seen in bvFTD, they tend to be seen in young individuals in whom motor manifestations are lacking and with no significant family history of either ALS or FTD (Lee et al. 2011).

Importantly, in 2011 large DNA repeats in *C9ORF72* were found as the major cause for FTD-ALS (deJesus-Hernandez et al. 2011; Renton et al. 2011). The fact that TDP-43, FUS, and *C9ORF72* all play a major role in DNA or RNA regulation suggests that an underlying mechanism involved with DNA or RNA injury or altered expression may link many of the most common forms of FTD-ALS.

DIFFERENTIAL DIAGNOSIS

While there are many patients who present with the constellation of FTD and ALS, there are many who start with bvFTD, nfvPPA, or ALS clinical syndromes, and only later do the FTD and ALS syndromes merge. The best predictors of FTD-ALS in an FTD patient are: family history of ALS, unexplained weight loss of motor bulk, shortness of breath, and pocketing of food. Conversely, in an ALS patient the presence of unexplained apathy, disengagement from decision making, disinhibition, or urinary or fecal incontinence may mark the beginnings of an FTD syndrome.

TREATMENT

Currently there are no FDA-approved medications for FTD-ALS syndrome. While these patients need the typical types of support that are available for ALS patients, they are often very resistant to help. The shortened life expectancy for these patients, less than 2 years from the time of diagnosis, reflects both the relentless nature of the disorder and the reluctance of families or physicians to invoke heroic measures in the ALS patient with a profound behavioral disorder.

FTD-ALS: CURRENT STATE AND RESEARCH ADVANCES

Clinical-Pathological Considerations

The links between FTD and ALS have forced both fields to think about the common biology associated with both conditions.

Approximately 25% of the patients with FTLD in the UCSF brain bank have TDP-43 type B neuropathology, although many of those patients never manifested ALS during life. FTD-ALS is one of the major clinical subtypes of FTD and is the most genetic of all the clinical syndromes.

Conversely, the presence of FTD clinical syndromes in an ALS cohort is debated, although there have been few such cohorts in whom there have been systematic analyses of their neuropsychiatric features. The personality and behavioral changes that precede bvFTD can be easy to miss, particularly in the setting of ALS, and even sophisticated programs can have difficulty capturing early features of frontal lobe dysfunction.

One group of patients in whom this fascinating association is seen are former National Football League players. Some former players develop chronic traumatic encephalopathy (CTE), while others develop ALS. While both groups show extensive aggregates of tau and TDP-43 in frontal and basal ganglia structures, the ALS patients extend the aggregates into the brainstem and spinal cord (McKee et al. 2010). This suggests that both the CTE and ALS groups of patients are generating a burden of neuropathology associated with similar molecules with the major differentiating feature between CTE and ALS being the aggregation of TDP-43 in the nuclei and motor neurons involved with movement.

A full-blown FTD syndrome (usually bvFTD) is present in less than 15% of ALS patients, but more subtle behavioral or language changes are far more common. Many of the patients with early FTD show psychiatric symptoms that may range from depression, apathy, cyclic euphoria and depression, and increased self-centeredness, to excessive sweetness or niceness. Cognitive slowing is another subtle manifestation of early FTD. These are symptoms that are rarely recognized as neurodegenerative, particularly in clinics focused around movement. Similarly, it is easy to miss a subtle nfvPPA or svPPA in a patient with dysarthria.

In a study by Chang (UCSF), patients with FTD and ALS showed extensive frontal atrophy that was more severe than both age-matched controls and patients with ALS without an FTD syndrome (Chang et al. 2005). Additionally, those patients with ALS in whom there was no evidence of FTD showed greater atrophy in the frontal regions than did age-matched controls. This finding suggested that even though they these patients had not yet manifested an FTD syndrome, they already were showing atrophy of the frontal cortex (Figure 5–1).

Ultimately, neuropathological studies that extensively evaluate frontal, basal ganglia, and thalamic structures will be needed to determine the co-occurrence of these conditions. With that said, it is clear that an effective treatment of ALS will require treating and protecting

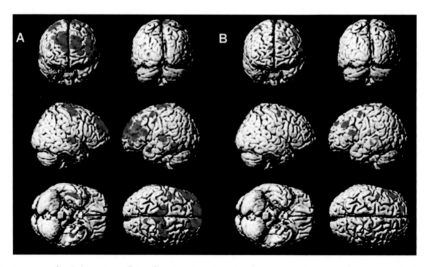

Figure 5–1. VBM results. **(A)** Regions of significant gray matter atrophy common to ALS and ALS/FTLD when compared to controls. **(B)** Regions of significant atrophy in ALS/FTLD greater than ALS and controls. (Chang et al. 2005.)

cortical, thalamic, and basal ganglia neurons, while the treatment of FTLD with underlying TDP-43 type B pathology will require strategies that protect the brainstem and spinal cord.

Molecular Considerations

The finding that TDP-43 forms the abnormal ubiquitin-bound aggregates in most cases of ALS and most of the non-tau forms of FTLD has transformed our understanding of these conditions. Soon after the discovery of TDP-43 in both sporadic FTD and ALS, patients were found in whom TDP-43 mutations led to familial forms of ALS and, in a few instances, FTD (Borghero et al. 2011). Additional molecular insights into FTD-ALS came with the discoveries that FUS aggregates were found in non-tau and non-TDP-43 subtypes of FTLD and could cause familial ALS (Kwiatkowski et al. 2009). Finally, showing that many cases of FTD-ALS were caused by a long DNA repeat mutation in *C9ORF72* suggested that DNA and RNA regulation represented a common pathway for these seeming diverse clinical syndromes and distinctive molecules (Bigio 2012, Rademakers 2012).

TARDBP is the precursor of TDP-43, the hyperphosphorylated and ubiquitinated protein found in FTD and ALS. *TARDBP* was first discovered to be a transcriptional repressor for HIV-1 transcription. TDP-43 is bound to fragments of DNA and RNA within the nucleus and has been proposed to play an important role in both suppression of DNA and RNA transcription and regulation and helped in the splicing of introns in pre-mRNA, converting it into mRNA (Buratti et al. 2011; Budini et al. 2011).

Feiguin and colleagues' (2009) work with drosophila showed that "flies lacking Drosophila TDP-43 appeared externally normal but presented deficient locomotive behaviors, reduced life span and anatomical defects at the neuromuscular junctions." Additionally, these phenotypes were rescued by expression of the human protein in a restricted group of neurons including motor neurons, supporting the idea that loss of function of TDP-43 rather than toxic gain of function is the mechanism for disease with FTD-ALS.

FUS is remarkably similar in activity to TDP-43. The N-terminal of *FUS* helps with transcriptional activation, and the C-terminal binds to both proteins and RNA. Both TDP and FUS are considered heterogeneous nuclear ribonucleoproteins (*hnRNPs*), and the sites in the nucleus that they bind and regulate appear to underlie their commonality in FTLD and ALS.

Animal models with TDP and FUS are just emerging but should eventually help to further our understanding of both FTLD and ALS. Guo and colleagues (Figure 5–2) showed that the A315T mutant has enhanced formation of aberrant TDP-43 species that are protease resistant and have sequence similarity to prion proteins (Guo et al 2011). This species formed amyloid fibrils in vitro that led to neuronal death

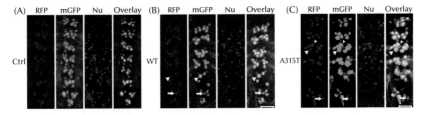

Figure 5–2. Expression of the A315T mutant causes more severe motor neuron (MN) damage. **(A)** Control flies have normal MNs with well-organized clusters in the ventral nerve cord (VNC). mGFP, membrane GFP; red fluorescent protein, RFP; Nu, Hoechst dye nuclear staining. **(B, C)** MNs in third-instar larvae of transgenic flies expressing hTDP-43 show cell death and morphological abnormality in MN clusters, especially in the last three VNC segments. MN damage is much more prominent in flies expressing the A315T mutant. Arrowheads mark swollen neurons with the mGFP area enlarged. Arrows mark MNs with fragmented or condensed nuclei and reduced mGFP signals. Quantification of MNs in the last three VNC segments indicates that 79 ± 5% of MNs expressing the A315T mutant, as compared to 32 ± 3% of those expressing wild-type (WT) TDP, show cell body swelling or condensed nuclei (with six flies in each group scored in three independent experiments). Fly genotypes: **(A)**, OK371-Gal4/UAS-mGFP/UAS-RFP; **(B)**, OK371-Gal4/UAS-mGFP/UAS-TDP-43-RFP; **(C)**, OK371-Gal4/UAS-mGFP/UAS-A315T TDP-43-RFP. Scale bars, 20 μm. (Guo et al. 2011.)

in primary cultures. The authors proposed the tantalizing hypothesis that TDP-43 has similarities with prions and might cause spread of the disease from one neuron to the next. Similarly, Ravits's exciting work (Ravits & LaSpada 2009) has demonstrated that ALS often spreads up and down the spinal cord from one region to the next, in a way that is reminiscent of prion disorders.

Wang and colleagues (Wang et al. 2011) showed that FUS and TDP-43 worked together in drosophila locomotion and influenced their ultimate life span. Drosophila mutants with disrupted FUS exhibited decreased speed and a shortened life span that could be rescued with wild-type human FUS but not FUS with ALS-causing mutations. A similar finding was found with TDP-43. These authors suggested that FUS acted together with and downstream of TDP-43 in a common genetic pathway in neurons. This finding established that FUS and TDP-43 function together in genetic regulation within the cell and suggests that their disruption may lead to ALS and FTD (Figure 5–3). With the links of *C9ORF72*, FUS, and TDP-43 to FTLD and ALS, there is a remarkable

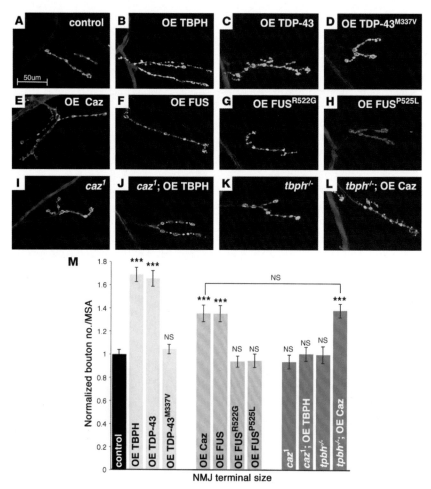

Figure 5–3. **(A–L)** Third instar NMJ terminals stained with anti-CSP (green) to label the presynapse and anti-HRP (red) to label the neuronal membrane at muscle 4, segment A3 for motor neuron overexpressing (OE) transgenic Caz, FUS, TBPH, TDP-43, and FUS or TDP-43 ALS mutants in wild-type (B–H) or tbph and caz1 mutants **(J and L)** driven in motor neurons by OK6-Gal4. The tbph–/– genotype is tbphΔ23/Df[2R]BSC660. Overexpression of wild-type TBPH, TDP-43, Caz, or FUS proteins induces NMJ expansion, while ALS mutant FUS or TDP-43M337V does not (B–H). Mutants of caz or tbph have normal NMJ morphology **(I and K)**. The NMJ expansion induced by expression of wild-type TDP-43 is completely suppressed in caz mutants **(J)**; however, the NMJ expansion induced by Caz overexpression is not suppressed in tbph mutants **(L)**. **(M)** Quantification of synapse terminal bouton number divided by muscle surface area for muscle 4 segment A3 normalized to control. Error bars represent SEM. °°°P < 0.001. (Wang et al. 2011.)

convergence of findings around DNA and RNA regulation and dysregulation as a common mechanism for both sets of conditions. More work is needed to understand why the frontal, brainstem, and spinal cord neurons are selectively vulnerable with FTLD and ALS.

Finally, in a cell model of TDP-43 mutations, overexpression of hTDP-43(M337V) led to toxicity that mimicked human forms of ALS with muscle atrophy, weakness, and fasciculations (Baloh et al. 2011). Uchida and colleagues were able to overexpress TDP-43 in the spinal cords of rats and cynomolgus monkeys. The authors demonstrated that the monkeys, but not the rats, developed a progressive motor neuron disease where TDP mislocalized from the nucleus to the cytoplasm (Uchida et al. 2012). These species differences may to help to explain why it has been so difficult to generate robust models of ALS with TDP-43 in mice.

Only recently have investigators shown the link between TDP-43, FUS, and ALS. The major debate remains as to whether it is the TDP-43 aggregate, spreading from cell to cell and causing neurotoxicity, that underlies FTD-ALS or whether it is the dysregulation of a multitude of genes when TDP-43 or FUS leaves the nucleus (Chen-Plotkin et al. 2010, Baloh et al. 2011, Guo et al. 2011, Lee et al. 2011). Over time this question will be answered. Understanding pathogenesis will be critical to the development of powerful therapies.

REFERENCES

Baloh RH. TDP-43: the relationship between protein aggregation and neurodegeneration in amyotrophic lateral sclerosis and frontotemporal lobar degeneration. FEBS J. 2011;278:3539–49.

Bigio EH. Motor neuron disease: the *C9ORF72* hexanucleotide repeat expansion in FTD and ALS. Nat Rev Neurol. 2012;8:249–50.

Bodansky A, Kim JM, Tempest L, Velagapudi A, Libby R, Ravits J. TDP-43 and ubiquitinated cytoplasmic aggregates in sporadic ALS are low frequency and widely distributed in the lower motor neuron columns independent of disease spread. Amyotroph Lateral Scler. 2010;11:321–7.

Borghero G, Floris G, Cannas A, Marrosu MG, Murru MR, Costantino E, Parish LD, Pugliatti M, Ticca A, Traynor BJ, Calvo A, Cammarosano S, Moglia C, Cistaro A, Brunetti M, Restagno G, Chiò A. A patient carrying a homozygous p.A382T TARDBP missense mutation shows a syndrome including ALS, extrapyramidal symptoms, and FTD. Neurobiol Aging. 2011;32:2327.e1–5.

Boxer AL, Mackenzie IR, Boeve BF, Baker M, Seeley WW, Crook R, Feldman H, Hsiung GY, Rutherford N, Laluz V, Whitwell J, Foti D, McDade E, Molano J, Karydas A, Wojtas A, Goldman J, Mirsky J, Sengdy P, Dearmond S, Miller BL, Rademakers R. Clinical, neuroimaging and neuropathological features of a new chromosome 9p-linked FTD-ALS family. J Neurol Neurosurg Psychiatry. 2011;82(2):196–203.

Brooks BR. El Escorial World Federation of Neurology criteria for the diagnosis of amyotrophic lateral sclerosis. Subcommittee on Motor Neuron Diseases/Amyotrophic Lateral Sclerosis of the World Federation of Neurology Research Group on Neuromuscular Diseases and the El Escorial "Clinical limits of amyotrophic lateral sclerosis" workshop contributors. J Neurol Sci. 1994;124 Suppl:96–107.

Budini M, Baralle FE, Buratti E. Regulation of gene expression by TDP-43 and FUS/TLS in frontotemporal lobar degeneration. Curr Alzheimer Res. 2011;8(3):237–45.

Buratti E, Baralle FE. TDP-43: new aspects of autoregulation mechanisms in RNA binding proteins and their connection with human disease. FEBS J. 2011;278(19):3530–8.

Chang JL, Lomen-Hoerth C, Murphy J, Henry RG, Kramer JH, Miller BL, Gorno-Tempini ML. A voxel-based morphometry study of patterns of brain atrophy in ALS and ALS/FTLD. Neurology. 2005;65:75–80.

Chen-Plotkin AS, Lee VM, Trojanowski JQ. TAR DNA-binding protein 43 in neurodegenerative disease. Nat Rev Neurol. 2010;6:211–20.

DeJesus-Hernandez M, Mackenzie IR, Boeve BF, Boxer AL, Baker M, Rutherford NJ, Nicholson AM, Finch NA, Flynn H, Adamson J, Kouri N, Wojtas A, Sengdy P, Hsiung GY, Karydas A, Seeley WW, Josephs KA, Coppola G, Geschwind DH, Wszolek ZK, Feldman H, Knopman DS, Petersen RC, Miller BL, Dickson DW, Boylan KB, Graff-Radford NR, Rademakers R. Expanded GGGGCC hexanucleotide repeat in noncoding region of *C9ORF72* causes chromosome 9p-linked FTD and ALS. Neuron. 2011;72:245–56.

Feiguin F, Godena VK, Romano G, D'Ambrogio A, Klima R, Baralle FE. Depletion of TDP-43 affects Drosophila motoneurons terminal synapsis and locomotive behavior. FEBS Lett. 2009;583(10):1586–92.

Geser F, Stein B, Partain M, Elman LB, McCluskey LF, Xie SX, Van Deerlin VM, Kwong LK, Lee VM, Trojanowski JQ. Motor neuron disease clinically limited to the lower motor neuron is a diffuse TDP-43 proteinopathy. Acta Neuropathol. 2011;121:509–17.

Goldman JS, Farmer JM, Wood EM, Johnson JK, Boxer A, Neuhaus J, Lomen-Hoerth C, Wilhelmsen KC, Lee VM, Grossman M, Miller BL. Comparison of family histories in FTLD subtypes and related tauopathies. Neurology. 2005;65:1817–9.

Guo W, Chen Y, Zhou X, Kar A, Ray P, Chen X, Rao EJ, Yang M, Ye H, Zhu L, Liu J, Xu M, Yang Y, Wang C, Zhang D, Bigio EH, Mesulam M, Shen Y, Xu Q, Fushimi K, Wu JY. An ALS-associated mutation affecting TDP-43 enhances protein aggregation, fibril formation and neurotoxicity. Nat Struct Mol Biol. 2011;18:822–30.

Huey ED, Ferrari R, Moreno JH, Jensen C, Morris CM, Potocnik F, Kalaria RN, Tierney M, Wassermann EM, Hardy J, Grafman J, Momeni P. FUS and TDP-43 genetic variability in FTD and CBS. Neurobiol Aging. 2012;33:1016.e9–17.

Koppers M, van Blitterswijk MM, Vlam L, Rowicka PA, van Vught PW, Groen EJ, Spliet WG, Engelen-Lee J, Schelhaas HJ, de Visser M, van der Kooi AJ, van der Pol WL, Pasterkamp RJ, Veldink JH, van den Berg LH. VCP mutations in familial and sporadic ALS. Neurobiol Aging. 2012;33:837.e7–13.

Kwiatkowski TJ Jr, Bosco DA, Leclerc AL, Tamrazian E, Vanderburg CR, Russ C, Davis A, Gilchrist J, Kasarskis EJ, Munsat T, Valdmanis P, Rouleau GA, Hosler BA, Cortelli P, de Jong PJ, Yoshinaga Y, Haines JL, Pericak-Vance MA, Yan J, Ticozzi N, Siddique T, McKenna-Yasek D, Sapp PC, Horvitz HR, Landers JE, Brown RH Jr. Mutations in the FUS/TLS gene on chromosome 16 cause familial amyotrophic lateral sclerosis. Science. 2009;323:1205–8.

Lee SE, Seeley WW, Poorzand P, Rademakers R, Karydas A, Stanley CM, Miller BL, Rankin KP. Clinical characterization of bvFTD due to FUS neuropathology. Neurocase. 2012;18(4):305–17.

Lillo P, Mioshi E, Zoing MC, Kiernan MC, Hodges JR. How common are behavioural changes in amyotrophic lateral sclerosis? Amyotroph Lateral Scler. 2011;12:45–51.

Lomen-Hoerth C, Anderson T, Miller BL. The overlap of amyotrophic lateral sclerosis and frontotemporal dementia. Neurology. 2002;59:1077–79.

Lomen-Hoerth C, Murphy J, Langmore S, Kramer JH, Olney RK, Miller BL. Are amyotrophic lateral sclerosis patients cognitively normal? Neurology. 2003;60:1094–97.

McKee AC, Gavett BE, Stern RA, Nowinski CJ, Cantu RC, Kowall NW, Perl DP, Hedley-Whyte ET, Price B, Sullivan C, Morin P, Lee HS, Kubilus CA, Daneshvar DH, Wulff M, Budson AE. TDP-43 proteinopathy and motor neuron disease in chronic traumatic encephalopathy. J Neuropathol Exp Neurol. 2010;69:918–29.

Neumann M, Rademakers R, Roeber S, Baker M, Kretzschmar HA, Mackenzie IR. 21. A new subtype of frontotemporal lobar degeneration with FUS pathology. Brain. 2009;132:2922–31.

Neumann M, Sampathu DM, Kwong LK, Truax AC, Micsenyi MC, Chou TT, Bruce J, Schuck T, Grossman M, Clark CM, McCluskey LF, Miller BL, Masliah E, Mackenzie IR, Feldman H, Feiden W, Kretzschmar HA, Trojanowski JQ, Lee VM. Ubiquitinated TDP-43 in frontotemporal lobar degeneration and amyotrophic lateral sclerosis. Science. 2006;314:130–3.

Olney RK, Murphy J, Forshew D, Garwood E, Miller BL, Langmore S, Kohn MA, Lomen-Hoerth C. The effects of executive and behavioral dysfunction on the course of ALS. Neurology. 2005;65(11):1774–7.

Rademakers R. C9orf72 repeat expansions in patients with ALS and FTD. Lancet Neurol. 2012;11:297–8R.

Rademakers R, Neumann M, Mackenzie IR. Advances in understanding the molecular basis of frontotemporal dementia. Nat Rev Neurol. 2012;8:423–34.

Ravits JM, La Spada AR. ALS motor phenotype heterogeneity, focality, and spread deconstructing motor neuron degeneration. Neurology. 2009;73:805–11.

Renton AE, Majounie E, Waite A, Simón-Sánchez J, Rollinson S, Gibbs JR, Schymick JC, Laaksovirta H, van Swieten JC, Myllykangas L, Kalimo H, Paetau A, Abramzon Y, Remes AM, Kaganovich A, Scholz SW, Duckworth J, Ding J, Harmer DW, Hernandez DG, Johnson JO, Mok K, Ryten M, Trabzuni D, Guerreiro RJ, Orrell RW, Neal J, Murray A, Pearson J, Jansen IE, Sondervan D, Seelaar H, Blake D, Young K, Halliwell N, Callister JB, Toulson G, Richardson A, Gerhard A, Snowden J, Mann D, Neary D, Nalls MA, Peuralinna T, Jansson L, Isoviita VM, Kaivorinne AL, Hölttä-Vuori M, Ikonen E, Sulkava R, Benatar M, Wuu J, Chiò A, Restagno G, Borghero G, Sabatelli M; ITALSGEN Consortium, Heckerman D, Rogaeva E, Zinman L, Rothstein JD, Sendtner M, Drepper C, Eichler EE, Alkan C, Abdullaev Z, Pack SD, Dutra A, Pak E, Hardy J, Singleton A, Williams NM, Heutink P, Pickering-Brown S, Morris HR, Tienari PJ, Traynor BJ. A hexanucleotide repeat expansion in C9ORF72 is the cause of chromosome 9p21-linked ALS-FTD. Neuron. 2011;72:257–68.

Sha S, Takada LT, Rankin KP, Yokoyama JS, Rutherford NJ, Fong JC, Khan B, Karydas A, Baker MC, DeJesus-Hernandez M, Pribadi M, Coppola G, Geschwind DH, Rademakers R, Lee SE, Seeley W, Miller BL, Boxer AL. Frontotemporal dementia due to C9ORF72 mutations: Clinical and imaging features. Neurology. 2012;79(10):1002–11.

Siddique T, Ajroud-Driss S. Familial amyotrophic lateral sclerosis, a historical perspective. Acta Myol. 2011;30(2):117–20.

Swarup V, Julien JP. ALS pathogenesis: recent insights from genetics and mouse models. Prog Neuropsychopharmacol Biol Psychiatry. 2011;35(2):363–9.

Strong MJ, Grace GM, Freedman M, Lomen-Hoerth C, Woolley S, Goldstein LH, Murphy J, Shoesmith C, Rosenfeld J, Leigh PN, Bruijn L, Ince P, Figlewicz D. Consensus criteria for the diagnosis of frontotemporal cognitive and behavioural syndromes in amyotrophic lateral sclerosis. Amyotroph Lateral Scler. 2009;10(3):131–46.

Takada LT, Pimentel MLV, DeJesus-Hernandez M, Fong JC, Yokoyama JS, Karydas A, Thibodeau MP, Rutherford NJ, Baker MC, Lomen-Hoerth C, Rademakers R, Miller BL. Frontotemporal dementia in a Brazilian kindred with the C9ORF72 mutation. Archives of Neurology. 2012;69(9):1149–53.

Uchida A, Sasaguri H, Kimura N, Tajiri M, Ohkubo T, Ono F, Sakaue F, Kanai K, Hirai T, Sano T, Shibuya K, Kobayashi M, Yamamoto M, Yokota S, Kubodera T, Tomori M, Sakaki K, Enomoto M, Hirai Y, Kumagai J, Yasutomi Y, Mochizuki H, Kuwabara S, Uchihara T, Mizusawa H, Yokota T. Non-human primate model of amyotrophic lateral sclerosis with cytoplasmic mislocalization of TDP-43. Brain. 2012;135(Pt 3):833–46.

Wang JW, Brent JR, Tomlinson A, Shneider NA, McCabe BD. The ALS-associated proteins FUS and TDP-43 function together to affect Drosophila locomotion and life span. J Clin Invest. 2011;121(10): 4118–26.

Chapter 6

Related Disorders: Corticobasal Degeneration and Progressive Supranuclear Palsy

OVERVIEW

Corticobasal degeneration (CBD) and progressive supranuclear palsy (PSP) are so strongly linked to each other and to clinical and pathological syndromes of frontotemporal dementia (FTD) that they are commonly considered FTD-spectrum diseases associated with abnormal movement. Additionally, CBD and PSP are characterized by tau pathology and thus are linked at a genetic and molecular level to frontotemporal lobar degeneration (FTLD) neuropathology (Feany & Dickson 1995).

Approximately 50% of patients with the nonfluent/agrammatic variant of primary progressive aphasia (nfvPPA) (Josephs et al. 2006) and many patients with the behavioral variant of FTD (bvFTD) show PSP or CBD changes post mortem (Rankin et al. 2011), while many, if not most, patients with PSP or CBD exhibit cognitive or behavioral deficits early in their illness (Boeve et al. 2003: Bak et al. 2010; Lee et al. 2011; Yatabe et al. 2011). With tau-related neurodegeneration, the basal ganglia and frontal circuitry are both selectively vulnerable (Saper et al. 1987), and this is responsible for the various presentations, such as motor and other behavioral and executive syndromes. As was first noted by Martin Albert, the degeneration of subcortical structures in the midbrain in PSP could lead to a dementia syndrome that he called "subcortical dementia" (Albert et al. 1974).

CORTICOBASAL DEGENERATION

CBD is an uncommon disorder, although its prevalence within the United States remains undetermined. It is rarely diagnosed correctly during life, and there are few disorders in neurology that have caused more confusion for clinicians. As is described in the nomenclature section (Chapter 1), most of the clinical descriptors for what are likely to predict CBD have been wrong. Asymmetric parkinsonian syndromes, myoclonus, visuospatial dysfunction, and apraxia of the upper extremity all represent signs purported to predict CBD, yet none of these findings have either sensitivity or specificity for CBD (Lee et al. 2011). Rather, many of these findings are characteristic of patients with Alzheimer's disease (AD). Most patients with CBD will fall into three categories: nfvPPA, bvFTD, or an executive motor syndrome.

Bradley Boeve introduced the term "corticobasal syndrome" (CBS) when he realized that many of the patients with CBS did not show classical CBD pathology (Boeve et al. 1999). It has only been in the last few years that our field has begun to realize that precisely predicting CBD neuropathology is very difficult, although separating patients with underlying AD has been made possible with amyloid imaging and CSF biomarkers (Rabinovici et al. 2011).

CASE HISTORY

A 68-year-old female started to notice trouble with her right foot. Soon afterward, she began to suffer from unexpected falls. Increasingly, the foot seemed to get stuck when she attempted to move. On several occasions, she complained that the foot moved when she wanted it to rest. While driving her car, she suddenly pushed the accelerator, crashing into a tree in her driveway. After this, she stopped driving. The problem continued to worsen, and she developed similar difficulties with the left foot. The right foot began to cramp and eventually took an inverted and flexed dystonic posture.

Falling became so frequent that she started to require the use of a wheelchair when leaving the home. Although a spinal cord process was suspected, extensive studies of the spinal cord revealed no detectable structural pathology, and CSF showed no evidence for inflammation. Oligoclonal banding was negative, and CSF A-beta and tau were normal.

Subtle difficulties in her right arm followed, and she complained of trouble properly placing her body into a chair. Both legs took a dystonic posture, and the patient complained of pain in the right foot. The pain was partially relieved by injections of botulinum toxin. Subtle problems with organization emerged, and she came to depend on her husband for preparing meals and looking after the family finances. A severe depression was evident, and the patient cried frequently, while dwelling on her future. The mood disorder only partially responded to high doses of antidepressants.

Past medical illnesses were unremarkable, and there was no family history of neurological disorders. A trial with levodopa/carbidopa did not improve any of the patient's motor problems.

On examination, the patient was a frightened appearing woman who was pleasant and cooperative. She frequently cried and beseeched her physicians to find a treatment for her illness. Basic neurological examination was unremarkable except for mildly increased tone in the right leg and dystonic posture of both feet. There was significant apraxia of the legs, and she was unable to move them to command. Occasional myoclonic jerks were evident in her right leg. There was a prominent grasp of the right hand and the hint of a grasp with the left hand. Cognitive testing was normal except for subtle problems with "d" generation. MRI showed marked Rolandic atrophy most severe in the supplementary motor region that was slightly worse on the left than the right. The atrophy spread into the frontal and parietal regions (Figure 6–1).

Her cognitive and motor difficulties worsened. Over the next year, she developed axial parkinsonism, worsening myoclonus and mild dysarthria of speech. Her depression was unremitting and unresponsive to multiple medication regimens. She died at age 72 years after six months in hospice.

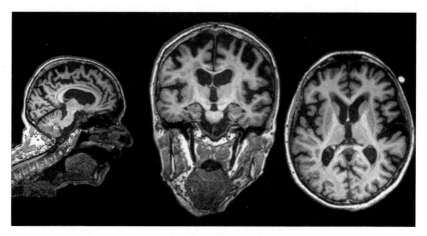

Figure 6–1. MRIs showing marked Rolandic atrophy, most severe in the supplementary motor region, slightly worse on the left than the right. The atrophy spreads into the frontal and parietal regions.

On autopsy, the classical findings of CBD were evident. There was extensive atrophy of the dorsal frontal and parietal regions. On H and E stains, there were multiple astrocytic plaques and coiled tangles within neurons. These aggregates stained positive for 4R tau. A neuropathological diagnosis of CBD was made.

Comment. Approximately one-third of patients with CBD pathology present with motor and executive control deficits, as in the case just described (Lee et al. 2011). While the classical descriptions of CBD have emphasized hand apraxia, more of our patients exhibit leg apraxia, or alien leg (Hu et al. 2005), likely due to the propensity of CBD to attack medial motor systems responsible for the control of leg movement (Lee et al. 2011).

Early in the course of the illness, our patient had features of an alien limb. Her leg was often unable to move to her command and moved without volition: on one occasion her foot involuntarily pressed on the car accelerator, causing an accident. Additionally, she developed a painful right foot dystonia. This dystonia responded well to botulinum toxin injection. Both alien foot and limb dystonia are common in CBD.

Because CBD spreads into dorsolateral and cingulate cortex, brain regions involved with executive control and drive, deficits on frontal-executive function, and marked apathy occur. With this clinical form of CBD, the presence of disinhibition and disordered social regulation is unusual, or emerges late, because ventral frontal and anterior temporal structures are typically spared.

CBD is associated with severe depression, often with preserved insight into the nature of the neurological condition (Geda et al. 2007). Many patients develop a profound sense of sadness and hopelessness, and require aggressive treatment with antidepressants. The depression and sense of despair in CBD is one of the most difficult components of this illness to treat. We have found depression particularly severe in the executive motor subtype of CBD.

CLINICAL FEATURES AND ANATOMY

As was described in Chapter 2, the study of FTD has helped define a clinical syndrome that best predicts CBD pathology. CBD appears to be a relatively uncommon disorder, and a recent study from rural Japan suggested that it had a prevalence of 9 per 100,000, roughly one-half of the prevalence for PSP.

Patients with CBD pathology typically present with one of three main clinical syndromes: bvFTD, nfvPPA, or an executive-motor (EM) disorder where motor abnormalities and abnormalities in executive control emerge together. In most patients with pathology-proven CBD, frontal behavioral or cognitive problems, not parietal or basal ganglia motor findings, dominate early stage disease. Imaging in patients with CBD tends to show atrophy in dorsal prefrontal and perirolandic cortex, striatum, and brainstem, with perirolandic atrophy being the key diagnostic marker (Figure 6–2).

There are still a small number of patients (1 of 18 in the UCSF case series) in whom a

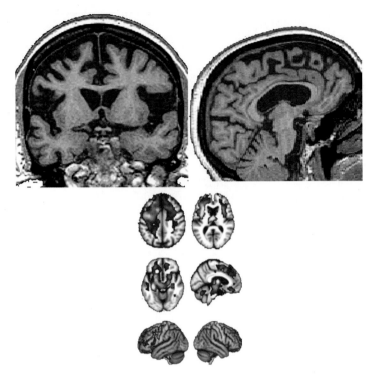

Figure 6–2. MRIs showing typical atrophy pattern seen in CBD, and VBM group analysis of CBD versus healthy controls. (MRI images courtesy of Suzee Lee, MD. VBM images adapted from Lee et al. 2011.)

posterior cortical atrophy syndrome turns out to show CBD neuropathology (Lee et al. 2011). Yet, most patients with posterior cortical atrophy have AD or Lewy body pathology, not CBD. It is still unknown whether or not there

are clinical features that will help to determine those posterior cortical atrophy patients who truly suffer from CBD.

Table 6–1 lists the features that best predict CBD contrasted with those more likely to

Table 6–1 Features That Best Predict Corticobasal Degeneration (CBD) Contrasted with Those More Likely to Predict Alzheimer's Disease (AD)

Clinical Feature	Corticobasal Degeneration	AD with or without Lewy Bodies
Apraxia	Oral-buccal	Ideomotor
Motor onset	Legs (alien foot)	Arm
Type of parkinsonism	Axial rigidity, modest or no response to L-dopa	Limb rigidity, modest response to L-dopa
Cognitive disorder	Frontal-executive	Visuospatial
Memory disturbance	Working memory	Episodic memory
Language disturbance	Nonfluent aphasia	Logopenic aphasia
Type of alien limb	Grasping groping dominant hand or oppositional nondominant hand	Parietal alien limb, upwardly drifting, profound neglect (usually left-sided)
Parietal sensory deficit	First symptom	Emerges later
Visual neglect	Unusual!	Common in AD and DLB
Asymmetric onset	Common	Common
Neuroimaging	Frontally predominant	Parietally predominant

Box 6.1 Diagnostic Criteria for Corticobasal Degeneration (CBD) (Boeve et al. 2003)

I. Core features

I.A. Insidious onset and progressive course
I.B. No identifiable cause (e.g., tumor, infarct)
I.C. Cortical dysfunction as reflected by at least one of the following:
    I.C.1. Focal or asymmetrical ideomotor apraxia
    I.C.2. Alien limb phenomenon
    I.C.3. Cortical sensory loss
    I.C.4. Visual or sensory hemineglect
    I.C.5. Constructional apraxia
    I.C.6. Focal or asymmetric myoclonus
    I.C.7. Apraxia of speech/nonfluent aphasia
I.D. Extrapyramidal dysfunction as reflected by at least one of the following:
    I.D.1. Focal or asymmetrical appendicular rigidity lacking prominent and sustained L-dopa response
    I.D.2. Focal or asymmetrical appendicular dystonia

II. Supportive investigations

II.A. Variable degrees of focal or lateralized cognitive dysfunction, with relative preservation of learning and memory, on neuropsychometric testing
II.B. Focal or asymmetric atrophy on computed tomography or magnetic resonance imaging, typically maximal in parietofrontal cortex
II.C. Focal or asymmetric hypoperfusion on single-photon emission computed tomography and positron emission tomography, typically maximal in parietofrontal cortex, basal ganglia, and/or thalamus

---

predict AD. Hence, current criteria for CBS should be followed with caution as the features of constructional apraxia, cortical sensory loss, visuospatial neglect, focal myoclonus, and focal limb apraxia are not highly specific for CBD neuropathology and often predict AD (Box 6.1).

The clinical progression for the typical CBD subtypes is variable. In our experience, the executive motor and nfvPPA groups survive around 5.6 years from the time of their first symptom, while the bvFTD and posterior cortical patients live closer to 8 years.

GENETIC AND PATHOLOGICAL CORRELATES

There is no currently highly specific genetic marker for CBD although approximately 90%
of Caucasians with CBD carry the H1H1 haplotype of tau (Conrad et al. 1997). By contrast, 70% of Caucasian controls are homozygous for H1. While nearly all Asians are H1H1, it is not yet known whether they are predisposed to CBD relative to Caucasians. The presence of an *ApoE4* allele increases the likelihood of either pure AD or at least comorbid Alzheimer pathology. Patients with *MAPT*, *GRN*, and *C9ORF72* mutations can present with nfvPPA, bvFTD, or an executive motor syndrome, the three prototypical CBD clinical syndromes, although usually a strong family history is present that has triggered the search for a genetic mutation.

Unfortunately there is still no specific marker for CBD, and patients suspected of having CBD can show CBD, AD, PSP, FTLD changes with TDP-43 type A inclusions, or Pick's disease. When frontal atrophy predominates,

CBD is more likely; when brainstem and subcortical atrophy predominate, PSP should be considered. Posterior extension of atrophy into precuneus and temporal-parietal cortex suggests underlying AD pathology.

The patient described in our history showed the classical neuropathological findings of CBD including 4R tau aggregates in neurons and glia and dystrophic neurites with 4R tau that form plaque-like structures within the cerebral cortex.

DIFFERENTIAL DIAGNOSIS

As has been noted, it is difficult to predict underlying CBD neuropathology. In the patient with nfvPPA who develops an alien right hand and dystonia, CBD is likely, although TDP-43 type A is possible. The variability of FTLD-spectrum neuropathologies associated with bvFTD make it hard to predict underlying CBD, but bvFTD patients with underlying CBD neuropathology often have less ventral atrophy than do the other forms of bvFTD, Hence they may be more apathetic with prominent executive loss but show less disinhibition than other bvFTD patients. In our experience, apraxia of the legs in the setting of a neurodegenerative condition is usually a manifestation of CBD and patients with prominent dorsal rolandic atrophy are more likely to show CBD.

Patients with CBS who exhibit asymmetric parkinsonism, visuospatial or naming deficits, hand apraxia, and myoclonus are more likely to show AD neuropathology. When CBS is caused by AD it is often seen in patients with early-age-of-onset disease. While the concept of CBS was valuable when it was first proposed, the value of a defining a clinical syndrome with low likelihood of demonstrating that neuropathology that it is purported to predict is dubious.

Other disorders with parkinsonian features and alpha-synuclein pathology including Parkinson's disease dementia, dementia with Lewy bodies, or multisystem atrophy can be mistaken for CBD. Unlike CBD, most patients with these disorders exhibit rapid eye movement (REM)–behavior disorder. Marked visuospatial deficits are more typical for the synucleinopathies than for CBD. Also, CBD does not typically cause autonomic dysfunction in contrast to the alpha-synucleinopathies.

Patients with prion disease can present with symptoms that suggest a CBD neuropathology, but usually differ clinically because their symptoms have evolved rapidly over months, not years. Additionally, patients with Creutzfeldt-Jakob disease usually exhibit cortical ribboning and basal ganglia hyperintensity on FLAIR and diffusion weighted imaging.

TREATMENT

While traditional treatments for Parkinson's disease have no proven efficacy for CBD, I will often try levodopa/carbidopa. With this therapy, in some patients there is a honeymoon period (usually short) where there is evidence for significant motor response. For patients with nfvPPA, speech therapy is valuable and usually appreciated greatly by the patient and family. Additionally, physical therapy will often help patients make small gains in gait and other motor functions and should be tried in nearly all patients. Because mood disorders are common in these patients, aggressive treatment with antidepressants should be tried.

CBD has no FDA-approved treatment, but there are aggressive efforts to find therapies for conditions where there are pathological aggregates of tau. Because PSP is more common, most of the clinical trials for 4R tau have been focused around PSP. If these therapies prove effective for PSP, it is likely that they will eventually find approval for CBD.

PROGRESSIVE SUPRANUCLEAR PALSY

Steele, Richardson, and Olszewski first described PSP in 1964 (Steele et al. 1964). The initial features of these patients include axial rigidity, vertical gaze palsy, frequent falls, pseudobulbar affect, frontal executive disabilities, and neuropsychiatric disturbances including depression, anxiety, and paranoia. Not initially noted in the early descriptions of PSP, it is now clear that many patients present with asymmetric frontal syndromes and can be diagnosed with nfvPPA or bvFTD. The current prediction for its prevalence is around 5 to 7 versus 18 per 100,000 (Litvan et al. 1996; Osaki et al. 2011).

CASE HISTORY

A wife brought her husband, a previously successful family practitioner, for assessment. In retrospect, the wife believed that his illness may have started around the time of her husband's retirement at age 65, when he became abnormally fatigued and began to sleep for 2-hour periods during the day. At age 68, the patient invested with a fraudulent company that he found on the Internet, and he lost $200,000 of his savings. Soon afterward, his wife had to take away his computer to prevent him from buying expensive items that he didn't need. Around the same time, he decided that he no longer needed to pay taxes, and he fired his accountant. Mild irritability emerged. The patient lost interest in most of his hobbies and stopped going out with friends.

During his 69th year, the patient's golf score handicap worsened by 10 points although he continued to play golf every day. He complained of difficulty reading. Several visits to the optometrist and replacing the lenses in his glasses did not improve his ability to read. Around the time of his visit he suffered a single fall on the golf course, failing to see a small tree stump over which he inadvertently tripped.

On examination the patient was pleasant but slow and had a prominent stare and hypererect posture. There was a mild dysarthria. He complained to the neurology team that there was no need for an evaluation, and he denied any cognitive or motor problems.

Cranial nerve examination revealed square wave jerks of the eyes, up and down gaze was decreased in movement by approximately 30 degrees. Both up and down gaze were markedly slowed, while there was only mild slowing of normal lateral gaze. Motor examination revealed mild axial rigidity with normal tone in the arms. His legs showed mildly increased tone. There was no tremor. Gait was hypererect and he could not perform tandem walk without falling.

MMSE was 30. Digit span was 6 forward and 3 backward. His verbal and visual memory were both normal, as were naming and visuospatial skills. Executive control was diminished, and he performed slowly on an alternating sequence task and made three errors. His "d" generation was six with three repetitions and three rule violations. Animal generation was 11. Design generation was three with six rule violations and two perseverations. On the antisaccade task, he made multiple incorrect gaze responses toward the stimulus but properly self-corrected (Figure 6–3).

His MRI scan revealed marked dorsal midbrain atrophy and a hummingbird sign (Figure 6–4). There was mild atrophy of the frontal regions bilaterally.

Over the next 2 years the patient's apathy greatly increased, and he often slept up to 16 hours a day. He played solitaire at the computer. Falls became prominent, but he was largely unaware of his motor difficulties. This led him to fall nearly every day, despite efforts by the family to get him to request help when he attempted to walk. On several occasions he fell forward without protecting his face and

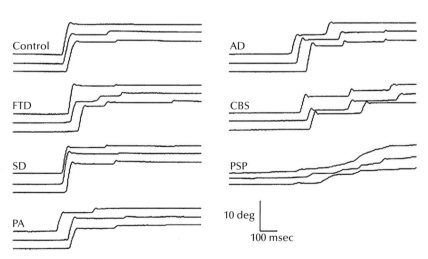

Figure 6–3. Upward saccade examples. Eye position versus time traces showing three representative, successive 10° upward saccades in a control subject and a patient from each of the diagnostic groups. (Boxer et al. 2008.)

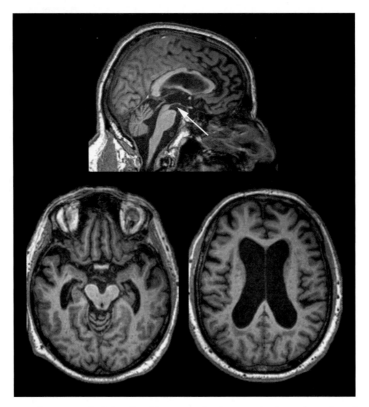

Figure 6–4. MRI scans showing marked dorsal midbrain atrophy, hummingbird sign (arrow), and mild atrophy of the frontal regions bilaterally.

actually suffered fractures of the ribs, the left radius, and mandible associated with three different falls. Frequent bouts of laughter and crying emerged that were diagnosed as pseudobulbar affect. At age 72 the patient died after falling onto his head on the cement while on a walk with his caregiver.

Autopsy revealed a large subdural hematoma with central herniation. The midbrain had dorsal atrophy. On microscopic study there were frequent globose tangles within neurons in frontal cortex, hippocampus, and midbrain tectum. Within these regions neurofibrillary tangles were visible. Additionally, thorny astrocytes were frequent in the subpial and subependymal layers of the frontal cortex. These inclusions stained positively for tau.

Comment. This elderly gentleman's illness began with fatigue. The fatigue was followed by poor decision-making and new deficits in executive control. Approximately one year later he had problems with ocular motility that interfered with his ability to read. As is often the case, the difficulty with reading that is due to the gaze disturbance of PSP was misdiagnosed as being caused by presbyopia. Soon afterward he suffered from a single fall.

Like many patients with PSP, our patient did not truly meet the probable PSP category of the National Institute of Neurological Disorders and Stroke (NINDS) research criteria, because there were not falls in the first year. While some patients begin with frequent falls in the first two years of the illness, many others like our patient have a cognitive or psychiatric syndrome that precedes the falls by years or even decades.

On neuropsychological testing, he showed classical findings of PSP with marked deficits in working memory (digit span backward of 3), inhibition (perseverative response on the antisaccade test and the design fluency task), and generation (low number of "d" words and designs), and inability to perform alternating sequences. Other cognitive domains including language and visuospatial skills were relatively spared, as is often the case in patients with mild to moderate PSP.

The parkinsonian features of the patient were not the typical pattern of idiopathic Parkinson's disease, as he did not have a tremor, cogwheel rigidity, or a stooped gait. There was no REM behavior syndrome as is seen in the synucleinopathies

(Dugger et al. 2012). The stare, square wave jerks, diminished vertical saccades, and axial but not limb rigidity on the neurological examination confirmed a diagnosis of PSP.

CLINICAL FEATURES AND ANATOMY

In Steele and colleagues' original description of PSP, they emphasized falls, supranuclear palsy, cognitive impairment, and swallowing disturbance. Often, falling is a prominent early symptom and any middle-aged to elderly patient with frequent unexplained falls should be evaluated for PSP (Box 6.2). Falls in these patients are due to a complex set of mechanisms including the vertical gaze disturbance, postural instability, motor rigidity and slowness, and poor insight into the gait instability. This constellation of problems leads to frequent, and sometimes very dangerous, unprotected falls with the patient landing awkwardly on their face or

---

Box 6.2 Diagnostic Criteria for Progressive Supranuclear Palsy (PSP) (Litvan et al. 1996)

III. Inclusion criteria

III.A. Possible: Gradually progressive disorder

III.B. Onset at age 40 or later

III.C. Either vertical (upward or downward gaze) supranuclear palsy OR both slowing of vertical saccades and prominent postural instability with falls in the first year of disease onset

III.D. No evidence of other diseases that could explain the foregoing features, as indicated by mandatory exclusion criteria

III.E. Probable: Vertical (upward or downward gaze) supranuclear palsy and prominent postural instability with falls in the first year of disease onset

III.F. Definite: Clinically probable or possible PSP and histopathologic evidence of typical PSP

IV. Exclusion criteria

IV.A. Possible: Gradually progressive disorder

IV.B. Onset at age 40 or later

IV.C. Either vertical (upward or downward gaze) supranuclear palsy OR both slowing of vertical saccades and prominent postural instability with falls in the first year of disease onset

IV.D. No evidence of other diseases that could explain the foregoing features, as indicated by mandatory exclusion criteria

IV.E. Probable: Vertical (upward or downward gaze) supranuclear palsy and prominent postural instability with falls in the first year of disease onset

IV.F. Definite: Clinically probable or possible PSP and histopathologic evidence of typical PSP

V. Supportive criteria

V.A. Symmetric akinesia or rigidity, proximal more than distal

V.B. Abnormal neck posture, especially retrocollis

V.C. Poor or absent response of parkinsonism to levodopa therapy

V.D. Early dysphagia and dysarthria

V.E. Early onset of cognitive impairment including at least two of the following: apathy, impairment in abstract thought, decreased verbal fluency, utilization or imitation behavior, or frontal release signs

back. We had one patient who insisted on running despite the fact that she fell nearly every time that she ran.

Marty Albert called PSP a subcortical dementia (Albert et al. 1974), emphasizing that the frontal lobes were disconnected from midbrain. Many patients begin with a frontal lobe syndrome where there are profound behavioral or executive changes due to disconnection of the frontal lobes from the basal ganglia. Additionally, in some cases of PSP the tau neuropathology spreads to the frontal regions, amplifying the frontal aspects of the presentation (Tsuboi et al. 2005). There are some patients who exhibit an nfvPPA syndrome as the first manifestation of their illness. This aphasia can often be distinguished from other causes for nfvPPA by the presence of a prominent dysarthria.

The vertical eye movement disturbance of PSP leads to difficulty with tracking words, but is often misunderstood to be a primary optical problem. Eye movement abnormalities can be the first manifestation of PSP, and some patients initially complain of difficulty with reading, leading to assessments by optometrists or ophthalmologists. Square-wave jerks and slowing of vertical saccades are early signs of PSP, and formal laboratory testing with oculography can help to seal the diagnosis of PSP (Boxer et al. 2012). Oculography demonstrates slowing, and sometimes restriction, of vertical more than horizontal gaze (Garbutt et al. 2008). Another eye movement symptom commonly seen in PSP is eyelid apraxia, and in some patients, the eyelids are involuntarily closed (Zadikoff et al. 2005). When this symptom is severe and persistent patients can spend most of the time with their eyes forced closed.

Less well understood are the psychiatric and sleep problems associated with PSP. The brainstem and cerebellum are extensively injured in PSP, and this can predispose to a protean range of symptoms from depression (Kim et al. 2009), euphoria, inappropriate risk-taking, anxiety, and addictive behaviors (Rankin et al. 2011). There can be abnormalities in getting to sleep and staying awake (Sixel-Döring et al. 2009), and these symptoms can have significant affects on the patient's quality of life.

David Williams from Australia has proposed dividing PSP syndromes into two major subtypes. For the first, which he calls "Richardson's syndrome" (RS), the typical PSP features are present including falls, cognitive dysfunction, supranuclear gaze palsy, abnormal saccadic/pursuit movements, and postural instability. This accounts for more than 50% of all PSP. The second subtype he calls "PSP-parkinsonism" (PSP-P) accounts for approximately one-third of all PSP. These individuals tend to present with atypical parkinsonian features that include asymmetric onset, tremor, bradykinesia, extra-axial dystonia and response to levodopa. Williams suggests that around 14% of cases are unclassifiable (Williams et al. 2005).

GENETIC AND PATHOLOGICAL CORRELATES

Like CBD, PSP is strongly linked to the H1H1 haplotype (Conrad et al. 1997; Webb et al. 2008), and approximately 90% of Caucasian patients carry this polymorphism, compared to approximately 70% of Caucasians without PSP. This haplotype seems to increase the production of 4R tau, possibly explaining its association with PSP.

The A152T genetic haplotype is an uncommon polymorphism in tau that may predispose someone to PSP, and some patients with *MAPT* mutations present with PSP-like or CBS-like phenotypes. Approximately 0.3% of healthy elderly controls carry this polymorphism, while close to 1% of FTD-spectrum patients are A152T carriers. In a series of eight individuals from the University of California, San Francisco (UCSF), two had PSP clinically, two others were suspected of CBD, one was diagnosed with nfvPPA, and another was diagnosed with bvFTD. Two had AD. The typical duration of illness for patients with PSP is around 4 years from the time of diagnosis to death.

Additionally, in a large genome-wide association study, polymorphisms in three genes, *STX6*, *EIF2AK3*, and *MOBP*, were associated with increased susceptibility to PSP. These genes encode proteins for vesicle-membrane fusion at the Golgi-endosomal interface, are involved with the endoplasmic reticulum unfolded protein response, and generate a myelin structural component (Höglinger et al. 2011). Further genetic studies are likely to find new genes associated with increased or decreased risk for PSP and CBD.

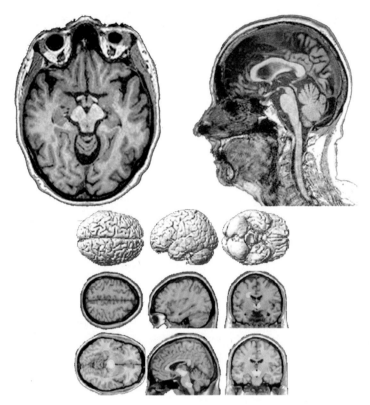

Figure 6–5. MRIs showing typical atrophy pattern seen in PSP, and VBM group analysis of PSP versus healthy controls. (MRI images courtesy of Adam Boxer, MD, PhD, and Lisa Voltarelli. VBM images adapted from Boxer et al. 2006.)

PSP is associated with brain atrophy (Massey et al. 2012) and grossly upon autopsy, patients with PSP show significant atrophy of the midbrain, basal ganglia, pons, and cerebellum (Figure 6–5). The pedunculopontine nucleus shows extensive neuronal loss and neurofibrillary tangles. The frontal lobes are variably involved. At a pathological level, PSP is associated with extensive gliosis and 4R tau aggregates that form globose-shaped tangles within the neuron and tufted aggregates with astrocytes.

DIFFERENTIAL DIAGNOSIS

When the diagnosis is wrong, the most common disease that is seen rather than PSP is CBD, another 4R tauopathy, and both CBD and PSP are associated with akinetic rigid forms of parkinsonism and gait disturbance. Furthermore, both nfvPPA and bvFTD can be the clinical manifestation of underlying neurodegeneration due to PSP or CBD. Early abnormalities

in vertical gaze strongly argue for PSP, while horizontal gaze abnormalities are more typical for CBD. While falls are more common in PSP, a subgroup of CBD patients develop problems with leg movement and fall in the early stages of their illness (Lee et al. 2011). Although some have suggested that CBD is more likely to be asymmetrical than PSP, asymmetry is not reliable for differentiating these two conditions (Lee et al. 2011). There are patients with the classical ophthalmoplegia of PSP who show CBD changes at autopsy, and patients with prominent falls and eye movement abnormalities who have CBD at neuropathology.

While PSP is a major cause for falls, cerebrovascular disease, Parkinson's disease, and peripheral nervous system problems are all causes of falling that are unrelated to PSP. The parkinsonian features of PSP are distinctive from Parkinson's disease because of the prominent axial rigidity, lack of tremor, and relative sparing of the arms. Yet, PSP patients are frequently misdiagnosed with Parkinson's disease.

Finally, it is important to remember that uncommon conditions including midbrain tumors, Whipple's disease, Gaucher's disease, Niemann-Pick-C, and mitochondrial disorders can sometimes cause prominent vertical gaze abnormalities and should be considered in any patient in whom PSP is diagnosed. Unlike PSP, Whipple's disease usually, but not always, presents with weight loss, diarrhea, and joint pain and neurologically is associated with oculomasticatory myorhythmia. Gaucher's and Niemann-Pick C disease often show hepatosplenomegaly and sometimes anemia is present.

TREATMENT

Treatment of PSP has proven to be difficult, and there are no FDA-approved therapies for this condition. While a robust and sustaining response to Sinemet is unusual with PSP, in some patients, dopamine repletion will have subtle effects on movement. Eyelid apraxia due to PSP will sometimes respond to Sinemet. Depression is common in these patients and they should be aggressively treated with antidepressants if a mood disorder emerges. Treatment of eyelid apraxia is perplexing, and while some patients improve with Sinemet, others get worse. The excessive sleep seen with PSP is difficult to control, although there are some patients in whom getting to sleep is a serious problem. Occasionally, the cautious treatment with a short-acting benzodiazepine or with a serotonin-modifying compound (Desyrel) will help with sleep without causing other side effects such as falling or excessive somnolence.

Physical therapy and exercise are valuable for maximizing motor function. Attention to the patient's tendency to fall or aspirate is required, because the patient is often unaware that he or she suffers from these problems. The eye of an occupational therapist will often help to make a house safer and both protect the patient from falling and diminish the impact of falls when they occur. Eating will need to be watched carefully. Swallowing studies help to predict the likelihood that a patient will aspirate. Thickening liquids and cutting solids into small pieces can diminish the likelihood of serious aspiration.

CBD AND PSP: CURRENT STATE AND RESEARCH ADVANCES

Clinical Dilemmas

While nearly all of the patients diagnosed with the PSP clinical syndrome at our center show PSP at neuropathology, CBD is still difficult to predict from the clinical syndrome. Unfortunately for both conditions, there are still many patients who are missed in the early stages of the illness when subtle frontal executive deficits or neuropsychiatric and behavior syndromes are present. Hopefully better markers for 4R tauopathies will emerge in the coming years that will allow recognition of both CBD and PSP at a time when the most effective therapies can be instituted.

While CSF markers are not yet able to predict either CBD or PSP, it seems likely that better CSF markers will emerge for these pure 4R tauopathies in the coming years. As this book is being written, there are a variety of groups working to develop ligands for tau that can be used to image patients with dementia. If these agents prove to be sensitive and specific, it will be possible to separate PSP and CBD from other forms of dementia where tau is not present and to follow the effectiveness of treatments for PSP and CBD (and other tauopathies).

New Discoveries on the Pathogenesis of CBD, PSP, and other Tauopathies

There is increasing evidence that tau spreads in a prion-like fashion from one cell to the next. Work by Clavaguera demonstrates that using transgenic mice, tau aggregates are visible 1 year after inoculation (Clavaguera et al. 2009). Similarly, in work from Marc Diamond's laboratory, an aggregated segment of tau initiated tau prion formation after it was introduced into cultured cells (Kfoury et al. 2012). In a recent review of prion-like mechanisms in neurodegeneration, Stanley Prusiner (Prusiner 2012) also suggested that the tauopathies associated with traumatic brain injury could spread via a prion-like mechanism and hypothesizes that "some of the variations in the clinical presentations of the tauopathies may be due to different prion strains, which represent distinct conformations."

Neuroimaging

Recent work spearheaded by William Seeley at UCSF has demonstrated the ability of resting state fMRI to both define the networks that are attacked by different neurodegenerative conditions and the mechanism for their spread. In work from Dr. Seeley's laboratory led by Raquel Gardner, the authors demonstrated diminished connectivity in dorsal midbrain and other structures in the brainstem, cerebellum, diencephalon, and basal ganglia. They suggested that the major abnormality involved disruption of corticosubcortical and cortical-brainstem circuits. Clinical severity correlated with severity of network disruption (personal communication).

This work offers great potential for the early diagnosis of PSP and differential diagnosis of this condition. Additionally, if this approach proves robust, there should be an opportunity to follow the progression of PSP for clinical trials with network connectivity mapping to determine the efficacy of specific compounds.

Additionally, a recent neuroimaging study by Zhou and colleagues (Zhou et al. 2012) in the Seeley laboratory using similar techniques has demonstrated that neurodegenerative disorders appear to spread along specific networks in a prion-like manner. This finding supports recent work by Marc Diamond at Washington University and others including Michelle Goedert (Goedert et al. 2010) that point to a prion-like spread by tau from cell to cell with tauopathies.

Hence, the combination of neuroimaging and basic biological approaches (see "Basic Biological Advances," below) are finding better ways to understand the pathogenesis of tauopathies while opening up new ways to follow progression and intervene with therapies. For example, targeting an intracellular protein like tau seemed daunting until the realization was made that tau sits in the synapse between neurons during the time of transmission. This makes antibody approaches far more appealing.

investigators have focused on animal models (worms, zebrafish, mice), tau spread, drug discovery, autophagy, clinical diagnosis and biomarkers, and induced pluripotent stem cells (iPSCs) to neurons, particularly as these animal models reflect on the A152T genetic polymorphism.

This group has helped to demonstrate the role of A152T in neurodegeneration. Transgenic mice with this mutation show a neurodegenerative phenotype (personal communication from Lennart Mucke and Eva and Eckhardt Mandelkow). Additionally, iPSCs have been generated from skin cells of A152T gene carriers. When iPSCs with the heterozygous mutation (152A/T) are differentiated into neurons, there is a major neurodegenerative phenotype. Furthermore, when a double mutation (152T/T) is created in those cells, the neurodegeneration is more severe, while when the mutation is corrected (152A/A) the neurodegenerative phenotype disappears (Yadong Huang, personal communication) (Figure 6–6).

Stan Prusiner has focused on a drug discovery effort to find compounds that lower tau, while Marc Diamond has looked for anti-tau antibodies. Tim Miller has focused the anti-oligonucleotide approach to lowering tau in animal models with the hope that this can be used in human tauopathies.

Li Gan from UCSF has demonstrated that tau acetylation may be critical for tau-related neurodegeneration (Min et al. 2010) (Figure 6–7). Ana Maria Cuervo and David Rubinzstein are exploring the use of autophagy compounds as a way to increase intracellular tau clearance (Figure 6–8). Schaeffer and colleagues (Schaeffer et al. 2012) have found that stimulating autophagy increases the clearance of tau in a mouse model, increasing the hope for this therapeutic approach in PSP and CBD.

This highly targeted effort is yielding novel insights into tau-related neurodegeneration and hopes to bring new treatments for tau into the clinic over the next few years.

Basic Biological Advances

A group of dedicated investigators supported by the Rainwater family have organized a collaborative network designed to find treatments for PSP and related tauopathies. The

Clinical Trials for Tauopathies

In recent years there has been a comprehensive effort to develop a clinical trials infrastructure for the treatment of tauopathies. While initial efforts attempted to include all of the

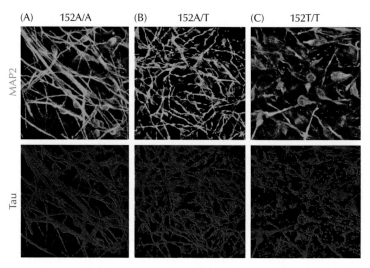

Figure 6–6. When a double mutation (*152T/T*) is created in neurons from induced pluripotent stem cells, the neurodegeneration is more severe, while when the mutation is corrected (*152A/A*) the neurodegenerative phenotype disappears.

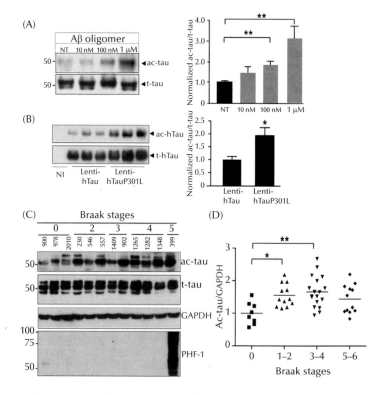

Figure 6–7. Tau acetylation is elevated under pathological conditions. (**A**) Tau acetylation was increased by low levels of Aβ oligomers in primary cortical neurons (DIV = 11). n = 5 from 3 experiments. °°, P = 0.003 (one-way ANOVA and Tukey-Kramer posthoc test). (**B**) Tau acetylation was associated with familial *MAPT* mutations in primary neurons (DIV = 13). Ac-tau/t-tau levels in neurons infected with Lenti-hTauwt were set as 1. n = 9 from three experiments. °, P = 0.013 (unpaired t test). (**C**) Representative western blots showing levels of ac-tau, t-tau, and hyperphosphorylated tau in human brains (Bm-22, superior temporal gyrus) at different Braak stages (0–5). (**D**) Ac-tau levels were elevated in patients with mild (Braak stages 1–2) to moderate (Braak stages 3–4) levels of tau pathology. n = 8–18 cases/Braak range. °, P < 0.05; °°, P < 0.01, one-way ANOVA Tukey-Kramer posthoc analyses. Values are means±SEM (A, B, D).

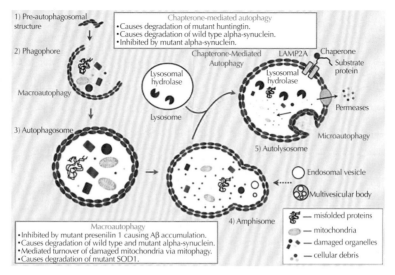

Figure 6–8. The autophagic process involves (1) Formation of pre-autophagosomal structures—a membrane source provides lipid bilayers for formation of a phagophore by a process known as "nucleation." (2) Phagophore/Isolation membrane formation—here a double membranous phagophore or isolation membrane derived from pre-autophagosomal structures sequester portions of cytosol, including organelles that leads to (3) the formation of autophagosomes. (4) Maturation phase—the completed autophagosomes during this step undergo maturation, which involves steps such as fusion with multivesicular bodies or endosomes to form an amphisome. (5) Docking and fusion—during this step the inner membrane compartment fuses with a lysosome, and its contents are degraded by lysosomal hydrolases. The three major forms of autophagy prevalent among common neurodegenerative disorders are macroautophagy, microautophagy, and chaperone-mediated autophagy (see text for the detailed description of the three types of autophagy and how they are associated with pathogenesis of common neurodegenerative disorders). (Banerjee et al. 2010.)

tauopathies ranging from PSP to CBD, tau mutations, and Pick's disease in a single trial, it quickly became clear that the clinical variability of these disorders prevented their inclusion under one umbrella. bvFTD due to CBD or Pick's disease is slower than nfvPPA or the executive motor syndrome of CBD. PSP has less distinctive atrophy than CBD or Pick's disease, impeding the possibility of using neuroimaging as a biomarker for these distinctive disorders. Finally, only the PSP clinical syndrome can predict a tauopathy, and PSP has a higher prevalence than the other tauopathies.

For these reasons, PSP has proven to be the most attractive target for clinical trials. Several trials for PSP have proven negative. GSK inhibitors including lithium (too toxic) and nypta (lack of efficacy) were negative. More recently, Dr. Adam Boxer from UCSF organized a large and cohesive clinical trials network for PSP and completed enrollment of more than 300 patients using NAP (davunetide), an eight-amino-acid peptide derived from activity-dependent neuroprotective protein (ADNP) (Gozes 2011). This compound was discovered and brought into clinical trials by Ilana Gozes at Tel Aviv University. Sadly, this compound did not show efficacy.

Other tau modifying trials are likely in the coming years and will likely include efforts to stabilize tau, prevent tau acetylation or phosphorylation, or clear tau from the brain with either antibodies or with autophagy-drive compounds.

REFERENCES

Albert ML, Feldman RG, Willis AL. The "subcortical dementia" of progressive supranuclear palsy. J Neurol Neurosurg Psychiatry. 1974;37(2):121–30.

Bak TH, Crawford LM, Berrios G, Hodges JR. Behavioural symptoms in progressive supranuclear palsy and frontotemporal dementia. J Neurol Neurosurg Psychiatry. 2010;81(9):1057–9.

Banerjee R, Beal MF, Thomas B. Autophagy in neurodegenerative disorders: pathogenic roles and therapeutic implications. Trends Neurosci. 2010;33:541–9.

Boeve BF, Lang AE, Litvan I. Corticobasal degeneration and its relationship to progressive supranuclear palsy and frontotemporal dementia. Ann Neurol. 2003;54 Suppl 5:S15–9.

Boeve BF, Maraganore DM, Parisi JE, Ahlskog JE, Graff-Radford N, Caselli RJ, Dickson DW, Kokmen E, Petersen RC. Pathologic heterogeneity in clinically diagnosed corticobasal degeneration. Neurology. 1999;53(4):795–800.

Boxer AL, Garbutt S, Seeley WW, Jafari A, Heuer HW, Mirsky J, Hellmuth J, Trojanowski JQ, Huang E, DeArmond S, Neuhaus J, Miller BL. Saccade abnormalities in autopsy-confirmed frontotemporal lobar degeneration and Alzheimer disease. Arch Neurol. 2012;69:509–17.

Boxer AL, Geschwind MD, Belfor N, Gorno-Tempini ML, Schauer GF, Miller BL, Weiner MW, Rosen HJ. Patterns of brain atrophy that differentiate corticobasal degeneration syndrome from progressive supranuclear palsy. Arch Neurol. 2006;63:81–6.

Clavaguera F, Bolmont T, Crowther RA, Abramowski D, Frank S, Probst A, Fraser G, Stalder AK, Beibel M, Staufenbiel M, Jucker M, Goedert M, Tolnay M. Transmission and spreading of tauopathy in transgenic mouse brain. Nat Cell Biol. 2009;11:909–13.

Conrad C, Andreadis A, Trojanowski JQ, Dickson DW, Kang D, Chen X, Wiederholt W, Hansen L, Masliah E, Thal LJ, Katzman R, Xia Y, Saitoh T. Genetic evidence for the involvement of tau in progressive supranuclear palsy. Ann Neurol. 1997;41(2):277–81.

Dugger BN, Boeve BF, Murray ME, Parisi JE, Fujishiro H, Dickson DW, Ferman TJ. Rapid eye movement sleep behavior disorder and subtypes in autopsy-confirmed dementia with Lewy bodies. Mov Disord. 2012;27(1):72–8.

Feany MB, Dickson DW. Widespread cytoskeletal pathology characterizes corticobasal degeneration. Am J Pathol. 1995;146:1388–96.

Garbutt S, Matlin A, Hellmuth J, Schenk AK, Johnson JK, Rosen H, Dean D, Kramer J, Neuhaus J, Miller BL, Lisberger SG, Boxer AL. Oculomotor function in frontotemporal lobar degeneration, related disorders and Alzheimer's disease. Brain. 2008;131:1268–81.

Geda YE, Boeve BF, Negash S, Graff-Radford NR, Knopman DS, Parisi JE, Dickson DW, Petersen RC. Neuropsychiatric features in 36 pathologically confirmed cases of corticobasal degeneration. J Neuropsychiatry Clin Neurosci. 2007;19(1):77–80.

Goedert M, Clavaguera F, Tolnay M. The propagation of prion-like protein inclusions in neurodegenerative diseases. Trends Neurosci. 2010;33:317–25.

Gozes I. NAP (davunetide) provides functional and structural neuroprotection. Curr Pharm Des. 2011;17:1040–4.

Höglinger GU, Melhem NM, Dickson DW, Sleiman PM, Wang LS, Klei L, Rademakers R, de Silva R, Litvan I, Riley DE, van Swieten JC, Heutink P, Wszolek ZK, Uitti RJ, Vandrovcova J, Hurtig HI, Gross RG, Maetzler W, Goldwurm S, Tolosa E, Borroni B, Pastor P; PSP Genetics Study Group, Cantwell LB, Han MR, Dillman A, van der Brug MP, Gibbs JR, Cookson MR, Hernandez DG, Singleton AB, Farrer MJ, Yu CE, Golbe LI, Revesz T, Hardy J, Lees AJ, Devlin B, Hakonarson H, Müller U, Schellenberg GD. Identification of common variants influencing risk of the tauopathy progressive supranuclear palsy. Nat Genet. 2011;43:699–705.

Hu WT, Josephs KA, Ahlskog JE, Shin C, Boeve BF, Witte RJ. MRI correlates of alien leg-like phenomenon in corticobasal degeneration. Mov Disord. 2005; 20(7):870–3.

Josephs KA, Duffy JR, Strand EA, Whitwell JL, Layton KF, Parisi JE, Hauser MF, Witte RJ, Boeve BF, Knopman DS, Dickson DW, Jack CR Jr, Petersen RC. Clinicopathological and imaging correlates of progressive aphasia and apraxia of speech. Brain. 2006; 129 (Pt 6):1385–98.

Kfoury N, Holmes BB, Jiang H, Holtzman DM, Diamond ML. Trans-cellular propagation of tau aggregation by fibrillar species. J Biol Chem. 2012;287:19440–51.

Kim WH, Lee YS, Jung SH, Choi HJ, Lee MJ, Kang MH, Kim CE, Lee JS, Bae JN. Major depressive disorder preceding the onset of progressive supranuclear palsy. Psychiatry Investig. 2009;6:112–4.

Lee SE, Rabinovici GD, Mayo MC, Wilson SM, Seeley WW, DeArmond SJ, Huang EJ, Trojanowski JQ, Growdon ME, Jang JY, Sidhu M, See TM, Karydas AM, Gorno-Tempini ML, Boxer AL, Weiner MW, Geschwind MD, Rankin KP, Miller BL. Clinicopathological correlations in corticobasal degeneration. Ann Neurol. 2011;70:327–40.

Litvan I, Mangone CA, McKee A, Verny M, Parsa A, Jellinger K, D'Olhaberriague L, Chaudhuri KR, Pearce RK. Natural history of progressive supranuclear palsy (Steele-Richardson-Olszewski syndrome) and clinical predictors of survival: a clinicopathological study. J Neurol Neurosurg Psychiatry. 1996;60:615–20.

Massey LA, Micallef C, Paviour DC, O'Sullivan SS, Ling H, Williams DR, Kallis C, Holton JL, Revesz T, Burn DJ, Yousry T, Lees AJ, Fox NC, Jäger HR. Conventional magnetic resonance imaging in confirmed progressive supranuclear palsy and multiple system atrophy. Mov Disord. 2012;27(14):1754–62.

Min SW, Cho SH, Zhou Y, Schroeder S, Seeley SS, Huang EJ, Shen Y, Masliah E, Alt F, Mukherjee C, Meyers D, Cole PA, Ott M, Gan L. Acetylation of tau inhibits its degradation and contributes to tauopathy. Neuron. 2010;67:953–66.

Osaki Y, Morita Y, Kuwahara T, Miyano I, Doi Y. Prevalence of Parkinson's disease and atypical parkinsonian syndromes in a rural Japanese district. Acta Neurol Scand. 2011;124(3):182–7.

Prusiner SB. A unifying role for prions in neurodegenerative disorders. Science. 2012;336:1511–3.

Rabinovici GD, Rosen HJ, Alkalay A, Kornak J, Furst AJ, Agarwal N, Mormino EC, O'Neil JP, Janabi M, Karydas A, Growdon ME, Jang JY, Huang EJ, Dearmond SJ, Trojanowski JQ, Grinberg LT, Gorno-Tempini ML, Seeley WW, Miller BL, Jagust WJ. Amyloid vs FDG-PET in the differential diagnosis of AD and FTLD. Neurology. 2011;77:2034–42.

Rankin KP, Mayo MC, Seeley WW, Lee S, Rabinovici G, Gorno-Tempini ML, Boxer AL, Weiner MW, Trojanowski JQ, DeArmond SJ, Miller BL. Behavioral variant frontotemporal dementia with corticobasal degeneration pathology: phenotypic comparison to bvFTD with Pick's disease. J Mol Neurosci. 2011;45:595–604.

Saper CB, Wainer BH, German DC. Axonal and transneuronal transport in the transmission of neurological disease: potential role in system degenerations, including Alzheimer's disease. Neuroscience. 1987;23(2):389–98.

Schaeffer V, Lavenir I, Ozcelik S, Tolnay M, Winkler DT, Goedert M. Stimulation of autophagy reduces neurodegeneration in a mouse model of human tauopathy. Brain. 2012;135(Pt 7):2169–7.

Sixel-Döring F, Schweitzer M, Mollenhauer B, Trenkwalder C. Polysomnographic findings, video-based sleep analysis and sleep perception in progressive supranuclear palsy. Sleep Med. 2009;10:407–15.

Steele JC, Richardson JC, Olszewski J. Progressive supranuclear palsy: A heterogeneous degeneration involving the brain stem, basal ganglia and cerebellum with vertical gaze and pseudobulbar palsy, nuchal dystonia and dementia. Arch Neurol. 1964;10:333–59.

Tsuboi Y, Josephs KA, Boeve BF, Litvan I, Caselli RJ, Caviness JN, Uitti RJ, Bott AD, Dickson DW. Increased tau burden in the cortices of progressive supranuclear palsy presenting with corticobasal syndrome. Mov Disord. 2005;20(8):982–8.

Webb A, Miller B, Bonasera S, Boxer A, Karydas A, Wilhelmsen KC. Role of the tau gene region chromosome inversion in progressive supranuclear palsy, corticobasal degeneration, and related disorders. Arch Neurol. 2008;65(11):1473–8.

Williams DR, de Silva R, Paviour DC, Pittman A, Watt HC, Kilford L, Holton JL, Revesz T, Lees AJ. Characteristics of two clinical phenotypes in pathologically proven progressive supranuclear palsy: Richardson's syndrome and PSP-parkinsonism. Brain. 2005;128:1247–58.

Yatabe Y, Hashimoto M, Kaneda K, Honda K, Ogawa Y, Yuuki S, Matsuzaki S, Tuyuguchi A, Kashiwagi H, Ikeda M. Neuropsychiatric symptoms of progressive palsy in a dementia clinic. Psychogeriatrics. 2011;11:54–9.

Zadikoff C, Lang AE. Apraxia in movement disorders. Brain. 2005;128(Pt 7):1480–97.

Zhou J, Gennatas ED, Kramer JH, Miller BL, Seeley WW. Predicting regional neurodegeneration from the healthy brain functional connectome. Neuron. 2012;73:1216–27.

Chapter 7

A Primer of FTLD Neuropathology

GENERAL FEATURES

"Frontotemporal lobar degeneration" (FTLD) is a pathological umbrella term encompassing several neuropathological entities characterized by superficial cortical microvacuolation accompanied by severe gliosis and neuronal loss. While the atrophy, neuronal loss, gliosis, and microvacuolization are nonspecific, the neuronal and glial aggregates are critical for understanding the pathological mechanism for these differing forms of FTLD. FTLD has its own set of unique pathological characteristics that help to define this increasingly diverse set of disorders (Mackenzie et al. 2011).

Additionally, frontotemporal gliosis, selective vulnerability of von Economo neurons, a propensity toward hippocampal sclerosis, and either tau-positive or TDP-43-positive neuronal inclusions are present in most cases (Mackenzie et al. 2011). The pathological findings seen in ALS, PSP, and CBD are commonly discovered in patients with classical FTD clinical syndromes (Liscic et al. 2008; Feany & Dickson 1996). The majority of FTLD-related pathology is idiopathic, although there are many cases associated with known mutations in specific FTLD-causing genes and a new set of genes that increase susceptibility to FTLD including the H1H1 haplotype (Webb et al. 2008) and the A152T tau gene (Coppola et al. 2012) and other polymorphisms (Höglinger et al. 2011) for tau-related neuropathology.

FTLD neuropathology seems to begin in the frontoinsular paralimbic regions (Seeley et al. 2008). Neuronal and synapse loss, gliosis, and neuronal and astrocytic aggregates are evident in these regions. Unlike Alzheimer's disease, FTLD is not associated with amyloid plaques or neurofibrillary tangles. The relatively young age of onset for many of these patients often means that the amyloid pathology associated with aging in general is absent. Similarly, Lewy body and vascular changes are usually absent (Forman et al. 2006).

Instead, FTLD brains show specific neuronal inclusions. The brain in approximately 40% of FTLD cases shows tau inclusions. The vast majority of other patients show aggregates that are tau-negative but TDP-43-positive. Approximately 5% of all FTLD cases are tau and TDP-43-negative but show inclusions to other proteins such as fused in sarcoma (FUS) (Urwin et al. 2010; Mackenzie et al. 2011).

A minority of patients will show mixtures of tau and TDP changes (Leverenz et al. 2007). In particular, argyrophilic grain disease (see "Argyrophilic Grain Disease" section below) can co-occur with other types of tau aggregates or with TDP-43 (Fujishiro et al. 2009). While some of these changes may be incidental, there are other cases where two distinctive pathologies drive two distinctive clinical syndromes.

Pathologically, at a gross morphologic level, atrophy is seen in the frontal and anterior temporal lobes. A four-point pathological staging system has been proposed that is based on the progressive atrophy that occurs across the different phases of the illness, and it correlates strongly with clinical symptomatology (Kril & Halliday 2011) (Figure 7–1). Microscopically the atrophy seen with FTLD is associated with any or all of the following: gliosis, inclusion bodies, swollen neurons, and microvacuolation. Increasingly, the focus of research is on whether the inclusions within neurons or glia consist of tau or TDP-43.

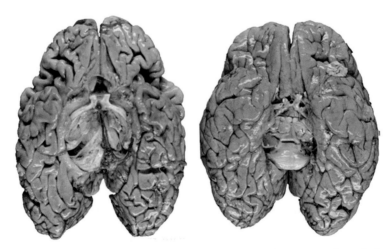

Figure 7–1. bvFTD versus normal brain. Note the atrophy of anterior temporal, anterior insular, and orbitofrontal regions, characteristic of bvFTD. (Image courtesy of Lea Grinberg, MD, PhD, and William Seeley, MD.)

OVERVIEW OF TAU-RELATED NEUROPATHOLOGY IN FTLD

Tau is a protein that binds to microtubules and is involved with the transportation of nutrients and proteins up and down the neuron, while helping to stabilize the cell's microtubules and thereby supports the neuron's three-dimensional structure (Mandelkow & Mandelkow 2012). In the normal adult human brain, tau is a soluble and predominantly axonal protein that is expressed as six isoforms, all of which are generated by the alternative splicing of the tau gene. Acetylation and hyperphosphorylation of tau can lead to pathological forms of tau that aggregate within and damage the neuron.

In humans, the tau isoforms found within the neuron are evenly divided between 4 repeat (4R) tau, where a long repeat at exon 10 is spliced into the tau protein, and 3R tau, where the tau lacks this extra repeat (Mandelkow & Mandelkow 2012, Kovacs et al. 2012). While the neurofibrillary changes found in Alzheimer's disease are associated with aggregates of both abnormally phosphorylated 3R and 4R tau, in most sporadic and familial forms of tau-positive FTLD, the tau aggregates are predominantly 4R tau. In fact, all of the major neurodegenerative FTLD syndromes with tau, with the exception of Pick's disease, have a predominance of 4R tau abnormal aggregates (Kovacs et al. 2012).

The tau gene (*MAPT*) is found on chromosome 17q21, and more than 50 different mutations have been associated with hereditary FTD linked to tau. This subtype of FTD is called "FTD with parkinsonism-linked to chromosome 17" (FTDP-17), because the FTD syndrome is associated with parkinsonism (Sima et al. 1996). While the original family described by Wilhelmsen and colleagues (Wilhelmsen et al. 1994) showed evidence for an amyotrophic lateral sclerosis (ALS) phenotype in a few members of this proband, the ALS phenotype appears to be rare with *MAPT* mutations.

MAPT mutations lead to disease via two major mechanisms, either by reducing the binding affinity of tau for microtubules, as occurs with most of the exon mutations, or by increasing production of 4R tau, as occurs with the *MAPT* intron mutations around exon 10

(Hong et al. 1998). Most patients with tau gene mutations develop an autosomal dominantly inherited syndrome with features of FTD, PSP, CBD, or rarely ALS, however, pathological and clinical heterogeneity is observed both among and within FTDP-17 families (Bugiani 2000). No tau mutations have so far been reported to cause familial forms of Alzheimer's disease, although as was noted in the last chapter, the A152T rare variant in tau predisposes people to both familial FTD-spectrum disorders and to familial forms of Alzheimer's disease.

OVERVIEW OF TDP-43- AND FUS-RELATED NEUROPATHOLOGY IN FTLD

An association between TDP-43 and FTLD was discovered more than 20 years after tau was linked to neurodegenerative disease (Neumann et al. 2006). Until TDP-43 was discovered as an FTLD and ALS protein, it was known that inclusions in more than 50% of FTLD cases were positive for ubiquitin, an unspecific cell death marker. For this reason, this group of FTD patients was given the name FTLD-U. Many such cases were associated with ALS, and for this reason, this subtype of FTD was called FTD-MND (motor neuron disease) or FTD-ALS.

In 2006 Manuela Neumann, working with John Trojanowski and Virginia Lee at the University of Pennsylvania, discovered that a hyperphosphorylated, ubiquitinated, and cleaved form of the TARDBP protein was the major disease protein in FTLD-U (Neumann et al. 2006). The same TDP-43 inclusions were also found in ALS patients without an FTD phenotype. Therefore, this discovery helped to further link FTD and ALS, suggesting that at a mechanistic level these two disorders were strongly related.

TDP-related FTLD has proven to be heterogeneous, and, in addition to FTD-ALS, these intracytoplasmic inclusions are seen in patients with progranulin mutations who almost never get ALS and in patients with TDP-43 mutations who usually get ALS but only rarely manifest a full-blown FTD syndrome. In addition, distinctive TDP-43 aggregates are seen in patients with the rare valosin mutations and occur in patients with *C9ORF72* mutations, a common cause for FTD, ALS, and FTD-ALS.

TDP-43 is still a relatively understudied protein that binds to both DNA and RNA and is involved with the regulation of transcription, mRNA splicing, and translational regulation. While abnormal aggregates of TDP-43 represent a common endpoint for patients with *GRN*, *TARDBP*, *C9ORF72*, and *VCP* mutations, the mechanism by which these aggregates lead to neurodegeneration may differ across FTLD subtypes. While progranulin appears to cause neurodegeneration by a distinctive mechanism associated with abnormal neuronal growth and excessive neuroinflammatory responses to brain injury (discussed in Chapter 8), *TARDBP* and *C9ORF72* seem to work by disrupting and poisoning nuclear function. Similarly, the other protein dysfunction associated with tau-negative FTLD FUS, likely causes disease by disrupting nuclear function. This mechanism is also discussed in Chapter 8.

GROSS ANATOMICAL AND MICROSCOPIC CHANGES IN FTLD

In FTLD, the gross changes feature a mild to severe decrease in overall brain weight, focal cortical atrophy, and ventricular enlargement (Figure 7–1). Atrophy is most severe in the paralimbic parts of the frontal lobes, anterior temporal lobes, basal ganglia, and, to a lesser extent, the brainstem. Thinning of the cortical ribbon and discoloration of white matter is common, and pallor and atrophy of the substantia nigra also occurs in the majority of cases. White matter degeneration is more extensive in FTLD-spectrum patients than in AD (Zhang et al. 2011). Synapse loss is significant, and neuronal loss is often accentuated in the frontoinsular region and superficial frontal and temporal areas. Arne Brun emphasized the predilection of neuronal loss in the first three layers of the frontal cortex (Brun 1987; Brun 2007), while Seeley and colleagues (Seeley et al. 2006) have suggested FTLD is associated with a selective vulnerability to von Economo neurons (see Von Economo Neurons section later in the chapter). In certain FTLD subtypes, particularly those with *C9ORF72* and *GRN* mutations, pathology is not only present in the frontotemporal regions, but it extends into more posterior brain regions.

Tau Aggregates

There are four major FTLD subtypes associated with tau aggregates: Pick's disease, CBD, PSP, and argyrophilic grain disease, all of which are discussed briefly here.

PICK'S DISEASE

Pick bodies were first described by Alzheimer in 1911. This pathological marker is characterized by silver-staining (argyrophilic) cytoplasmic neuronal inclusions (Pick bodies) that result in swollen and structurally distorted neurons called Pick cells (Gans 1922). These inclusions tend to be seen in the dentate gyrus and CA1 and subicular regions of the hippocampus, amygdala, paralimbic cortex, ventral temporal lobes, and less commonly in the anterior frontal and dorsal temporal regions. Pick bodies are composed of filaments of the tau protein, often 3R tau, although 4R tau can be present (Figure 7–2).

Pick's disease is rarely if ever seen in familial forms of FTLD and usually presents as a sporadic bvFTD syndrome with massive atrophy of the ventral frontal and temporal regions. All patients with FTLD-related neuropathology were considered to be a variant of Pick's disease until the 1980s, when Arne Brun demonstrated that only approximately 20% of all FTLD-spectrum cases had classical silver-staining Pick-like inclusions (Brun 1987). There have been cases of the nonfluent/agrammatic variant of primary progressive aphasia (nfvPPA) and the semantic variant of PPA (svPPA) that are due to Pick's neuropathology. In Pick's disease, motor problems tend to develop later in the disease course. The etiology for Pick's disease remains unknown.

PSP AND CBD

PSP and CBD have many clinical and pathological similarities, and the clinical overlap can make it difficult to accurately separate the two disorders during life. PSP and CBD are associated with behavioral, frontal-executive, and extrapyramidal changes, clinical abnormalities that are due to the selective vulnerability of frontal-subcortical and the basal ganglia circuits with both conditions (Boeve et al. 2003; Shelley et al. 2009). Additionally, neurons, astrocytes, and oligodendrocytes accumulate

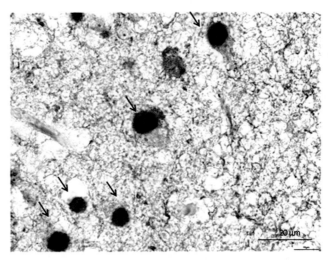

Figure 7–2. Middle frontal gyrus showing Pick bodies (arrows). Pick bodies, located predominantly in the superficial cortical layers, are small, round, neuronal cytoplasmic inclusions. Immunohistochemistry for hyperphosphorylated tau. (Image courtesy of Lea Grinberg, MD, PhD, and William Seeley, MD.)

abnormal aggregates of 4R tau and both CBD and PSP patients have an overrepresentation of the H1H1 tau haplotype (Conrad et al. 1997).

There are significant differences between the two conditions. PSP has a predilection for the subcortical structures including the midbrain, pons, and cerebellum, while CBD tends to spare these regions, at least early in the illness. The early involvement of supranuclear gaze due to this midbrain degeneration is a highly valuable way to differentiate PSP from CBD and is a strong predictor of underlying PSP pathology. Another difference between the two conditions is that the spatial patterns of the tau aggregations are slightly different with PSP compared to CBD. PSP is associated with globose tangles (Figure 7–3) and thorny astrocytes (Figure 7–4), while CBD leads to a coiled shaped tangle in neurons (coiled bodies) (Figure 7–5) and thread-like aggregates of tau that accumulate in a plaque-like form that are called astrocytic plaques (Feany & Dickson 1996) (Figure 7–6). Whether these subtle neuropathological differences are meaningful at a mechanistic level or will require differences in therapeutic strategies is unknown, but the fact that both disorders are 4R tauopathies with similar genetic risk factors suggests that they are strongly linked, and treatment for one is likely to be helpful for the other.

ARGYROPHILIC GRAIN DISEASE

The fourth, and most poorly understood, but most frequent, tau-related subtype of FTD is called argyrophilic grain disease (AGD). The clinical syndromes associated with AGD are diverse and range from mild cognitive impairment with a slow progression to the behavioral variant of FTD (bvFTD) or PSP. AGD often is seen in association with other neuropathological diseases, and this has made it hard to determine the clinical-pathological correlates of this entity. It is estimated that AGD is seen in approximately 5% of all patients with dementia (Thal et al. 2005).

In one study from Fujino and colleagues, AGD occurred in 26% of 239 Alzheimer's disease cases (Fujino et al. 2005), and Soma and colleagues (Soma et al. 2012) found that 38% of patients with sporadic ALS also had AGD neuropathology. By contrast, in another study 60% of patients with AGD also had TDP-43 (Fujishiro et al. 2009). It is also seen in PSP and CBD (Fujino et al. 2005).

AGD has a predilection for the medial temporal lobe and leads to small aggregates of 4R tau in neuronal dendrites (Figure 7–7). Because of AGD's slow progression, Lea Grinberg at the University of California, San Francisco (UCSF) has suggested that this form of tau may be less toxic than other types of aggregates,

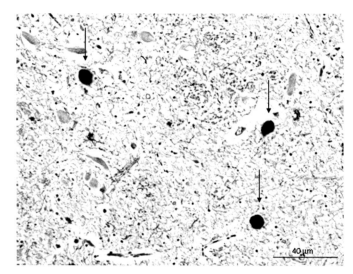

Figure 7–3. Insular cortex shows globose tangles (arrows) seen in PSP. These tangles differ from the flame-shaped tangles seen in AD. Immunohistochemistry for hyperphosphorylated tau. (Image courtesy of Lea Grinberg, MD, PhD, and William Seeley, MD.)

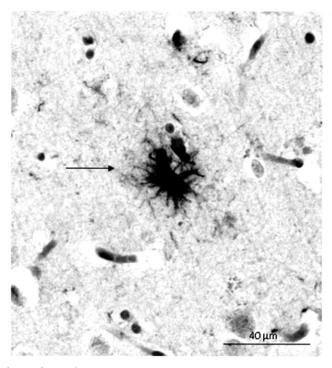

Figure 7–4. Precentral gyrus shows a thorny astrocyte (arrow), a glial cytoplasmic inclusion subtype seen in some patients with PSP. Immunohistochemistry for hyperphosphorylated tau. (Image courtesy of Lea Grinberg, MD, PhD, and William Seeley, MD.)

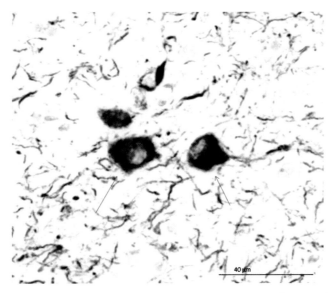

Figure 7–5. Precentral gyrus shows corticobasal bodies (arrows), neuronal cytoplasmic inclusions, seen in CBD. Immunohistochemistry for hyperphosphorylated tau. (Image courtesy of Lea Grinberg, MD, PhD, and William Seeley, MD.)

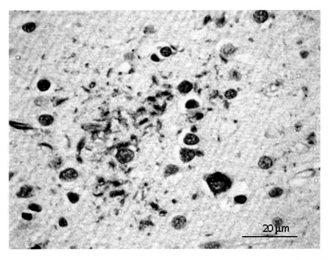

Figure 7–6. Precentral gyrus shows an astrocytic plaque, characteristic of CBD. Immunohistochemistry for hyperphosphorylated tau. (Image courtesy of Lea Grinberg, MD, PhD, and William Seeley, MD.)

and that it may possibly be a protective form of tau (personal communication). The concept of protective aggregates has a precedence in Huntington's disease, where Steve Finkbeiner and colleagues at UCSF demonstrated that cells with Huntington aggregates lived longer than those with soluble Huntington protein (Arrasate et al. 2004). In the coming years more work will be needed to better understand the risk factors (beyond old age) for AGD and how this pathological aggregate affects the brain and influences disease course.

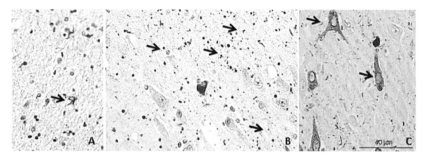

Figure 7–7. Neuropathological features of argyrophilic grain disease. **(A)** coiled body (arrow) in an oligodendrocyte in the white matter adjoining the entorhinal cortex. **(B)** Argyrophilic grains spread in the neuropil of region CA1 of the hippocampus. **(C)** Pre-tangles (arrows) in the region CA2 of the hippocampus. (Image courtesy of Lea Grinberg, MD, PhD, and William Seeley, MD.)

FTLD with Ubiquitin- and TDP-43-Positive Inclusions

TDP-43 normally resides within the nucleus, but in FTLD the TDP-43 leaves the nucleus and aggregates within the cytoplasm of neurons and glia in an ubiquitinated and hyperphosphorylated form (Buratti & Barale 2011). It is still actively debated whether the primary mechanism for TDP-43-related neurodegeneration is the toxicity of the cytoplasmic aggregates or the altered regulation of DNA and RNA caused by the mislocalization of the TDP-43 from the nucleus (Polymenidou et al. 2012).

A new international system has harmonized the classification of FTLD neuropathology with four major subtypes: A, B, C, and D (Mackenzie et al. 2011). Type A TDP-43 aggregates are seen in patients with *GRN* mutations, in some patients with seemingly sporadic bvFTD or nfvPPA (Armstrong & Cairns 2011), and in some patients with *C9ORF72* mutations (William Seeley, personal communication). Type A neuropathology is associated with dystrophic neurites, neuronal cytoplasmic TDP-43 inclusions, and sometimes with lentiform neuronal intranuclear inclusions (Figure 7–8). These distinctive intranuclear aggregates were first described by Ian Mackenzie at the

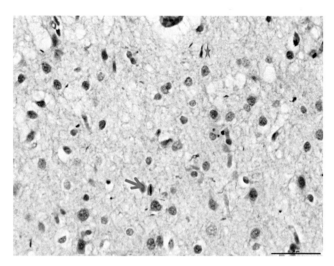

Figure 7–8. Superficial layer of middle temporal gyrus showing changes characteristic of TDP-type A. This subtype features short neurites and threads (red star), and glial and neuronal inclusions, predominantly in superficial layers. In some cases, lentiform nuclear inclusions (arrow) are seen. Immunohistochemistry for TDP-43. (Image courtesy of Lea Grinberg, MD, PhD, and William Seeley, MD.)

University of British Columbia in familial cases with FTD, leading him to hypothesize that they represented a subgroup of patients with a unique genetic form of FTLD. This observation was a critical step in the discovery of *GRN* mutations.

TDP-43 type B is typical for patients with FTD and ALS (FTD-MND). The majority of patients with FTD-MND show this distinctive subtype of TDP-43 neuropathology. In brains with this pattern of disease there is a loss of nuclear TDP and there are extensive neuronal cytoplasmic inclusions (Figure 7–9). This was once classified as FTD-MND or FTLD-U but now subsumes the vast majority of patients of FTD with ALS and family cases with a history for both FTD and ALS.

Type C is seen with svPPA and rarely with other FTD clinical subtypes. In the UCSF neuropathology series this pattern of TDP aggregation is nearly always the pattern seen in patients with svPPA. This TDP subtype shows long dystrophic neurites in the superficial cortical layers with diffuse TDP aggregates but few neuronal inclusions (Figure 7–10).

Finally, valosin-mutations are associated with bvFTD, inclusion body myositis, and Paget's disease of bone (Koppers et al. 2012). At pathology these patients show TDP type D neuropathology with dystrophic neurites and

abnormal intranuclear inclusions but rarely cytoplasmic inclusions. Some patients with this rare genetic mutation go on to develop ALS.

Clinical phenotyping has proven remarkably powerful for predicting TDP subtypes, particularly for svPPA (nearly always TDP-43C) and FTD-MND (nearly always TDP-43B). When the bvFTD syndrome is tau-negative it is typically associated with TDP-43A (evenly divided between *GRN* mutation carriers and sporadic cases), and when nfvPPA is associated with TDP-43 (not tau) pathology, it is also usually type A.

At the time of this publication, *C9ORF72* had been discovered as the major gene responsible for familial forms of FTD and ALS, and it is likely that there will be still further modifications in the TDP-43 classification based on the unique nuclear inclusions identified with this subtype of FTLD. While most *C9ORF72* mutation carriers have been classified as TDP-43B, we also have patients with a TDP-43 A-type pattern. Two unique aspects of these cases are the presence of RNA nuclear aggregates and the presence of frequent ubiquitin-positive, TDP-43-negative aggregates in the dentate granule cells.

These diverse patterns and etiologies for TDP-43 neuropathology suggest that different neuropathological patterns may require

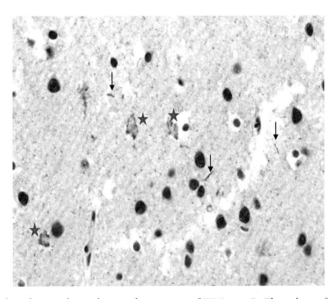

Figure 7–9. Middle frontal gyrus shows changes characteristic of TDP-type B. This subtype features moderate numbers of neuronal cytoplasmic inclusions (stars) in superficial and deep cortical layers but few dystrophic neurites (arrows). Immunohistochemistry for TDP-43. (Image courtesy of Lea Grinberg, MD, PhD, and William Seeley, MD.)

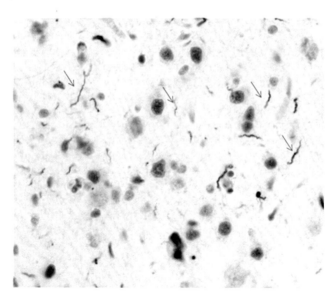

Figure 7–10. Middle temporal gyrus shows changes characteristic of TDP-type C. This subtype features long and thin dystrophic neurites (arrows) and very few neuronal cytoplasmic inclusions. Immunohistochemistry for TDP-43. (Image courtesy of Lea Grinberg, MD, PhD, and William Seeley, MD.)

different therapies, although it is still possible that a single TDP-43 modifying therapy will treat all of these FTLD subtypes.

Progranulin deficiency leads to approximately one-half of the TDP-43 type A cases. Raising brain progranulin is a logical and potentially highly efficacious therapy for the familial and possibly sporadic forms of TDP-43 type A pathology. Whether similar approaches will help the patients with TDP-43 type A pathology in whom progranulin mutations are not present is unknown. Also, recognizing such cases ante mortem is not yet possible, so even if these cases represent a progranulin deficient form of FTD, identifying such cases would be problematic.

It is unlikely that the type B cases will respond to such an approach, and FTD-MND is not yet linked in any way to progranulin deficiency or progranulin mutations. TDP-43 type B neuropathology is commonly associated C9ORF72 mutations, so the FTD-MND subgroup might require strategies focused around abnormal mRNA expression (see Chapter 8).

Most TDP-43 type C cases are sporadic patients with svPPA. Recent work led by Zac Miller at UCSF and Tony Wyss-Coray at Stanford University suggests that autoimmunity may play a role in many cases of svPPA (TDP-43 type C). These patients might require

still different therapeutic approaches that focused around specific changes in inflammatory protein cascades and abnormalities in lymphocyte signaling.

Finally, TDP-43 type D cases are due to valosin mutations suggesting still another distinctive mechanism for FTLD-neuropathology related to mitochondrial dysfunction and alterations in autophagy. This mechanism might require entirely different therapeutic approaches.

FTLD with Tau- and TDP-43-Negative but FUS-Positive Inclusions

Approximately 5% of patients with bvFTD show aggregates that are tau and TDP negative but stain positively for the FUS protein (Neumann et al. 2009). The clinical spectrum of FUS-positive FTD is still being actively studied, but most such cases have been under the age of 60 years and have suffered from bvFTD (Urwin et al. 2010). In the initial descriptions of these patients, many showed disinhibition, psychosis, and loss of empathy for others. Motor abnormalities appeared only late in the course of the illness, and none of the patients exhibited ALS. Imaging showed ventral frontal and caudate atrophy. Mutations in FUS can cause familial ALS, but most FUS-positive FTLD is not associated with a family history of FTD or ALS, and most FUS-positive FTLD patients never exhibited ALS during life.

FUS is a DNA- and RNA-binding protein, has functions that parallel those of TDP-43, and is likely involved with transcription, mRNA splicing, and translational regulation (Ito & Suzuki 2011). FUS mutations can cause familial forms of ALS and rarely bvFTD syndromes. Like TDP-43, FUS normally resides within the nucleus, but in FTLD the FUS leaves the nucleus and aggregates within the cytoplasm of neurons (Figure 7–11).

The N-terminal piece of *FUS* is involved with the activation of transcription, while the C-terminus binds proteins, DNA and RNA. Specific transcription factors recognize FUS. In addition, recognition sites for the transcription factors AP2, GCF, and Sp1 have been identified in FUS. FUS binds single- and double-stranded DNA and RNA and recognizes specific RNA repeat motifs (King et al. 2012). It is also recognized to be the hnRNP P2 protein, a part of a complex that helps with the maturation of pre-mRNA. Also, FUS is similar to the Ewing's sarcoma protein and the TATA-binding protein making up a family of homologous DNA/RNA proteins (Couthouis et al. 2012). Yet, these two proteins remain in the nucleus in FUS-related neurodegeneration, while FUS does not (Mackenzie & Neumann 2012).

While genetic mutations in *FUS* can lead to ALS (and bvFTD), these patients only aggregate FUS, while sporadic forms of FTLD without known mutations aggregate the other FET proteins including TATA and Ewing's Sarcoma protein (Neumann et al. 2011). The unique functions and vulnerability of FUS in the setting of FTD-ALS remains uncertain, but, as with TDP-43, the abnormalities in DNA and RNA signaling appear to be central to this relatively new subtype of FTLD.

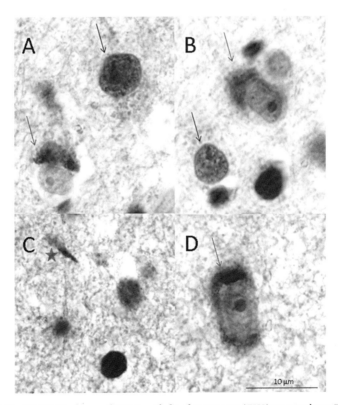

Figure 7–11. (A–B) The FTLD-U subtype of FTLD with fused in sarcoma (FUS) protein shows FUS-positive neuronal cytoplasmic inclusions. **(C)** Short thick dystrophic neurites. **(D)** Often, nuclear or C-shaped perinuclear (arrow) inclusions are seen. (Image courtesy of Lea Grinberg, MD, PhD, and William Seeley, MD.)

SQSTM1 and FTLD

The laboratory of Teepu Siddique discovered another FLTD neuropathological subtype (Siddique & Ajroud-Driss 2011). In 2011 their group looked at 546 patients with familial (n = 340) or sporadic (n = 206) ALS and screened them all for *SQSTM1* mutations. They found 10 novel *SQSTM1* mutations (nine heterozygous missense and one deletion) in 15 patients (6 with familial ALS and 9 with sporadic ALS) (Fecto et al. 2011). While the clinical phenotype of these patients related to FTD remains to be determined, this appears to be a form of FTD-ALS related to the p62 protein, and aggregation of this protein is evident in patients with FTD-ALS. The p62 scaffold protein is involved in cell signaling, receptor internalization, and protein turnover (Figure 7–12).

C9ORF72 patients have p62-positive but TDP-43-negative inclusions in hippocampus and cerebellum. More work is needed to understand how the p62 protein is involved in FTLD-related neurodegeneration.

Dementia Lacking Distinctive Histopathology (DLDH)

This category of FTLD where there is frontotemporal gliosis without known protein aggregates has practically disappeared as the various proteins associated with FTLD (tau, TDP-43, FUS, and p62) have been identified. The rare mutation *CHMP2B* still leads to an FTLD neuropathological picture without known proteins aggregates (Gydesen et al. 2002).

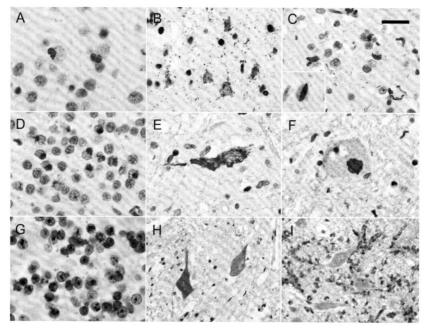

Figure 7–12. Neuropathological features associated with the *C9ORF72* mutation. All cases showed compact and granular TDP-43-immunoreactive neuronal cytoplasmic inclusions in the neocortex, typical of FTLD-TDP type B (**A**). Granular neuronal pre-inclusions in neocortex layer II were common (**B**). A subset of cases had compact neuronal cytoplasmic inclusions, short neurites, and rare lentiform neuronal intranuclear inclusions (inset) in layer II neocortex, consistent with FTLD-TDP type A (**C**). Compact and granular neuronal cytoplasmic inclusions in hippocampal dentate granule cells were a consistent feature (**D**). Lower motor neurons contained neuronal cytoplasmic inclusions with granular, filamentous (**E**), or compact Lewy body–like morphology (**F**). Small neuronal cytoplasmic inclusions and short neurites in the granule cell layer of the cerebellar cortex were immunoreactive for ubiquitin and p62, but negative for TDP-43 (**G**). Increased cytoplasmic staining of some lower motor neurons was seen in cases of ALS, both with and without the *C9ORF72* mutation (**H**). In all cases of FTLD (with and without the *C9ORF72* mutation) hippocampal pyramidal neurons were surrounded by coarse punctate staining, consistent with enlarged presynaptic terminals (**I**). Immunohistochemistry for TDP-43 (**A–F**), ubiquitin (**G**), and *C9ORF72* (**H** and **I**). Scale bars: **A, D–F, H** and **I** = 25 μm; **B** and **C** = 30 μm; **G** = 12 μm. (Hsiung et al. 2012.)

SPECIAL FEATURES OF FTLD PATHOLOGY

Hippocampal Sclerosis

Hippocampal sclerosis is a neuropathological entity that is characterized by extensive and highly focal neuronal loss and gliosis in the subiculum and CA1 region of the hippocampus. The association between hippocampal sclerosis and hypoxia and metabolic insults such as hypoglycemia or status epilepticus is well established and is associated with a severe, sometimes isolated amnesia.

In recent years it has become apparent that hippocampal sclerosis is commonly seen associated with brain aging and neurodegeneration. First this neuropathological abnormality was linked to a slow form of Alzheimer's disease. In general, the likelihood of hippocampal sclerosis increases with aging, and at least 10% of individuals over the age of 85 show this finding at autopsy. In the very old, when hippocampal sclerosis is present, this change is usually associated with TDP-43 aggregates. Clinically, many of these individuals show a slowly progressive amnestic syndrome, although some exhibit bvFTD-type behaviors.

Additionally, FTLD-spectrum disorders are associated with a high frequency of hippocampal sclerosis, particularly cases with TDP-43 neuropathology. The mechanism for this coassociation is unknown, but in many instances patients with hippocampal sclerosis and TDP-43 exhibit significant problems with memory in addition to their behavioral syndromes. In one study by Dennis Dickson and his group (Amador-Ortiz et al. 2007), 20% of patients with pathologically confirmed Alzheimer's disease showed hippocampal sclerosis, while 70% of those individuals with hippocampal sclerosis also had ubiquitinated aggregates suggesting an FTLD-spectrum disorder. In another study by Peter Nelson and colleagues at the University of Kentucky (Nelson et al. 2011), approximately 10% of patients over 85 had hippocampal sclerosis, and in the 106 patients with this finding, aberrant TDP-43 immunohistochemistry was seen in 89.9% of those patients with hippocampal sclerosis but only 9.7% of hippocampal sclerosis negative patients. Over age 95 the risk for demonstrating hippocampal sclerosis skyrocketed. These findings link FTLD-related pathology to a very old cohort of patients and suggests that we may be underestimating the true prevalence of FTLD due to the infrequent clinical or neuropathological diagnosis of this condition in the old and the very old.

Von Economo Neurons

Originally the great neuroanatomist Betz described these structurally distinctive neurons, yet it was von Economo who brought attention to these cells that carry his name, von Economo neurons (VENs). In 1929 von Economo reported his work on these large bipolar apical neurons, also called spindle cells based on their unusual shape. VENs sit in layer 5 of the frontoinsular region with 30% greater density in the right than the left side of the brain. They appear strongly related to a structurally similar cell with a forked dendritic end that are called fork cells and appear built to carry information quickly from one brain area to another (Seeley et al. 2012).

In 1999 John Allman at the California Institute of Technology brought new interest to these neurons when he and his group discovered that they were present in the anterior cingulate cortex in great apes but no other primates (Nimchinsky et al. 1999). Additionally, he discovered that these cells were of highest density in humans. Later it was learned that African and Asian elephants (Hakeem et al. 2009) and a wide variety of whales ranging from humpback, fin, killer, sperm to beluga, as well as the bottlenose and Risso's dolphin all have VENs in this same frontoinsular region (Butti et al. 2009). More recently, small numbers of VENs have been found in macaques (Evrard et al. 2012).

These neurons developed most extensively in big-brained, highly social species (Figure 7–13). The cells sit in phylogenetically old parts of the ventral frontal and insular cortex that are involved with processing physiologically relevant internal signals related to feeding and pain, yet clearly have unique functions related to the interpretations of these signals that are required for these highly social and intelligent species. Although correlation does not equal causation, it may be relevant that species with these cells have the ability to recognize their own face in a mirror (Plotnik et al.

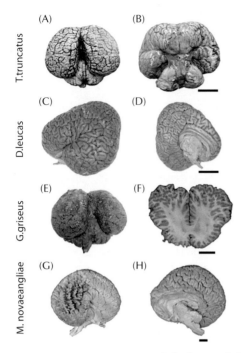

Figure 7–13. Macroscopic views of the brains of the cetacean species analyzed in the present study. Dorsal (**A**) and ventral (**B**) views of the brain of a bottlenose dolphin; lateral (**C**) and midline (**D**) views of the left hemisphere of the brain of a beluga whale; dorsal view (**E**) and coronal slab at the level of the genu of the corpus callosum (**F**) of the brain of a Risso's dolphin; lateral (**G**) and midline view (**H**) of the right hemisphere of the brain of a humpback whale. Note the large size of the brains and the complex gyral pattern. The lateral aspect of the parietal lobe of the humpback whale brain sustained damage when the specimen was removed from the skull (**G**). This, however, did not affect the present study. The brains are not shown to scale. Scale bars = 3 cm. (Butti et al. 2009.)

2006; Delfour & Marten 2001). By contrast, the more primitive members of their phyla do not have these neurons.

The function and even connections of the VENs remain under study, but these cells do connect to dorsolateral frontal, frontopolar, and amygdalar structures. While speculative, Allman and colleagues suggest that anterior cingulate VENs connect to the frontopolar region and possibly help to modify emotionally salient information that can be acted on by the broad expanse of the dorsolateral prefrontal cortex to which these cells seem to connect.

William Seeley at UCSF demonstrated in 2006 that VENs appeared to be the first cell to degenerate in bvFTD (Seeley et al. 2006)

(Figure 7–14). In contrast, in Alzheimer's disease these cells were spared, even late in the illness. Additionally, he and colleagues showed that fork cells were also involved in FTLD cases (Kim et al. 2012). This remarkable set of observations suggests that these phylogenetically late neurons may be the site where bvFTD begins. Both tau and TDP-43 forms of FTLD involve VENs, although mechanistically it remains unknown why these cells are selectively attacked early in FTLD process. Similarly, the clinical manifestation associated with dysfunction in VENs (presumably the first clinical stage in the pathogenesis of FTLD) is unknown.

VENs seem to be critically important to FTLD, particularly when the clinical manifestation is associated with bvFTD. Additionally, they are phylogenetically new and hold fascinating mysteries regarding our brain's unique anatomy, compared to other species. Understanding the physiology, anatomical connections, genetic profile, and features that increase their selective vulnerability in FTLD will be important if effective therapies emerge to protect these delicate cells.

FTLD NEUROPATHOLOGY: CURRENT STATE AND RESEARCH ADVANCES

FTLD has gone from a simple homogeneous disorder with frontotemporal gliosis and atrophy to a disorder associated with a newly discovered set of molecules that spread along specific circuits in a prion-like fashion. PSP, CBD, and AGD are 4R tauopathies, with a predilection for frontoinsular, limbic, and basal ganglia and brainstem circuits. Pick's disease is a 3R tauopathy with a predilection for the ventral frontoinsular region. All of these disorders attack frontoinsular and basal ganglia, but tend not to cause motor neuron disease. Treatment for one of these tauopathies is likely to trigger treatment for them all.

The FTLD disorders associated with abnormal aggregates of TDP-43 are diverse. Patients with progranulin mutations show characteristic lentiform nuclear aggregates of TDP-43 and cytoplasmic TDP as well. This is called TDP-43 type A. In this case, the translocation of TDP-43 seems to be in response to a

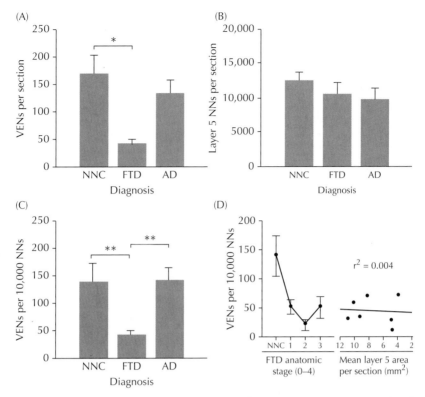

Figure 7–14. Severe, selective, disease-specific, and early loss of von Economo neurons (VENs) in frontotemporal dementia (FTD). **(A)** VENs per section were reduced by 74% in FTD compared with nonneurological control subjects (NNC) (*p < 0.005, Tukey's test after F-test for three-group analysis of variance [ANOVA]). **(B)** Layer 5 neighboring neurons (NNs), in contrast, showed a mild, statistically nonsignificant reduction in FTD, similar to that seen in AD. **(C)** VEN per 10,000 NN estimates indicated selective VEN depletion in FTD compared with NNC subjects and patients with AD (**p < 0.05, Tukey's tests after F-test for three-group ANOVA). **(D)** Even mild stages of FTD-related atrophy were accompanied by marked VEN dropout. Mean Layer 5 area per anterior cingulate cortex (ACC) section, used here as a local marker for disease severity, had no bearing on the VEN/10,000 NN ratio, further suggesting that VEN selectivity occurred across FTD stages. Results are shown as means ± standard error of the mean. (Seeley et al. 2006.)

deficiency of progranulin, and correction of that deficiency might allow the neurons under stress from low progranulin to return to their normal state. Similar neuropathology occurs in some patients with bvFTD and nfvPPA in whom no progranulin mutation was evident. Additionally, we have seen this type A neuropathological pattern in some patients with *C9ORF72* mutations. Whether these patients are progranulin deficient in some way remains unknown. Progranulin deficiency is a powerful model for understanding how TDP-43 responds to stress.

TDP-43 type B is the typical neuropathological picture of ALS and FTD-ALS and of some patients with just FTD. It can occur in patients with or without mutations in *C9ORF72* (Murray et al. 2011). There is

much to be learned about the pathogenesis of TDP-43 type B. It is clear that finding a treatment for this form of TDP-43opathy will require a better understanding of how TDP-43 moves from the nucleus to the cytoplasm and a better understanding of its role in the regulation of DNA and RNA processing. The molecules associated with FTD-ALS are TDP-43, FUS, and *C9ORF72*. All seem to be involved in DNA and RNA regulation. TDP-43 and FUS have multiple potential mechanisms, and it is not yet clear whether they spread in a prion-like fashion from cell to cell or whether the dysregulation of RNA and DNA processing is central to their pathogenesis. It appears that the road to the treatment of ALS and FTD with a propensity to ALS is through these unique proteins.

TDP-43 type C is the third major form of TDP-43 neuropathology and seems only distantly related to Types A and B. These patients suffer from svPPA, experience a slow neurodegenerative course and rarely develop ALS. Recent work at UCSF suggests that these patients have a strong autoimmune signal and understanding the role of immunological cascades in svPPA represents a future challenge for the field.

Finally, both the tau and TDP-43 forms of FTD-ALS selectively attack von Economo neurons, and the selective vulnerability of these cells may be a clue to the treatment of all forms of FTLD. As the genetic features of these cells become better understood, modeling them in the test tube may become possible, facilitating therapies that are targeted to protect the von Economo neurons, thereby protecting the brain from this condition.

What Is the Role of TDP-43 in Non-FTLD Degenerative Conditions?: Alzheimer's Disease and Chronic Traumatic Encephalopathy

One recent and important discovery is that TDP-43 aggregates are not solely restricted to patients with FTLD syndromes. It is now apparent that approximately one-half of patients with Alzheimer's disease and one-quarter of patients with mild cognitive impairment have TDP-43 aggregates. The presence of TDP-43 may even be higher when alpha-synuclein is present (Rauramaa et al. 2011). The medial temporal lobe represents a site where TDP-43 is high in patients with Alzheimer's disease, although they are also present in the frontal lobes (Kadokura et al. 2009).

While some have argued that this is the co-occurrence of two neuropathologies, others believe that the presence of one protein may trigger the other. Importantly, Nelson and colleagues at the University of Kentucky have demonstrated that TDP-43 correlates independently from plaques or hippocampal sclerosis as a marker for Alzheimer's disease (Nelson et al. 2010). In the coming years it is likely that TDP-43 will begin to garner the same attention that amyloid β-42 and tau have generated in the past. It is an important, yet still poorly understand compound that is expressed in the setting of a multitude of neurodegenerative disorders.

Another fascinating association with TDP-43 is with chronic traumatic encephalopathy (CTE), a neurodegenerative condition (or set of conditions) that can emerge after head trauma. Ann McKee at Boston University found widespread aggregates of TDP-43 in 10 of 12 patients who died with CTE. Regions that were most severely affected included the frontal and temporal cortices, medial temporal lobe, basal ganglia, diencephalon, and brainstem. Three of the 12 suffered a clinical syndrome suggestive of ALS, and in these individuals the TDP-43 inclusions extended to the spinal cord (McKee et al. 2010). This work strongly links CTE to ALS and FTLD and suggests that head injury might be a risk for ALS with TDP-43. The other major protein that aggregates in CTE is tau. Hence, the two major FTLD proteins both accumulate in this head-trauma related neurodegenerative disorder.

Basic Mechanisms in TDP-43, FUS, and *C9ORF72*

TDP-43 and FUS are fascinating molecules that appear to be mobilized in the setting of stress, moving out of the nucleus to the cytoplasm, into "stress granules" that are associated with the endoplasmic reticulum (Ito & Suzuki 2011). Within the nucleus they also have an important role in regulating DNA, RNA, and pre-mRNA (Buratti & Baralle 2011). It is clear that when these proteins are mutated, neurodegenerative conditions emerge.

Recent work has focused around the concept that TDP-43 and FUS are RNA-binding proteins that have RNA recognition motifs (King et al. 2012). These motifs have aggregation susceptibilities that may make them prion-like and prone to pathological aggregation. FUS is the second most prone to aggregation of all these proteins, and TDP-43 ranks 10th.

Additionally, FUS is considered a member of the FET family of proteins (Mackenzie & Neumann 2012; Couthouis et al. 2012). These proteins associate with the transcription factor II and RNA polymerase II. Finally, A2/BI another protein with an RNA recognition motif is predicted to engage GGGGCC (the repeat in

C9ORF72) and also is sequestered in RNA foci in another RNA-mediated neurodegenerative syndrome, fragile X-tremor-ataxia syndrome. These new sets of proteins will be extensively studied to better determine whether and how they interact with FUS and other FTLD proteins. At a mechanistic level much is still to be learned about the TDP-43, FUS, and C9 proteins to better determine their role in FTD and ALS.

Does FTLD Spread in a Prion-like Fashion?

Stanley Prusiner at UCSF first introduced the concept that neurodegenerative disorders could spread from cell to cell via misfolded proteins in his studies of Jakob-Creutzfeldt disease (Prusiner 1982). His recent update on this topic (Prusiner 2012) summarized new data to suggest that many of the neurodegenerative conditions might actually spread in a similar manner. While none of the neurodegenerative diseases are as invasive as prions, there is now extensive data to support the idea that Lewy bodies, amyloid-β-42, and tau can move from one region in the brain to another in a prion-like manner and accelerate neuropathology in animal models. The data supporting this mechanism for other neurodegenerative conditions will not be discussed here, although we do discuss evidence for FTLD-spectrum conditions.

Recently, it has been discovered that each neurodegenerative disease hits specific brain networks and spreads along these pathways versus a diffuse hit to the brain. For the first time, there is clinical data to support the idea that a prion-like mechanism is a feasible explanation for how neurodegeneration spreads across the large neuronal networks in the brain. An imaginative research study by Helen Zhou, William Seeley, and colleagues at UCSF (Zhou et al. 2012) looked at four hypotheses for the spread along specific networks: "nodal stress, transneuronal spread, trophic failure, and shared vulnerability." Using graph theoretical analyses in healthy subjects, the authors found that brain areas with "higher total connectional flow and, more consistently, shorter functional paths to the epicenters, showed greater disease-related vulnerability." They suggested that this best supported a "transneuronal spread model of network-based vulnerability."

Molecular studies are also beginning to support this idea. Bess Frost working in Marc Diamond's laboratory (Frost et al. 2009) demonstrated that tau aggregates were taken up by cultured cells and were able to induce fibrillization of intracellular full-length tau. In turn, these fibrils "were able to seed fibril formation of recombinant tau monomer in vitro and newly aggregated intracellular tau transferred between co-cultured cells." In more recent work from the Diamond laboratory (Kfoury et al. 2012) the authors concluded, "Thus, propagation of tau protein misfolding among cells can be mediated by release and subsequent uptake of fibrils that directly contact native protein in recipient cells."

Michel Goedert and Maria Spillantini (Goedert & Spillantini 2011) have recently suggested that tau may have different strains, a concept strongly supported with prion disease. These different strains spread with varying virulence and form distinctive aggregates. Similarly, Goedert suggests (Goedert et al. 2010) that intracellular inclusions of tau, α-synuclein, Huntington, and superoxide dismutase 1, all spread through the nervous system in a prion-like fashion.

Currently, animal models of tauopathy and TDP-43 forms of FTLD are being extensively studied for transmissibility in a number of laboratories including the Prusiner laboratory at UCSF. The evidence is mounting that the neuropathology of FTLD and related disorders are associated with a prion-like spread of misfolded proteins to the adjacent cells within a functional network. Subsequently, the misfolded protein causes structural changes in the uninfected cell. Understanding these prion-like mechanisms is a critical step toward developing new therapies for FTLD.

FTD PATHOLOGY GLOSSARY

A listing of commonly used FTLD terms can be found in Box 7.1.

Box 7.1 Frontotemporal Dementia Neuropathology Glossary

Astrocytic plaques: Aggregates of tau found in corticobasal degeneration.

Atrophy: Wasting away or shrinking. Many neurodegenerative disorders are associated with loss of tissue, giving the appearance of atrophy on the MRI.

Cellular inclusion: Any aggregate not ordinarily found within a cell.

Frontotemporal dementia (FTD): The umbrella term for the clinical syndromes of behavioral variant frontotemporal dementia (bvFTD), semantic variant PPA (svPPA) and nonfluent/agrammatic variant primary progressive aphasia (nfavPPA). These syndromes share involvement of the frontal and temporal lobes of the brain. This term is sometimes used to refer specifically to bvFTD.

Frontotemporal lobar degeneration (FTLD): The term that describes the specific pathological diseases that result in FTD syndromes. Subtyping is based on the specific proteins found within neuronal inclusions.

FUS: Fused in Sarcoma is a DNA- and RNA-binding protein likely involved with transcription, mRNA splicing, and translational regulation. FUS mutations can cause familial forms of ALS, and rarely bvFTD syndromes.

Gliosis: A process leading to scars in the central nervous system that involves the production of a dense fibrous network of glia in areas of damage. Gliosis is a prominent feature of many diseases of the central nervous system, including frontotemporal dementia, Alzheimer's disease, multiple sclerosis, and stroke.

Globose tangles: Rounded accumulations of tau in neuronal cytoplasm found in progressive supranuclear palsy pathology.

Neurofibrillary tangle: Pathological clusters of the abnormally phosphorylated tau protein that are found within neurons.

Neuronal inclusion: Any small intracellular body found within a neuron (nerve or brain cell).

Pick bodies: A rounded neuronal cytoplasmic inclusion that stains positive for silver. It is made up of the protein tau and seen in less than 10% of patients with FTD.

Pick cells: Neurons swollen by cytoplasmic neuronal inclusions.

Pick's disease: A neurodegenerative disease characterized by silver-staining (argyrophilic) cytoplasmic neuronal inclusions (Pick bodies) Pick's disease usually presents as behavioral variant frontotemporal dementia but less commonly leads to an nfvPPA or svPPA syndrome.

Progranulin: Progranulin is a cellular protein encoded by *GRN*.

Tau: A protein in the body that stabilizes the cytoskeleton and aids cellular transportation. It is encoded by *MAPT*.

TDP-43: Transactive response (TAR)-DNA-binding protein 43 is a cellular protein encoded by *TARDBP*.

Thorny astrocytes: Astrocytes with abnormal aggregates of 4R tau seen in progressive supranuclear palsy.

Von Economo neurons: Large, bipolar neurons in layer 5b of the anterior cingulate, and frontoinsular cortices of great apes (humans, gorillas, chimpanzees, bonobos, and orangutans), dolphins, whales, and elephants.

REFERENCES

Amador-Ortiz C, Lin WL, Ahmed Z, Personett D, Davies P, Duara R, Graff-Radford NR, Hutton ML, Dickson DW. TDP-43 immunoreactivity in hippocampal sclerosis and Alzheimer's disease. Ann Neurol. 2007;61:435–45.

Armstrong RA, Cairns NJ. Spatial patterns of TDP-43 neuronal cytoplasmic inclusions (NCI) in fifteen cases of frontotemporal lobar degeneration with TDP-43 proteinopathy (FTLD-TDP). Neurol Sci. 2011;32(4):653–9.

Arrasate M, Mitra S, Schweitzer ES, Segal MR, Finkbeiner S. Inclusion body formation reduces levels of mutant huntingtin and the risk of neuronal death. Nature. 2004;431(7010):805–10.

Boeve BF, Lang AE, Litvan I. Corticobasal degeneration and its relationship to progressive supranuclear palsy and frontotemporal dementia. Ann Neurol. 2003;54 Suppl 5:S15–9.

Brun A. Frontal lobe degeneration of non-Alzheimer type. I. Neuropathology. Arch Gerontol Geriatr. 1987;6(3):193–208.

Brun A. Identification and characterization of frontal lobe degeneration: historical perspective on the development of FTD. Alzheimer Dis Assoc Disord. 2007;21(4):S3–4.

Bugiani O. FTDP-17: phenotypical heterogeneity within P301S. Ann Neurol. 2000;48(1):126.

Buratti E, Baralle FE. TDP-43: new aspects of auto-regulation mechanisms in RNA binding proteins and their connection with human disease. FEBS J. 2011;278(19):3530–8.

Butti C, Sherwood CC, Hakeem AY, Allman JM, Hof PR. Total number and volume of Von Economo neurons in the cerebral cortex of cetaceans. J Comp Neurol. 2009;515:243–59.

Conrad C, Andreadis A, Trojanowski JQ, Dickson DW, Kang D, Chen X, Wiederholt W, Hansen L, Masliah E, Thal LJ, Katzman R, Xia Y, Saitoh T. Genetic evidence for the involvement of tau in progressive supranuclear palsy. Ann Neurol. 1997;41(2):277–81.

Coppola G, Chinnathambi S, Lee JJ, Dombroski BA, Baker MC, Soto-Ortolaza AI, Lee SE, Klein E, Huang AY, Sears R, Lane JR, Karydas AM, Kenet RO, Biernat J, Wang LS, Cotman CW, Decarli CS, Levey AI, Ringman JM, Mendez MF, Chui HC, Le Ber I, Brice A, Lupton MK, Preza E, Lovestone S, Powell J, Graff-Radford N, Petersen RC, Boeve BF, Lippa CF, Bigio EH, Mackenzie I, Finger E, Kertesz A, Caselli RJ, Gearing M, Juncos JL, Ghetti B, Spina S, Bordelon YM, Tourtellotte WW, Frosch MP, Vonsattel JP, Zarow C, Beach TG, Albin RL, Lieberman AP, Lee VM, Trojanowski JQ, Van Deerlin VM, Bird TD, Galasko DR, Masliah E, White CL, Troncoso JC, Hannequin D, Boxer AL, Geschwind MD, Kumar S, Mandelkow EM, Wszolek ZK, Uitti RJ, Dickson DW, Haines JL, Mayeux R, Pericak-Vance MA, Farrer LA; Alzheimer's Disease Genetics Consortium, Ross OA, Rademakers R, Schellenberg GD, Miller BL, Mandelkow E, Geschwind DH. Evidence for a role of the rare p.A152T variant in MAPT in increasing the risk for FTD-spectrum and Alzheimer's diseases. Hum Mol Genet. 2012;21:3500–12.

Couthouis J, Hart MP, Erion R, King OD, Diaz Z, Nakaya T, Ibrahim F, Kim HJ, Mojsilovic-Petrovic J, Panossian S, Kim CE, Frackelton EC, Solski JA, Williams KL, Clay-Falcone D, Elman L, McCluskey L, Greene R, Hakonarson H, Kalb RG, Lee VM, Trojanowski JQ, Nicholson GA, Blair IP, Bonini NM, Van Deerlin VM, Mourelatos Z, Shorter J, Gitler AD. Evaluating the role of the FUS/TLS-related gene EWSR1 in amyotrophic lateral sclerosis. Hum Mol Genet. 2012;21:2899–911.

Delfour F, Marten K. Mirror image processing in three marine mammal species: killer whales (Orcinus orca), false killer whales (Pseudorca crassidens) and California sea lions (Zalophus californianus). Behav Processes 2001;53(3):181–90.

Evrard HC, Forro T, Logothetis NK. Von Economo neurons in the anterior insula of the macaque monkey. Neuron. 2012;74(3):482–9.

Feany MB, Dickson DW. Neurodegenerative disorders with extensive tau pathology: a comparative study and review. Ann Neurol. 1996;40:139–48.

Fecto F, Yan J, Vemula SP, Liu E, Yang Y, Chen W, Zheng JG, Shi Y, Siddique N, Arrat H, Donkervoort S, Ajroud-Driss S, Sufit RL, Heller SL, Deng HX, Siddique T. SQSTM1 mutations in familial and sporadic amyotrophic lateral sclerosis. Arch Neurol. 2011;68:1440–6.

Forman MS, Farmer J, Johnson JK, Clark CM, Arnold SE, Coslett HB, Chatterjee A, Hurtig HI, Karlawish JH, Rosen HJ, Van Deerlin V, Lee VM, Miller BL, Trojanowski JQ, Grossman M. Frontotemporal dementia: clinicopathological correlations. Ann Neurol. 2006;59(6):952–62.

Frost B, Jacks RL, Diamond MI. Propagation of tau misfolding from the outside to the inside of a cell. J Biol Chem. 2009;284(19):12845–52.

Fujino Y, Wang DS, Thomas N, Espinoza M, Davies P, Dickson DW. Increased frequency of argyrophilic grain disease in Alzheimer disease with 4R tau-specific immunohistochemistry. J Neuropathol Exp Neurol. 2005;64(3):209–14.

Fujishiro H, Uchikado H, Arai T, Hasegawa M, Akiyama H, Yokota O, Tsuchiya K, Togo T, Iseki E, Hirayasu Y. Accumulation of phosphorylated TDP-43 in brains of patients with argyrophilic grain disease. Acta Neuropathol. 2009;117(2):151–8.

Gans A. Betrachtungen über Art und Ausbreitung des krankhaften Prozesses in einem Fall von Pickscher Atrophie des Stirnhirns. Ztschr f d gse Neurol u Psychiatr. 1922;80:10–28.

Goedert M, Clavaguera F, Tolnay M. The propagation of prion-like protein inclusions in neurodegenerative diseases. Trends Neurosci. 2010;33(7):317–25.

Goedert M, Spillantini MG. Pathogenesis of the tauopathies. J Mol Neurosci. 2011;45(3):425–31.

Gydesen, S., Brown, J. M., Brun, A., Chakrabarti, L., Gade, A., Johannsen, P., Rossor, M., Thusgaard, T., Grove, A., Yancopoulou, D., Spillantini, M. G., Fisher, E. M. C., Collinge, J., Sorensen, S. A. Chromosome 3 linked frontotemporal dementia (FTD-3). Neurology. 2002;59:1585–94.

Hakeem AY, Sherwood CC, Bonar CJ, Butti C, Hof PR, Allman JM. Von Economo neurons in the elephant brain. Anat Rec (Hoboken). 2009;292(2):242–8.

Höglinger GU, Melhem NM, Dickson DW, Sleiman PM, Wang LS, Klei L, Rademakers R, de Silva R, Litvan I,

Riley DE, van Swieten JC, Heutink P, Wszolek ZK, Uitti RJ, Vandrovcova J, Hurtig HI, Gross RG, Maetzler W, Goldwurm S, Tolosa E, Borroni B, Pastor P; PSP Genetics Study Group, Cantwell LB, Han MR, Dillman A, van der Brug MP, Gibbs JR, Cookson MR, Hernandez DG, Singleton AB, Farrer MJ, Yu CE, Golbe LI, Revesz T, Hardy J, Lees AJ, Devlin B, Hakonarson H, Müller U, Schellenberg GD. Identification of common variants influencing risk of the tauopathy progressive supranuclear palsy. Nat Genet. 2011;43:699–705.

Hong M, Zhukareva V, Vogelsberg-Ragaglia V, Wszolek Z, Reed L, Miller B, Geschwind D, Bird T, McKeel D, Goate A, Morris J, Wilhelmsen K, Schellenberg GD, Trojanowski J, Lee V. Mutation-specific functional impairments in distinct tau isoforms of hereditary FTDP-17. Science. 1998;282(5395):1914–17.

Ito D, Suzuki N. Conjoint pathologic cascades mediated by ALS/FTLD-U linked RNA-binding proteins TDP-43 and FUS. Neurology. 2011;77(17):1636–43.

Kadokura A, Yamazaki T, Lemere CA, Takatama M, Okamoto K. Regional distribution of TDP-43 inclusions in Alzheimer disease (AD) brains: their relation to AD common pathology. Neuropathology. 2009;29:566–73.

Kfoury N, Holmes BB, Jiang H, Holtzman DM, Diamond MI. Trans-cellular propagation of Tau aggregation by fibrillar species. J Biol Chem. 2012;287(23):19440–51.

Kim EJ, Sidhu M, Gaus SE, Huang EJ, Hof PR, Miller BL, DeArmond SJ, Seeley WW. Selective frontoinsular von Economo neuron and fork cell loss in early behavioral variant frontotemporal dementia. Cereb Cortex. 2012;22:251–9.

King OD, Gitler AD, Shorter J. The tip of the iceberg: RNA-binding proteins with prion-like domains in neurodegenerative disease. Brain Res. 2012;1462:61–80.

Koppers M, van Blitterswijk MM, Vlam L, Rowicka PA, van Vught PW, Groen EJ, Spliet WG, Engelen-Lee J, Schelhaas HJ, de Visser M, van der Kooi AJ, van der Pol WL, Pasterkamp RJ, Veldink JH, van den Berg LH. VCP mutations in familial and sporadic ALS. Neurobiol Aging. 2012;33:837.e7–13.

Kovacs GG, Rozemuller AJ, van Swieten JC, Gelpi E, Majtenyi K, Al-Sarraj S, Troakes C, Bódi I, King A, Hortobágyi T, Esiri MM, Ansorge O, Giaccone G, Ferrer I, Arzberger T, Bogdanovic N, Nilsson T, Leisser I, Alafuzoff I, Ironside JW, Kretzschmar H, Budka H. Neuropathology of the hippocampus in FTLD-Tau with Pick bodies: A study of the BrainNet Europe Consortium. Neuropathol Appl Neurobiol. 2012 Apr 4.[Epub ahead of print]

Kril JJ, Halliday GM. Pathological staging of frontotemporal lobar degeneration. J Mol Neurosci. 2011;45(3):379–83.

Leverenz JB, Yu CE, Montine TJ, Steinbart E, Bekris LM, Zabetian C, Kwong LK, Lee VM, Schellenberg GD, Bird TD. A novel progranulin mutation associated with variable clinical presentation and tau, TDP-43 and alpha-synuclein pathology. Brain. 2007;130 (Pt 5):1360–74.

Liscic RM, Grinberg LT, Zidar J, Gitcho MA, Cairns NJ. ALS and FTLD: two faces of TDP-43 proteinopathy. Eur J Neurol. 2008;15:772–80.

Mackenzie IR, Munoz DG, Kusaka H, Yokota O, Ishihara K, Roeber S, Kretzschmar HA, Cairns NJ, Neumann M. Distinct pathological subtypes of FTLD-FUS. Acta Neuropathol. 2011;121(2):207–18.

Mackenzie IR, Neumann M. FET proteins in frontotemporal dementia and amyotrophic lateral sclerosis. Brain Res. 2012;1462:40–3.

Mackenzie IR, Neumann M, Baborie A, Sampathu DM, Du Plessis D, Jaros E, Perry RH, Trojanowski JQ, Mann DM, Lee VM. A harmonized classification system for FTLD-TDP pathology. Acta Neuropathol. 2011;122(1):111–3.

Mandelkow EM, Mandelkow E. Biochemistry and cell biology of tau protein in neurofibrillary degeneration. Cold Spring Harb Perspect Med. 2012;2(7):a006247.

McKee AC, Gavett BE, Stern RA, Nowinski CJ, Cantu RC, Kowall NW, Perl DP, Hedley-Whyte ET, Price B, Sullivan C, Morin P, Lee HS, Kubilus CA, Daneshvar DH, Wulff M, Budson AE. TDP-43 proteinopathy and motor neuron disease in chronic traumatic encephalopathy. J Neuropathol Exp Neurol. 2010;69:918–29.

Murray ME, DeJesus-Hernandez M, Rutherford NJ, Baker M, Duara R, Graff-Radford NR, Wszolek ZK, Ferman TJ, Josephs KA, Boylan KB, Rademakers R, Dickson DW. Clinical and neuropathologic heterogeneity of c9FTD/ALS associated with hexanucleotide repeat expansion in C9ORF72. Acta Neuropathol. 2011;122:673–90.

Nelson PT, Abner EL, Schmitt FA, Kryscio RJ, Jicha GA, Smith CD, Davis DG, Poduska JW, Patel E, Mendiondo MS, Markesbery WR. Modeling the association between 43 different clinical and pathological variables and the severity of cognitive impairment in a large autopsy cohort of elderly persons. Brain Pathol. 2010;20:66–79.

Nelson PT, Schmitt FA, Lin Y, Abner EL, Jicha GA, Patel E, Thomason PC, Neitner JH, Smith CD, Santacruz KS, Sonnen JA, Poon LW, Gearing M, Green RC, Woodard JL, Van Eldik LJ, Kryscio RJ. Hippocampal sclerosis in advanced age: clinical and pathological features. Brain. 2011;134(5): 1506–18.

Neumann M, Bentmann E, Dormann D, Iawaid A, DeJesus-Hernandez M, Ansorge O, Roeber S, Kretzschmar HA, Munoz DG, Kusaka H, Yokota O, Ang LC, Bilbao J, Rademakers R, Haass C, Mackenzie IR. FET proteins TAF15 and EWS are selective markers that distinguish FTLD with FUS pathology from amyotrophic lateral sclerosis with FUS mutations. Brain. 2011;134(pt9):2595–609.

Neumann M, Sampathu DM, Kwong LK, Truax AC, Micsenyi MC, Chou TT, Bruce J, Schuck T, Grossman M, Clark CM, McCluskey LF, Miller BL, Masliah E, Mackenzie IR, Feldman H, Feiden W, Kretzschmar HA, Trojanowski JQ, Lee VM. Ubiquitinated TDP-43 in frontotemporal lobar degeneration and amyotrophic lateral sclerosis. Science. 2006;314:130–3.

Neumann M. Rademakers R, Roeber S, Baker M, Kretzschmar HA, Mackenzie IR. A new subtype of frontotemporal lobar degeneration with FUS pathology. Brain. 2009;132(Pt 11):2922–31.

Nimchinsky EA, Gilissen E, Allman JM, Perl DP, Erwin JM, Hof PR. A neuronal morphologic type unique to humans and great apes. Proc Natl Acad Sci USA. 1999;96(9):5268–73.

Plotnik JM, de Waal FB, Reiss D. Self-recognition in an Asian elephant. Proc Natl Acad Sci USA. 2006;103(45): 17053–7.

Polymenidou M, Lagier-Tourenne C, Hutt KR, Bennett CF, Cleveland DW, Yeo GW. Misregulated RNA processing in amyotrophic lateral sclerosis. Brain Res. 2012;1462:3–15.

Prusiner SB. Cell biology. A unifying role for prions in neurodegenerative diseases. Science. 2012;336(6088): 1511–3.

Prusiner SB. Novel proteinaceous infectious particles cause scrapie. Science. 1982;216(4542):136–44.

Rauramaa T, Pikkarainen M, Englung E, Ince PG, Jellinger K, Paetau A, Alafuzoff I. TAR-DNA binding protein-43 and alterations in the hippocampus. J Neural Transm. 2011;118:683–9.

Seeley WW, Carlin DA, Allman JM, Macedo MN, Bush C, Miller BL, DeArmond SJ. Early frontotemporal dementia targets neurons unique to apes and humans. Ann Neurol. 2006;60:660–7.

Seeley WW, Crawford R, Rascovsky K, Kramer JH, Weiner M, Miller BL, Gorno-Tempini ML. Frontal paralimbic network atrophy in very mild behavioral variant frontotemporal dementia. Arch Neurol. 2008;65(2):249–55.

Seeley WW, Merkle FT, Gaus SE, Craig AD, Allman JM, Hof PR, Economo CV. Distinctive neurons of the anterior cingulate and frontoinsular cortex: a historical perspective. Cereb Cortex. 2012;22(2):245–50.

Shelley BP, Hodges JR, Kipps CM, Xuereb JH, Bak TH. Is the pathology of corticobasal syndrome predictable in life? Mov Disord. 2009;24:1593–9.

Siddique T, Ajroud-Driss S. Familial amyotrophic lateral sclerosis, a historical perspective. Acta Myol. 2011;30:117–20.

Sima AA, Defendini R, Keohane C, D'Amato C, Foster NL, Parchi P, Gambetti P, Lynch T, Wilhelmsen KC. The neuropathology of chromosome 17-linked dementia. Ann Neurol. 1996;39(6):734–43.

Soma K, Fu YJ, Wakabayashi K, Onodera O, Kakita A, Takahashi H. Co-occurrence of argyrophilic grain disease in sporadic amyotrophic lateral sclerosis. Neuropathol Appl Neurobiol. 2012;38(1):54–60.

Thal DR, Schultz C, Botez G, Del Tredici K, Mrak RE, Griffin WS, Wiestler OD, Braak H, Ghebremedhin E. The impact of argyrophilic grain disease on the development of dementia and its relationship to concurrent Alzheimer's disease-related pathology. Neuropathol Appl Neurobiol. 2005;31(3):270–9.

Urwin H, Josephs KA, Rohrer JD, Mackenzie IR, Neumann M, Authier A, Seelaar H, Van Swieten JC, Brown JM, Johannsen P, Nielsen JE, Holm IE; FREJA Consortium, Dickson DW, Rademakers R, Graff-Radford NR, Parisi JE, Petersen RC, Hatanpaa KJ, White CL 3rd, Weiner MF, Geser F, Van Deerlin VM, Trojanowski JQ, Miller BL, Seeley WW, van der Zee J, Kumar-Singh S, Engelborghs S, De Deyn PP, Van Broeckhoven C, Bigio EH, Deng HX, Halliday GM, Kril JJ, Munoz DG, Mann DM, Pickering-Brown SM, Doodeman V, Adamson G, Ghazi-Noori S, Fisher EM, Holton JL, Revesz T, Rossor MN, Collinge J, Mead S, Isaacs AM. FUS pathology defines the majority of tau- and TDP-43-negative frontotemporal lobar degeneration. Acta Neuropathol. 2010; 120:33–41.

Webb A, Miller B, Bonasera S, Boxer A, Karydas A, Wilhelmsen KC. Role of the tau gene region chromosome inversion in progressive supranuclear palsy, corticobasal degeneration, and related disorders. Arch Neurol. 2008;65(11):1473–8.

Wilhelmsen KC, Lynch T, Pavlou E, Higgins M, Nygaard TG. Localization of disinhibition-dementia-parkinsonism-amyotrophy complex to 17q21-22. Am J Hum Genet. 1994;55:1159–65.

Zhang Y, Schuff N, Ching C, Tosun D, Zhan W, Nezamzadeh M, Rosen HJ, Kramer JH, Gorno-Tempini ML, Miller BL, Weiner MW. Joint assessment of structural, perfusion, and diffusion MRI in Alzheimer's disease and frontotemporal dementia. Int J Alzheimers Dis. 2011;2011:546871.

Zhou J, Gennatas ED, Kramer JH, Miller BL, Seeley WW. Predicting regional neurodegeneration from the healthy brain functional connectome. Neuron. 2012;73(6):1216–27.

Chapter 8

FTD Genes

OVERVIEW

Frontotemporal dementia (FTD) has a significant genetic component, and approximately 40% of patients exhibit a family history for dementia, a neuropsychiatric syndrome, or movement disorder, and 10% have an autosomal dominant history that suggests an underlying single gene cause of illness (Chow et al. 1999). An autosomal dominant form of FTD should be considered when three or more family members are affected in successive generations, with two individuals who are first-degree relatives of the third.

Many, but not all, of the disease-causing genes associated with FTD are now known. With the discovery of each new gene comes a plethora of new insights into the molecular basis and pathogenesis of the various forms of FTD. Additionally finding new genes facilitates the study of patients who are in the earliest stage of their illness—gene carriers who are often many decades away from the onset of formal dementia. Knowing the genes that lead to FTD has facilitated the development of animal models that are based on these mutations. In turn, these powerful model systems allow investigators to explore the pathogenesis of FTD and test compounds that might slow down or even stop the degenerative process.

The three genes most frequently implicated in FTD, listed in decreasing order of frequency in the UCSF samples are *C9ORF72*, tau (*MAPT*), and progranulin (*GRN*). The clinical features of patients with mutations in these genes and mutations in other genes less

131

frequently associated with FTD, including *VCP*, *CHMP2B*, *TARDBP*, *FUS*, *EXT2*, *SQSTM1*, and *UBQLN2* will be described in this chapter. Similarly, the basic biology of these genes and the proteins that they produce will be discussed. Finally, there will be a brief discussion of genes including apolipoprotein E4 (apoE-ε4) and catechol-o-methyltransferase (COMT) that appear to modify the presentation and possibly progression of FTD-spectrum disorders.

GENES IMPLICATED IN FTD

Listed below are the genes known to harbor pathogenic mutations for FTD:

- **MAPT** on chromosome 17 encodes the microtubule-associated protein tau. Tau is involved with the assembly and maintenance of microtubules (Hong et al. 1998). Both exon and intron mutations in *MAPT* can lead to FTD, progressive supranuclear palsy (PSP), or corticobasal degeneration (CBD) syndromes (Hutton et al. 1998; Spillantini et al. 1998; Clark et al. 1998).
- **GRN** on chromosome 17 encodes progranulin, a glycoprotein that functions as an autocrine growth factor. It can be processed into smaller peptides called granulins that appear to be involved with proinflammatory pathways (Baker et al. 2006; Rademakers et al. 2007; Ward & Miller, 2011).
- **C9ORF72** on chromosome 9 encodes a protein of unknown function, called *C9orf72*. There are two isoforms of the *C9orf72* protein with apparent molecular masses of 55 kDA and 25 kDA. A hexanucleotide repeat expansion in a noncoding region of *C9ORF72* is the most common cause for the familial forms of both FTD and ALS and FTD-ALS. Additionally, it accounts for approximately 5% of sporadic cases of FTD and ALS (Millecamps et al. 2012; DeJesus-Hernandez et al. 2011; Renton et al. 2011).
- **TARDBP** on chromosome 1 encodes the 43 kDa transactive response (TAR) DNA-binding protein (TDP-43). Mutations in this gene are rare and usually cause pure ALS syndromes, but there are a few examples of mutations in TDP-43 that also lead to FTD and extrapyramidal syndromes (Borghero et al. 2011; Mosca et al. 2012).

- **VCP** on chromosome 9 encodes valosin-containing protein. Mutations in this gene cause inclusion body myositis with Paget's disease of bone. Only about one-third to half of patients with *VCP* mutations develop an FTD syndrome (Watts et al. 2007). ALS is also associated with mutations in *VCP* (Johnson et al. 2010).
- **FUS** on chromosome 16 is the second most common mutation associated with familial ALS (Kwiatkowski et al. 2009). Like TDP-43, this gene produces a protein that regulates both DNA and RNA expression. While most patients with mutations in *FUS* manifest ALS, there are patients who develop FTD as well (Yan et al. 2010; Huey et al. 2012). Additionally, mutations may also be a risk for familial essential tremor (Merner et al. 2012).
- **CHMP2B** on chromosome 3 encodes charged multivesicular body protein 2B (also known as chromatin modifying protein 2B). Mutations in this gene are a rare cause of FTD and have been observed primarily in related families of Danish descent (Lindquist et al. 2008).
- **SQSTM1** on chromosome 5 encodes ubiquitin-binding protein p62, also known as sequestosome 1. Mutations in this gene were recently identified as a cause of familial and sporadic ALS. There are still very few reports about this gene but it appears that a dementia syndrome is associated with this gene in addition to the ALS (Fecto et al. 2011).
- **UBQLN2** on the X chromosome encodes ubiquilin-2, a gene product involved in ubiquitin-mediated protein degradation. Mutations in this gene, which cause ALS with or without dementia, are inherited in an X-linked pattern. (Deng et al. 2011)

Other genetic mutations have been associated with FTD, but their links to this disorder are more poorly understood. These mutations involve the genes dynactin (*DCTN1*) (Münch et al. 2005; Vilariño-Güell et al. 2009), *TREM-2* (Ken Kosik, personal communication), and exostosin2 (*EXT-2*) (Narvid et al. 2009). While dynactin, *TREM-2*, and *EXT2* may be responsible for a few cases of FTD, their presence in clinical populations is uncommon. Table 8–1 lists the clinical and molecular features of the eight major genes known to cause FTD.

Table 8–1 Genes Responsible for Frontotemporal Dementia (FTD)

Gene	Protein	Function	Syndrome	Brain Inclusion
C9ORF72	Unknown	Unknown	FTD, ALS, or FTD-ALS	TDP type A or TDP type B and RNA nuclear aggregates
MAPT	Tau	Microtubule stabilization	FTD, PSP, CBD	Tau aggregates and tangles
GRN	Progranulin	Growth factor, inflammation	FTD, CBD, PD, AD	TDP type A
TARDBP	TDP43	DNA, RNA modulation	ALS, rarely FTD	?
VCP	ATP-binding	Intracellular transport	Paget's, IBM, FTD (ALS?)	TDP type D
ESCRT2	ESCRT2	Form and sort endosome cargo	FTD	Unknown
EXT2		Protein processing	Osteosarcomas, myopathy, and FTD	

MAPT

TAU OVERVIEW

Tau was discovered in 1975 by cell biologist Marc Kirschner and his team (Weingarten et al. 1975). Tau is a microtubule-associated protein that helps to assemble and stabilize microtubules while simultaneously facilitating axonal transport along the neuron and maintaining neuronal structure.

In humans, tau has six isoforms that are generated in neurons via alternative splicing. The isoforms differ depending on whether they have 29- or 58- amino-acid inserts in the amino-terminal region or contain a 31-amino acid repeat in the carboxy-terminal region. Exon 10 encodes this carboxy-terminal inclusion that is associated with three different tau isoforms, all of which have four repeats. Neurons have approximately equal concentrations of the 3R and 4R tau isoforms with a slightly greater concentration of 3R tau in cortex. In patients with tau mutations in or around exon 10, most of the neuropathological aggregates consist of 4R tau, while in those with mutations outside that region both 3 and 4R aggregations are seen.

In the early to early to mid-1980s, a variety of investigators including Bernadino Ghetti (Ghetti & Gambetti 1983), Andre Delacourte (Delacourte & Defossez 1986), Peter Davies and Ben Wolozin (Wolozin et al. 1986), Ken Kosik and Dennis Selkoe (Kosik et al. 1986), and J. P. Brion (Brion et al. 1986) determined that there were strong links between tau and dementia. Tau is a major component of the neurofibrillary tangle in Alzheimer's disease (AD), the globose tangle and tufted astrocyte in PSP, the coiled neuron and astrocytic plaque in CBD, the Pick body in Pick's disease, and the argyrophilic grains in argyrophilic grain disease (Feany & Dickson 1996).

TAU CLINICAL GENETICS

In 1994 Kirk Wilhelmsen and Timothy Lynch linked a family with a frontal dementia, parkinsonism, and amyotrophy to a region on chromosome 17 (17q21-22) (Wilhelmsen et al. 1994). Soon afterward approximately 15 families with a non-AD familial dementia were linked to this same region on chromosome 17. In 1998, Hutton and colleagues demonstrated FTD-causing mutations within the exons 9-13, a region of tau that is involved with microtubule binding, and in IVS10 (intervening sequence 10), an intron involved in alternative splicing of mRNA transcripts (Hutton et al. 1998).

The spectrum of disease seen with *MAPT* mutations was broad, with the majority of patients exhibiting a bvFTD syndrome, although others were diagnosed with nonfluent/agrammatic variant of primary progressive aphasia (nfvPPA), semantic variant of PPA (svPPA), PSP, or CBD. Remarkably, these *MAPT* mutations displayed significant variability in clinical expression, even among individuals within a family who shared the same mutation. For example, Bugiani (Bugiani et al. 1999) described a family with CBD in one generation and FTD in another. In addition, the clinical phenotypes associated with *MAPT* mutations could not be easily distinguished from those observed in sporadic disease with underlying tau neuropathology. Wszolek characterized a large family with a loop shaped intron mutation between exons 9 and 10 in whom many of the family members developed a PSP-like illness (Clark et al. 1998). In addition to the neuropsychiatric syndromes associated with these mutations, it is now accepted that there is a schizophrenia-like presentation in some patients with tau mutations (Khan et al. 2012).

Much has been learned about *MAPT* gene carriers since the initial studies, and more than 44 distinctive mutations have been reported in 132 different families. Patients with *MAPT* mutations tend to present clinically at around age 50, and these mutations account for approximately 5% of autosomal dominant FTD. *MAPT* mutations are rarely observed in the absence of a family history of FTD, dementia, or parkinsonism (Seelaar et al. 2001).

Many gene carriers exhibit a long prodrome with psychiatric illness before developing a frank dementia. The types of psychiatric problems we have seen include addictive behaviors, anxiety, risk-taking, depression (and sometimes suicide), loss of emotional connections with family and friends, and a tendency toward social isolation. Often, this prodrome slowly devolves into deteriorating work and social function. In some of our patients, before a dementia emerges, the prominent presence of psychiatric symptoms leads to a diagnosis of borderline personality disorder, schizophrenia, or bipolar illness.

In a 2001 study of a Quebec family who carried the *P301L* mutation, Dan Geschwind, Ziad Nasreddine, and colleagues demonstrated that gene carriers were already exhibiting frontal executive deficits in their 20s, decades before they were likely to manifest dementia (Geschwind et al. 2001). While not all the families with a *MAPT* mutation that we have studied show an early abnormality in executive function in gene carriers, its presence can be a clue to the gene status of the patient.

It is our impression that mutation carriers are less likely to seek out their gene status than are noncarrier siblings, reflecting suspiciousness and even paranoia as well as a tendency toward denial of illness—anosognosia. These psychiatric disorders together suggest that very early in life literally many decades before the onset of dementia, *MAPT* gene mutation carriers may already be showing clinical manifestations of their illness.

Jonathan Rohrer and colleagues at Queen Square have shown that the brains of *MAPT* patients tend to exhibit symmetrical anterior frontotemporal degeneration; asymmetric FTD syndromes are less common with these mutations (Rohrer & Warren 2011).

Because the basal ganglia degenerates along with cortical structures in *MAPT* mutation carriers, some patients begin with a parkinsonian-type syndrome that includes falls, staring, or axial rigidity. An ophthalmoplegia suggestive of PSP is very common. In the later stages of the illness, patients become bedridden and have problems with aspiration.

Early recognition of brain dysfunction is being sought for the gene mutations that cause FTD. While some patients already with *MAPT* mutations show atrophic patterns suggestive of early bvFTD before they are symptomatic, this is unusual. More commonly, patients begin with subtle psychiatric symptoms (Khan et al. 2012) but exhibit normal findings on structural imaging. An imaging biomarker such as functional MRI might help to determine when a therapy should be introduced. William Seeley and Suzee Lee at UCSF and John van Swieten in Holland are exploring the use of connectivity mapping to detect changes in the fronto-insular, anterior temporal, and ventral striatal circuits that tau mutations appear to attack in the early stages of disease (Zhou et al. 2012) (Figure 8–1).

TAU BASIC BIOLOGY

Two distinctive mechanisms have been hypothesized for how *MAPT* mutations cause disease. With IVS10 splice site mutations, tau mRNA transcripts are preferentially spliced, which disrupts the 1:1 ratio between 3R and 4R isoforms of tau in favor of 4R (Hutton et al. 1998). The 4R isoform binds poorly to microtubules and shows an abnormal affinity for self-aggregation in neurons and glia. Most of the disease-causing exon mutations are found within exons 9, 10, 11, or 12, associated with microtubule binding sites. Missense mutations in these exons seem to lead to abnormal microtubule binding (Hutton et al. 1998; Clark et al. 1998; Poorkaj

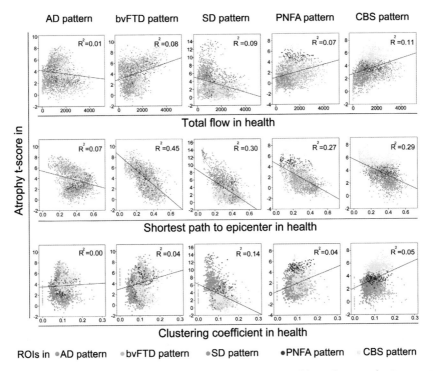

Figure 8–1. Transnetwork Graph Theoretical Connectivity Measures in Health Predict Atrophy Severity in Disease. **Row 2:** ROIs showing greater disease-related atrophy were those featuring shorter functional paths, in the healthy brain, to the disease-associated epicenters (p < 0.05 familywise error corrected for multiple comparisons for AD, bvFTD, SD, PNFA, and CBS). **Rows 1 and 3:** Inconsistent weaker or nonsignificant relationships were observed between total flow or clustering coefficient and disease-related atrophy. (Zhou et al. 2012.)

et al. 1998 Spillantini et al. 1998). This, in turn, causes destabilization of the neuron's structure and function and ultimately neuronal death.

In addition to pathogenic mutations, there are other *MAPT* genotypes that are overrepresented in FTD-spectrum disorders. These genotypes reflect normal genetic variation. *MAPT* is located within one of two haplotypes, called H1 and H2, which are segments of DNA variants (or polymorphisms) that tend to be inherited together as discrete units, across which recombination is suppressed or selected against (Fung et al. 2005). The H2 haplotype is found nearly exclusively in Caucasians and was created as the result of an ancient inversion event involving a DNA span of 100 kb. The H1/H1 genotype is observed in approximately 90% of Caucasian patients with PSP and CBD, while only 60–70% of healthy controls are H1 homozygotes (Conrad et al. 1997; Baker et al. 1999). This suggests an increased susceptibility to PSP and CBD among individuals with the H1/H1 genotype. The mechanism for

increased susceptibility is unknown, but this polymorphism may increase the amount of 4R tau expressed by the neuron (Myers et al. 2007).

Similarly, A152T, a rare variant in the tau gene on exon 7, present in approximately 0.3% of controls and about 0.8–1% of FTLD-spectrum disorders, predisposes individuals to nfvPPA, CBD, PSP, and bvFTD. The relative risk for gene carriers is similar to the risk of apoE-ε4) for AD. The mechanism for this susceptibility to FTD-spectrum disorders is under active study, but this rare tau variant seems to be associated with increased expression of 4R tau and also has a tendency to fragment into toxic oligomers that poison neuronal functions.

Additionally, this A152T polymorphism also increases an individual's susceptibility to AD by approximately twofold. To date, this is the only tau polymorphism with a clear association with both FTD spectrum disorders and AD (Coppola et al. 2012). In the study of patients with this polymorphism, it appears that those with FTD get the illness at a younger age (50s and 60s) while the patients who develop AD are much older (70s).

TAU THERAPEUTIC APPROACHES

There have been a variety of therapeutic approaches considered for patients with tau-related neurodegeneration. The philanthropy-supported Tau Consortium is exploring better ways to treat FTD-related syndromes. Tau mutation carriers represent the ideal group to explore therapies because they can be followed from asymptomatic into early symptomatic phases of their disease when treatment is more likely to be effective.

Because tau acetylation followed by phosphorylation may begin the neurodegenerative process, compounds that block or reverse these enzymatic steps are being considered (Min et al. 2010). Other approaches focus on stabilizing microtubules. Salicylate blocks tau acetylation (Li Gan, personal communication), while epothilon B (Zhang et al. 2012) seems to stabilize tau and is being considered as a therapy for PSP. The GSK-inhibitors NYPTA and lithium have been tried in clinical trials for AD and PSP, but these trials have been stopped because they have proven too toxic (lithium) and not efficacious (NYPTA). Similarly, the tau stabilizing compound davunetide (Gold 2012) failed to prove efficacious in a 300-person placebo-controlled trial for PSP.

Ken Kosik and colleagues have focused on cyclin dependent kinase 5 (CDK5) (Kosik & Shimura 2005), a protein that is involved in the phosphorylation of tau. When this protein is silenced there is diminished phosphorylation of tau in neurons and there is a decrease in neurofibrillary tangles in the hippocampus of triple transgenic mice (Piedrahita et al. 2010).

Additionally, in animal models the suppression of tau production or removal of tau (by antibodies) can markedly alleviate, if not prevent, the development of clinical disease (Roberson et al. 2007). Initially there were concerns that antibody therapies would not work because tau was intracellular, but new evidence that tau is present in the synaptic space between neurons (Kfoury et al. 2012) gives hope to the idea that antibodies might be able to remove tau from the brain, diminishing its spread and toxicity. This has opened the possibility for a multitude of therapeutic approaches focused around the clearance of tau by different antibodies that will likely be tried in the near future.

Over the past decade there has been important research that has helped to understand the way that the cell metabolizes tau. Tau is an unfolded protein that is highly soluble, but Eva Mandelkow and Eckhardt Mandelkow note as well "the large number of structural conformations and biochemical modifications (phosphorylation, proteolysis, glycosylation, and others), [and] the multitude of interaction partners (mainly microtubules, but also other cytoskeletal proteins, kinases, and phosphatases, motor proteins, chaperones, and membrane proteins)" (Mandelkow & Mandelkow 2012).

It is now known that the heat shock proteins are responsible for preventing unfolded proteins like tau from aggregating and injuring the neuron (Abisambra et al. 2011). The chaperone system that involves the proteins carboxy terminus of Hsc70 interacting protein (CHIP) and heat shock protein 70 (HSP70) helps bring tau to the proteasome. The BCL2-associated athanogene 2 (BAG2)/HSP70 chaperones help bring tau from the microtubule to the proteasome for degradation (Carrettiero et al. 2009). Dan Finley at Harvard has explored better ways of clearing tau via the proteasome (Finley 2011; Dange et al. 2011), while Michele Goedert at Cambridge has studied the removal of tau via autophagy (Schaeffer et al. 2012; Schaeffer & Goedert 2012). These approaches offer the opportunity to bring new therapies for tau-related neurodegeneration. FTD-spectrum disorders like PSP and CBD represent an exciting target for tau-therapies because, unlike AD, the disease is caused solely by tau.

GRN

OVERVIEW

After *MAPT* mutations were discovered as a cause for FTD, other families remained whose illness displayed linkage to chromosome 17 but were not associated with *MAPT* mutations. Many investigators speculated that pathogenic mutations in the promoter region of *MAPT* had thus far eluded detection. Yet, in 2006, parallel publications from Mayo Clinic led by Matt Baker, Rosa Rademakers, and Michael Hutton (Baker et al. 2006) and from the University of Antwerp in Belgium led by Christine van Broekhoeven (Cruts et al. 2006) demonstrated that these chromosome 17–linked families carried a mutation in *GRN*, that was found in a DNA span only 1 kb away from the *MAPT* locus. The close proximity of these two genes that were associated with FTD appeared to be a remarkable coincidence.

Mutations in *GRN* are the only pathogenic alleles that seem to cause disease via haploinsufficiency. Indeed, haploinsufficiency rarely causes neurodegenerative disease. The most common *GRN* mutation, p.R493X, is a nonsense mutation (Rademakers et al. 2007), which results in the introduction of a stop codon that results in premature truncation of the mRNA transcript and its subsequent nonsense-mediated decay. Other pathogenic alleles include frameshift or promoter region mutations, which also lead to the functional loss of one *GRN* allele. Measurement of blood *GRN* mRNA (Coppola et al. 2006) or plasma progranulin levels (Finch et al. 2009) shows that peripheral concentrations are less than 50% of normal. These diminished levels of mRNA and protein, make *GRN* mutation carriers a group of patients in whom a robust peripheral biomarker is available for clinical trials.

A fascinating recent clinical report has linked progranulin deficiency to neuronal ceroid lipufuscinosis. Smith and colleagues described a brother and a sister in their early twenties with a rapidly progressive dementia with myoclonic seizures, retinal dystrophy, and cerebellar ataxia. MRI from both showed mild cerebellar atrophy (Smith et al. 2012). Electron microscopy from a skin biopsy suggested neuronal ceroid lipufuscinosis with "fingerprint profiles in membrane-bound structures in eccrine-secretory cells and in endothelium." After extensive genetic profiling, it was determined that both the brother and sister were homozygous for a c.813_816del (p.Thr272Serfs°10) mutation in the *GRN* gene. Progranulin levels were absent in peripheral blood, supporting a complete loss of the progranulin protein.

Because neuronal ceroid lipofuscinosis is a disorder associated with extensive aggregation of lipofuscin that develops secondary to abnormal lysosomal processing, the presence of lipufuscinosis in two progranulin deficient siblings suggests that progranulin is involved with lysosomal functions. Lipofuscin is membrane-bound waste material within the cell, and it accumulates when there is incomplete lysosomal degradation of damaged mitochondria. Lipofuscin appears to accumulate within nondividing cells like neurons, and its presence may impair the ubiquitin and proteasome pathway (Gray & Woulfe 2005).

Smith and her colleagues suggested that the GRN homozygosity "results in microglial activation, increased ubiquitination, and excess lipopigment deposition" (Smith et al. 2012). This data from humans is congruent with data from homozygous progranulin deficient mice showing that there is abnormal autofluorescent lipopigment in neurons (Ahmed et al. 2010). Whether the lipufuscinosis is unique to homozygotes, or represents a more generalized defect in lysosomal function that also occurs in *GRN* heterozygotes as well, is still being studied. Further studies of lipofuscin in human tissues of patients with *GRN* mutations and in animal models of *GRN* deficiency will be needed to better understand the role of lipofuscin in this form of FTLD.

PROGRANULIN CLINICAL GENETICS

The deficiency of progranulin causes a circuit-specific neurodegenerative condition with a propensity to attack the frontoinsular region. To date, 69 different *GRN* mutations have been reported in 231 families. *GRN* mutations are responsible for 5–10% of all cases of FTLD and 13–25% of familial cases (Boeve & Hutton 2008; Gass et al. 2006; Rademakers et al. 2007). Patients with *GRN* mutations tend to be older than those with *MAPT* mutations, and in a large Dutch cohort, the typical age-of-diagnosis was 62 years (Seelaar et al. 2011). Unlike *MAPT* and *C9ORF72* mutations, which display near 100% penetrance by age 70, approximately 10% of *GRN* mutation carriers remain asymptomatic by age 70 years and do not suffer from dementia (Seelaar et al. 2011). This variability in the age-of-onset complicates genetic counseling for individuals who carry *GRN*, because there is a high degree of uncertainty as to whether the gene carrier will ever get FTD.

There are a variety of genetic factors that are known to either diminish or increase the likelihood that a gene carrier will develop a dementia. Finch, Rademakers, and colleagues have demonstrated that the minor allele variant in

TMEM106 can delay the age of onset for FTD or even prevent the disease (Finch et al. 2011). In their series of patients with *GRN* mutations, carriers of the minor allele were severely underrepresented and tended to present later in life. This minor allele may help to increase progranulin expression in the normal chromosome, thereby protecting patients with this normal variant from FTD. The minor *TMEM106* variant may be a factor in why some patients do not exhibit FTD by age 70.

Additionally, Rademakers and colleagues have found another common genetic variant (rs5848), in the untranslated region of *GRN* that is a binding-site for a microRNA called (miR-659) that may change the susceptibility for FTLD of the non-tau subtype (Hsiung et al. 2011). In a series of pathology confirmed patients with FTLD with ubiquitin inclusions patient carriers homozygous for the T-allele of rs5848 had an approximately twofold increased risk for this clinical subtype of FTLD compared to homozygous C-allele carriers. The authors suggested that the microRNA-659 more efficiently bound to the T than to the C allele, thereby suppressing *GRN* expression more efficiently.

While most *GRN* mutations lead to a bvFTD syndrome, other patients begin with nfvPPA, svPPA, CBD, Parkinson's disease, and sometimes AD (Rademakers et al. 2007). Sleegars and colleagues suggest that *GRN* mutations may also be a risk factor for AD, although the mechanism for this association is unknown (Sleegers et al. 2010). We have seen the coassociation of AD in two *GRN* mutation carriers under the age of 60 and have hypothesized that a progranulin deficiency also predisposes to AD (David Perry, personal communication). This may account for the higher number of AD diagnoses in cohorts of *GRN* mutation carriers.

Unlike *MAPT* mutations, which cause relatively symmetrical neurodegeneration, *GRN*-associated disease can be asymmetrical, predominantly affecting one hemisphere while sparing the other (Rohrer & Warren 2011). Also, neurodegeneration associated with *GRN* mutations is more likely to be associated with parietal and even occipital atrophy than is typical for sporadic FTD. *GRN* mutations do not appear to be associated with ALS, but patients do go on to develop parkinsonian features as the disease progresses.

When the disease attacks the right hemisphere, a progressive sociopathy with loss of emotional warmth and disinhibition can be the dominant syndrome. By contrast, when the left hemisphere is involved the patients usually present with executive problems or PPA. A highly asymmetric neurodegenerative pattern in a patient with a familial form of FTD strongly suggests the presence of a *GRN* mutation (Rohrer & Warren 2011).

As with the other FTD-related mutations, there is often a long psychiatric prodrome with addictive behaviors, social decline, and, sometimes, cognitive deficits and movement abnormalities that precede the onset of dementia. Hallucinations may be particularly common in *GRN* mutation carriers (Le Ber et al. 2008), and we have seen patients diagnosed with borderline personality disorder, antisocial personality disorder, bipolar illness, and even schizophrenia.

PROGRANULIN BASIC BIOLOGY

The full-length progranulin protein is a ~70-kDa glycoprotein of 7.5 tandem, cysteine-rich modules that are called granulins. The unprocessed progranulin protein seems to have growth factor features and increases cell proliferation and survival. Additionally, it may be neuroprotective via anti-inflammatory effects. By contrast, the granulins that are cleaved from progranulin work as pro-inflammatory molecules (Hu et al. 2010; Ward & Miller 2011).

The regulation of progranulin is under active study. The holoprotein is broken down into smaller granulin molecules by serine proteases such as elastase. A protein called "secreted leukocyte protease inhibitor" is secreted by neurotrophils and macrophages and inhibits the breakdown of progranulin (Grobmyer et al. 2000). High levels of full-length progranulin are found in wounds of secreted leukocyte protease inhibitor deficient mice, supporting its role in protecting the body from inflammation (Zhu et al. 2002).

Progranulin is produced across body and brain and seems to act on neurons via the sortilin receptor (Hu et al. 2010). When the brain is injured, glia produce progranulin and granulins. There is microglial activation with release of cytokines and other inflammatory proteins including TNF-α. Progranulin has an antagonizing effect on the TNF-α receptor and modulates inflammation via this mechanism (Cenik et al. 2012).

Aimee Kao has demonstrated in progranulin deficient worms that there is an accelerated apoptosis. Additionally, she found that macrophages cultured from progranulin knockout mice displayed increased rates of apoptotic-cell phagocytosis (Kao et al. 2011). This interesting data set links progranulin deficiency to accelerated cellular death via an inflammatory mechanism.

This dual role of progranulin has been demonstrated in progranulin deficient mice. Bob Farese and Lauren Herl Martens have shown an exaggerated inflammatory response in progranulin knockout mice. In their models, the bacterial-derived endotoxin lipopolysaccharide (LPS) combined with interferon-gamma stimulates a massive increase in microglial activation and cytokine release (Figure 8–2).

In addition to its role in inflammation, progranulin is involved with neuronal growth and protection. Andrew Bateman who first discovered progranulin (Bateman et al. 1990) showed that this protein is located within compartments of the secretory pathway including the Golgi apparatus (Toh et al. 2011). Transfection of progranulin in motor neurons triggered the appearance of dendrites, and its presence helped these cells to survive serum deprivation for up to two months via an antiapoptotic mechanism (Ryan et al. 2009). Progranulin deficient mice show a marked decrease in synaptic density (Petkau et al. 2012). Similarly, in studies by Tapia and colleagues (Tapia et al. 2011), lowering the progranulin levels in rat primary hippocampal cultures reduced neural connectivity by decreasing neuronal arborization and length as well as synapse density.

Hence there are at least two metabolic pathways that are important for the neurodegenerative process. One pathway is mediated via the whole progranulin protein that is a growth factor for neurons, while the other is mediated via the granulins that are pro-inflammatory (Toh et al. 2011, Ward & Miller 2011). These two mechanisms, growth and inflammation, are mediated by different pathways. Sortilin appears to be the neuronal receptor for the whole progranulin molecule (Hu et al. 2010) and may help to bring progranulin into and out of the neuron, while the inflammatory pathway may be stimulated by the granulins.

PROGRANULIN THERAPEUTIC APPROACHES

Understanding of the pathogenesis of FTD due to *GRN* mutations has been greatly facilitated by the Consortium for Frontotemporal Dementia established by Bob Farese, Lennart Mucke, and myself at UCSF and Joachim Herz at the University of Texas at Dallas. This consortium has created cell-culture, induced pluripotent stem cells (iPSCs) derived neurons, worm, and mouse models of FTD. Figure 8–3 demonstrates some of the model systems that are helping to tease out the role of inflammation versus neuronal death associated with FTD.

These new discoveries have offered great excitement for potential therapeutic interventions in gene carriers. One approach to the treatment of FTD related to progranulin would

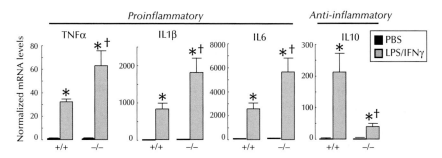

Figure 8–2. The models of Bob Farese and Lauren Herl Martens show an exaggerated inflammatory response in progranulin knockout mice. In their models, the bacterial-derived endotoxin lipopolysaccharide (LPS) combined with interferon-gamma stimulates a massive increase in microglial activation and cytokine release. The figure shows quantitative data measuring the mRNA of cytokines in phosphate buffered saline or stimulated primary microglia derived from the mice. (Image courtesy of Lauren Herl Martens.)

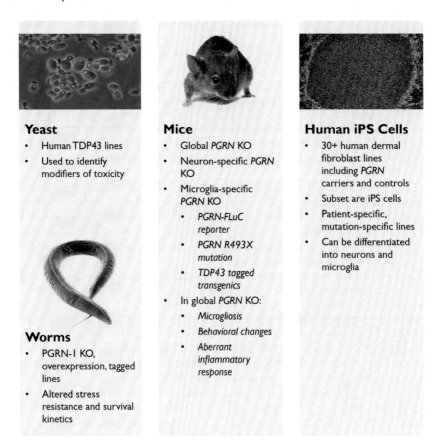

Yeast
- Human TDP43 lines
- Used to identify modifiers of toxicity

Worms
- PGRN-1 KO, overexpression, tagged lines
- Altered stress resistance and survival kinetics

Mice
- Global *PGRN* KO
- Neuron-specific *PGRN* KO
- Microglia-specific *PGRN* KO
  - *PGRN-FLuC reporter*
  - *PGRN R493X mutation*
  - *TDP43 tagged transgenics*
- In global *PGRN* KO:
  - *Microgliosis*
  - *Behavioral changes*
  - *Aberrant inflammatory response*

Human iPS Cells
- 30+ human dermal fibroblast lines including *PGRN* carriers and controls
- Subset are iPS cells
- Patient-specific, mutation-specific lines
- Can be differentiated into neurons and microglia

Figure 8–3. Models of progranulin.

be to increase the production of this protein by either upregulating expression of the normal allele or correcting expression of the pathogenic allele with medications that read through a nonsense mutation, for example (Cenik et al. 2011). There is still uncertainty with regard to whether progranulin deficiency works via an inflammatory mechanism or through a growth factor deficiency. This distinction is important because if inflammation is important, anti-TNF compounds could prove effective. By contrast, if the growth factor activity of progranulin is critical, more effective approaches would require stimulating sortilin by elevating brain progranulin or via other receptor agonists. In preliminary work with Tony Wyss-Coray, the major proteomic signals that differentiate *GRN* human carriers and mice with *GRN* deficiency is that TNF-α is significantly raised, offering a potential target for anti-inflammatory approaches.

Our program has had little success in compounds that are designed to read through nonsense mutations but has made significant progress in the development of medications that seem to increase progranulin expression. The histone deacetylase inhibitor (HDAC) vorinostat markedly increases progranulin levels in cell culture and iPSCs (Cenik et al. 2011) (Figure 8–4), and a clinical trial using a similar compound that crosses the blood-brain barrier is being considered for a multicenter trial at the time of this publication.

C9ORF72

OVERVIEW

In 2000 Bob Brown and colleagues showed linkage to chromosome 9q21-122 for families with FTD and ALS (Hosler et al. 2000). It took

(A)

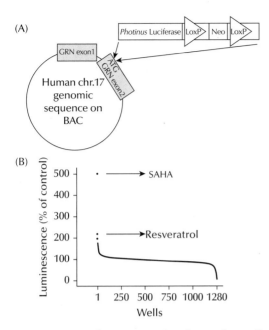

(B)

Figure 8–4. Luciferase reporter-based HTS for small molecule enhancers of progranulin expression. (A) schematic representation of a bacterial artificial chromosome (BAC)-based reporter construct. Luciferase coding sequence was inserted into exon 2 of the human GRN gene, replacing the original start codon with the first codon of luciferase cDNA. chr.17, chromosome 17. © The American Society for Biochemistry and Molecular Biology. (B) results from screening 1200 compounds composing the Prestwick Chemical Library®. Neuro-2a cells stably expressing the reporter were treated with the compounds at 2.5 µm for 24 h, and luciferase activity was measured afterward. Arrows indicate the compounds that resulted in the top two highest activities.

11 more years before a mutation was discovered in 2011 by two groups working in collaboration, one based at NIH led by Bryan Traynor (Renton et al. 2011), the other at Mayo Clinic led by Rosa Rademakers (deJesus-Hernandez et al. 2010).

The *C9ORF72* mutation can cause FTD, ALS, or the combination of the two (FTD-ALS) (Byrne et al. 2012; Chiò et al. 2012; Takada et al. 2012). The mean age of onset is 56 years, and this is the most common genetic abnormality in both familial FTD and familial ALS (22.5%). The mutation is a large expansion of a hexanucleotide (GGGGCC) repeat in a noncoding region of *C9ORF72* (deJesus-Hernandez et al. 2011). Expansions associated with disease are estimated to have a size of greater than 700 repeats, as compared to the fewer than 23 repeats that are found in

healthy individuals. It is still unknown whether the underlying pathogenesis of this mutation involves a loss of a function, a gain of function, or both, and whether the abnormal repeats can bind to and interfere with gene expression.

A gain of function mutation is proposed to mediate disease through the aggregation of long mRNA transcripts into abnormal RNA foci (deJesus-Hernandez et al. 2011). The mRNA aggregates accumulate in cortical and motor neurons, and it seems likely that this is an RNA-mediated neurodegenerative disease akin to the pathogenesis of myotonic muscular dystrophy or fragile X-associated tremor and ataxia syndrome (FXTAS) (Millecamps et al. 2012). Todd and Paulson have described this mechanism for neurodegeneration in an excellent recent review (Todd & Paulson 2010). The underlying mechanism of both syndromes involves transcriptional alterations that generate antisense transcripts, which lead to aberrant mRNA splicing and processing and activation of abnormal signaling cascades.

C9ORF72 CLINICAL GENETICS

In the UCSF clinical series, 28 of 412 FTD-spectrum patients carried the C9 mutation (Sha et al. 2012). There were no patients with a primary diagnosis of AD or Parkinson's disease, and nfvPPA and svPPA were also absent in our first series. Therefore, bvFTD was far and away the most common dementia phenotype, and all C9 positive patients had a clinical syndrome of bvFTD, ALS, or FTD-ALS. C9-positive bvFTD patients had more delusions and aggression as presenting symptoms and worse working memory, but milder disinhibition, eating, and aberrant motor behavior at the first evaluation as compared to C9 negative bvFTD cases.

Imaging can be distinctive in C9-related FTD and may not show the typical findings of bvFTD. In particular, there is often more dorsal frontal and parietal (C9-positive FTD-ALS), thalamic, and cerebellar atrophy in C9-positive bvFTD cases as compared to C9-negative bvFTD cases (Sha et al. 2012). Whether the thalamic or cerebellar atrophy is clinically significant remains undetermined. To date, few of our patients have shown cerebellar motor abnormalities, although some of the dysregulation of mood and behavior in C9-related bvFTD may be related to midline cerebellar dysfunction.

Most patients with this mutation began the disease process with a neuropsychiatric disorder that eventually evolved into a bvFTD syndrome. The progression from a psychiatric condition to a frank dementia can be quite extended, and we have described two patients in whom a psychiatric prodrome with features of borderline personality disorder and bipolar illness or sociopathy remained stable for nearly a decade (Khan et al. 2012).

Similarly, the ALS with C9 appears to be longer in duration that non-C9 cases. In one series, the ALS was more likely to be bulbar in onset than nongenetic forms of ALS. Additionally, the ALS can be complicated by dystonia, changes in ocular motility, and rigidity (Takada et al. 2012). Hence, the ALS can be atypical in that it is complicated by motor changes that extend beyond the lower motor and upper motor neurons into the basal ganglia and midbrain. It remains to be determined whether the presence of parkinsonism in a patient with ALS may be a clue that the disorder is genetic and should trigger a search for C9 mutations.

The lag between the onset of a psychiatric disorder and formal dementia or ALS can be long, even many decades. This delay is going to make the management of these patients complex, and determining with individuals and families whether or not to obtain genetic testing will require careful consideration.

C9ORF72 THERAPEUTIC APPROACHES

Treating the *C9ORF72* mutation may prove to be difficult, and to date the other diseases with RNA-mediated neurodegeneration, FXTAS and myotonic dystrophy, have no effective treatments. Delivery of a therapy into the brain and spinal cord may also prove difficult, even if the proper compound existed. Small molecules that silence RNA are being considered as therapies for myotonic dystrophy and might work for *C9ORF72* mutations (Guan & Disney 2012). Studies by Tim Miller using anti-oligonucleotide approaches have shown promise in patients with *SOD* mutations and ALS, and similar approaches might have efficacy for C9 (Miller & Cleveland 2003). More work with model systems will be needed in the coming decades to determine what therapies will be feasible and effective.

Valosin-Containing-Protein ATPase (VCP)

Mutations in *VCP* cause neuronal inclusions made of ubiquitin and TDP-43. VCP is a structural protein that has a wide variety of functions, particularly in intracellular trafficking and energy metabolism. *VCP* mutations are associated with an autosomal dominant condition called inclusion body myopathy associated with Paget's disease of bone (PDB) and/or FTD (IBMPFD) (Watts et al. 2007). Approximately 80% of individuals have a family history of the condition, with 20% appearing to be the first affected individual in the family. Among individuals who meet diagnostic criteria for IBMPFD, nearly 100% have an identified mutation in *VCP*. No other conditions are known to be associated with changes in *VCP*. This mutation is extremely rare and should be considered when there is a history of Paget's disease or inclusion body-myositis in a patient with a bvFTD syndrome.

TARDBP

TARDBP mutations lead to inclusions consisting of ubiquitin and TDP-43 in cells of the brain and nervous system. TDP-43 is normally only found in the nucleus of a cell, but in its abnormal form is found in the working area of the cell outside the nucleus. *TARDBP* mutations have been identified in individuals with sporadic and familial ALS and in a few cases of FTD (Borghero et al. 2011; Mosca et al. 2012). These are extremely rare mutations, and genetic testing to look for changes in *TARDBP* is available on a research basis only.

FUS

Like *TARDBP*, mutations in *FUS* most commonly cause ALS (Kwiatkowski et al. 2009). Mutations lead to abnormal aggregates of *FUS* inside and outside of the nucleus. Like *TARDBP*, *FUS* mutations rarely cause familial FTD, and genetic testing is only available in research settings.

CHMP2B

CHMP2B mutations are an extremely rare cause of familial FTD and may be specific to a few families (Lindquist et al. 2008). *CHMP2B* encodes a protein that recycles or destroys old receptors on the cell surface of the cell. It is unclear at this point whether the mutation increases or decreases function, but it does lead to inclusions made of ubiquitin but not TDP-43 in brain cells. *CHMP2B* mutations are associated with FTD, FTD-ALS, and ALS. Currently, testing for *CHMP2B* mutations is available on a research basis only.

SQSTM1 and Ubiquilin-2

These two new mutations were discovered at the end of 2011. Most of the data on these two genes associates them with ALS, although both seem to have a propensity toward causing a frontal type dementia. The SQSTM1 protein or P62 binds to ubiquitin; although the mechanism for neurodegeneration related to FTD and to ALS still remains mysterious, SQSTM1 may interact with TDP-43 within the nucleus (Tanji et al. 2012).

Siddique and colleagues (Fecto et al. 2011; Deng et al. 2011) suggest that both may act at the level of protein degradation pathways within the cell body and at the synapse. If true, further work on stimulating protein degradation in these diseases either through the proteasome or via autophagy pathways may prove efficacious for these subtypes of FTD and ALS.

GENES THAT MODIFY FTD EXPRESSION

Studies now under way suggest there are genes that can modify the presentation of FTD, even though they are not specifically causal. Apolipoprotein E ε-4 is a potent risk factor for AD (Bachman et al. 2003) and possibly other neurodegenerative conditions such as Parkinson's disease (Kiyohara et al. 2011), but is not a potent risk factor for FTD (Chow et al. 1999). In a study by Agosta and colleagues at UCSF (Agosta et al. 2009), apoE4 gene carriers

with FTD were compared to FTD patients who did not carry apoE4. In the E4-positive group, the atrophy in the frontal lobes was greater than the atrophy that was found in the E4-negative patients. There was no statistical difference between the two groups in the parietal regions. This study suggested that the presence of an E4 gene accelerated the pathology within the brain regions attacked by the FTD process.

In a related publication Vossel and colleagues (Vossel et al. 2012), studied two individuals who carried the C9ORF72 mutation and died with FTD-ALS. One of the patients was an apoE-ε4 homozygote while the other was a heterozygote. The patient with two E4s had a more severe cognitive and behavioral phenotype, and greater atrophy in the frontotemporal and insular regions. At a molecular level there were apoE fragments and aggregates in the anterior cingulate cortex that were more abundant in the homozygote. The authors concluded, "although differences seen in a sibling pair could arise due to chance, these findings raise the possibility that apoE4 exacerbates brain pathology in FTLD through formation of neurotoxic apoE fragments and interactions with TDP-43."

In another publication, Gennatas and colleagues (Gennatas et al. 2012) explored the influence of brain dopamine on neurodegeneration patterns in dementia cohorts that included patients with FTD. Catechol-O-methyltransferase polymorphisms for valine and methionine can influence the concentration of brain dopamine in prefrontal cortex and brainstem. Catechol-O-methyltransferase inactivates catecholamine neurotransmitters including dopamine, epinephrine, and norepinephrine, and individuals who carry the valine polymorphism metabolize these neurotransmitters approximately four times more rapidly than those with the methionine polymorphism. Hence, valine carriers have less prefrontal and brainstem dopamine.

Including healthy controls and patients with bvFTD, AD, and svPPA, 252 subjects were compared. MRI showed more severe atrophy in the subjects carrying the valine polymorphism in ventromedial prefrontal cortex, bilateral dorsal midinsula, left dorsolateral prefrontal cortex, and right ventral striatum. Methionine allele carriers showed greater VTA volumes than age-matched controls. Gray matter intensities within COMT-related brain regions correlated with cognitive and behavioral deficits. Hence, it appears that patients who have low brain dopamine during life may develop accelerated neurodegeneration in the FTD-networks. There must be many other genetic susceptibility factors that can either increase or decrease a patient's susceptibility to FTD, but research into this area is just beginning.

MANAGEMENT AND GENETIC COUNSELING

Single gene mutations that cause FTD are inherited in an autosomal dominant manner, meaning each child of an affected parent has a 50% chance of inheriting the change and also developing the condition. Currently, seven genes have been implicated in autosomal dominant FTD. It is possible additional genes will be identified in the future. Therefore, the absence of detecting a mutation in one of the known genes may not reduce risk for family members, particularly in the context of a family history that reflects an autosomal dominant inheritance pattern of FTD, dementia, parkinsonism, and/or motor neuron disease.

Deciding whether or not to obtain genetic testing is difficult for the family and the physician. Consideration of genetic testing for an individual who is asymptomatic (called *predictive genetic testing*) raises distinct and complex psychosocial issues, as compared to the consideration of testing for an individual who is symptomatic (called *diagnostic genetic testing*). In accordance with international standards of medical ethics that are adapted from guidelines set forth for Huntington's disease, both predictive and diagnostic genetic testing should be offered in concert with pretest genetic counseling (Guidelines for Huntington's disease 1994). Pretest genetic counseling should help individuals appreciate the risks, benefits, and limitations of testing. It should help individuals anticipate the impact of genetic testing on themselves, family members, and on their interpersonal relationships. For individuals who are cognitively or behaviorally impaired, genetic counseling should involve a healthcare proxy, legal guardian, or next-of-kin. It has become clear that many patients who carry

genetic mutations have a long prodrome that may influence social relationships, work, and decision-making. Because no treatment is currently available for any of the genetic forms of FTD, many people defer knowing. Doing no harm is a fundamental philosophical tenet of medicine, and telling one family member the results of genetic testing can have widespread implications for a multitude of close and distant relatives.

Still, there are legitimate reasons why a patient might want to know if they are a gene carrier. Decisions about whether or not to have children, when to retire, and how to plan for the future can be influenced by this knowledge, so for this reason many centers, including our own at UCSF, do offer gene testing for appropriate cases. Individuals who wish to learn the potential cause of FTD in their family should be offered genetic counseling, irrespective of but especially in the presence of a suggestive family history.

Mutations in the *C9ORF72*, *MAPT*, and *GRN* are the most common genetic causes of FTD. Clinical genetic testing for *MAPT*, *GRN*, *C9ORF72*, and *VCP* is available. Genetic testing should be undertaken with careful consideration and in the context of genetic counseling (Guidelines for Huntington's disease 1994). At tertiary medical centers a genetic counselor or other genetics professional should be available to offer genetic counseling and facilitate testing. Assessing family history is a key component of genetic counseling, and to that end, the clinician should obtain a detailed three-generation pedigree that queries for the presence of FTD, ALS, other dementias, parkinsonism, and psychiatric conditions.

Because of the variability in how these diseases present, a careful analysis of family, medical, and social history can help clarify whether an affected person has a sporadic or genetic form of FTD. Even when there appears to be an autosomal dominant pattern of FTD within a family, the exact genetic cause may not be known.

REFERENCES

Abisambra JF, Jinwal UK, Jones JR, Blair LJ, Koren J 3rd, Dickey CA. Exploiting the diversity of the heat-shock protein family for primary and secondary tauopathy therapeutics. Curr Neuropharmacol. 2011;9(4):623–31.

Agosta F, Vossel KA, Miller BL, Migliaccio R, Bonasera SJ, Filippi M, Boxer AL, Karydas A, Possin KL, Gorno-Tempini ML. Apolipoprotein E epsilon4 is associated with disease-specific effects on brain atrophy in Alzheimer's disease and frontotemporal dementia. Proc Natl Acad Sci U S A. 2009;106(6):2018–22.

Ahmed Z, Sheng H, Xu YF, Lin WL, Innes AE, Gass J, Yu X, Wuertzer CA, Hou H, Chiba S. Accelerated lipofuscinosis and ubiquitination in granulin knockout mice suggest a role for progranulin in successful aging. Am J Pathol. 2010;77:311–24.

Bachman DL, Green RC, Benke KS, Cupples LA, Farrer LA; MIRAGE Study Group. Comparison of Alzheimer's disease risk factors in white and African American families. Neurology. 2003;60(8):1372–4.

Baker M, Litvan I, Houlden H, Adamson J, Dickson D, Perez-Tur J, Hardy J, Lynch T, Bigio E, Hutton M. Association of an extended haplotype in the tau gene with progressive supranuclear palsy. Hum Mol Genet. 1999;8:711–5.

Baker M, Mackenzie IR, Pickering-Brown SM, Gass J, Rademakers R, Lindholm C, Snowden J, Adamson J, Sadovnick AD, Rollinson S, Cannon A, Dwosh E, Neary D, Melquist S, Richardson A, Dickson D, Berger Z, Eriksen J, Robinson T, Zehr C, Dickey CA, Crook R, McGowan E, Mann D, Boeve B, Feldman H, Hutton M. Mutations in progranulin cause tau-negative frontotemporal dementia linked to chromosome 17. Nature. 2006;442:916–9.

Bateman A, Belcourt D, Bennett H, Lazure C, Solomon S. Granulins, a novel class of peptide from leukocytes. Biochem Biophys Res Commun. 1990;173:1161–8.

Boeve BF, Hutton M. Refining frontotemporal dementia with parkinsonism linked to chromosome 17: introducing FTDP-17 (MAPT) and FTDP-17 (PGRN). Arch Neurol. 2008;65(4):460–4.

Borghero G, Floris G, Cannas A, Marrosu MG, Murru MR, Costantino E, Parish LD, Pugliatti M, Ticca A, Traynor BJ, Calvo A, Cammarosano S, Moglia C, Cistaro A, Brunetti M, Restagno G, Chiò A. A patient carrying a homozygous p.A382T TARDBP missense mutation shows a syndrome including ALS, extrapyramidal symptoms, and FTD. Neurobiol Aging. 2011;32:2327.e1–5.

Brion JP, Flament-Durand J, Dustin P. Alzheimer's disease and tau proteins. Lancet. 1986;2(8515):1098.

Bugiani O, Murrell JR, Giaccone G, Hasegawa M, Ghigo G, Tabaton M, Morbin M, Primavera A, Carella F, Solaro C, Grisoli M, Savoiardo M, Spillantini MG, Tagliavini F, Goedert M, Ghetti B. Frontotemporal dementia and corticobasal degeneration in a family with a P301S mutation in tau. J Neuropathol Exp Neurol. 1999;58(6):667–77.

Byrne S, Elamin M, Bede P, Shatunov A, Walsh C, Corr B, Heverin M, Jordan N, Kenna K, Lynch C, McLaughlin RL, Iyer PM, O'Brien C, Phukan J, Wynne B, Bokde AL, Bradley DG, Pender N, Al-Chalabi A, Hardiman O. Cognitive and clinical characteristics of patients with amyotrophic lateral sclerosis carrying a C9orf72 repeat expansion: a population-based cohort study. Lancet Neurol. 2012;11:232–40. Erratum in: Lancet Neurol. 2012;11:388.

Carrettiero DC, Hernandez I, Neveu P, Papagiannakopoulos T, Kosik KS. The cochaperone BAG2 sweeps paired helical filament- insoluble tau from the microtubule. J Neurosci. 2009;29(7):2151–61.

Cenik B, Sephton CF, Cenik BK, Herz J, Yu G. Progranulin: a proteolytically processed protein at the crossroads of inflammation and neurodegeneration. J Biol Chem. 2012;287(39):32298–306.

Cenik B, Sephton CF, Dewey CM, Xian X, Wei S, Yu K, Niu W, Coppola G, Coughlin SE, Lee SE, Dries DR, Almeida S, Geschwind DH, Gao FB, Miller BL, Farese RV Jr, Posner BA, Yu G, Herz J. Suberoylanilide hydroxamic acid (vorinostat) up-regulates progranulin transcription: Rational therapeutic approach to frontotemporal dementia. J Biol Chem. 2011;286:16101–8.

Chiò A, Borghero G, Restagno G, Mora G, Drepper C, Traynor BJ, Sendtner M, Brunetti M, Ossola I, Calvo A, Pugliatti M, Sotgiu MA, Murru MR, Marrosu MG, Marrosu F, Marinou K, Mandrioli J, Sola P, Caponnetto C, Mancardi G, Mandich P, La Bella V, Spataro R, Conte A, Monsurrò MR, Tedeschi G, Pisano F, Bartolomei I, Salvi F, Lauria Pinter G, Simone I, Logroscino G, Gambardella A, Quattrone A, Lunetta C, Volanti P, Zollino M, Penco S, Battistini S; ITALSGEN consortium, Renton AE, Majounie E, Abramzon Y, Conforti FL, Giannini F, Corbo M, Sabatelli M. Clinical characteristics of patients with familial amyotrophic lateral sclerosis carrying the pathogenic GGGGCC hexanucleotide repeat expansion of C9ORF72. Brain. 2012;135(Pt 3):784–93.

Chow TW, Miller BL, Hayashi VN, Geschwind DH. Inheritance of frontotemporal dementia. Arch Neurol. 1999;56(7):817–22.

Clark LN, Poorkaj P, Wszolek Z, Geschwind DH, Nasreddine ZS, Miller B, Li D, Payami H, Awert F, Markopoulou K, Andreadis A, D'Souza I, Lee VM, Reed L, Trojanowski JQ, Zhukareva V, Bird T, Schellenberg G, Wilhelmsen KC. Pathogenic implications of mutations in the tau gene in pallido-ponto-nigral degeneration and related neurodegenerative disorders linked to chromosome 17. Proc Natl Acad Sci U S A. 1998;95:13103–07.

Conrad C, Andreadis A, Trojanowski JQ, Dickson DW, Kang D, Chen X, Wiederholt W, Hansen L, Masliah E, Thal LJ, Katzman R, Xia Y, Saitoh T. Genetic evidence for the involvement of tau in progressive supranuclear palsy. Ann Neurol. 1997;41:277–81.

Coppola G, Chinnathambi S, Lee JJ, Dombroski BA, Baker MC, Soto-Ortolaza AI, Lee SE, Klein E, Huang AY, Sears R, Lane JR, Karydas AM, Kenet RO, Biernat J, Wang LS, Cotman CW, Decarli CS, Levey AI, Ringman JM, Mendez MF, Chui HC, Le Ber I, Brice A, Lupton MK, Preza E, Lovestone S, Powell J, Graff-Radford N, Petersen RC, Boeve BF, Lippa CF, Bigio EH, Mackenzie I, Finger E, Kertesz A, Caselli RJ, Gearing M, Juncos JL, Ghetti B, Spina S, Bordelon YM, Tourtellotte WW, Frosch MP, Vonsattel JP, Zarow C, Beach TG, Albin RL, Lieberman AP, Lee VM, Trojanowski JQ, Van Deerlin VM, Bird TD, Galasko DR, Masliah E, White CL, Troncoso JC, Hannequin D, Boxer AL, Geschwind MD, Kumar S, Mandelkow EM, Wszolek ZK, Uitti RJ, Dickson DW, Haines JL, Mayeux R, Pericak-Vance MA, Farrer LA; Alzheimer's Disease Genetics Consortium, Ross OA, Rademakers R, Schellenberg GD, Miller BL, Mandelkow E, Geschwind DH. Evidence for a role of the rare p.A152T variant in MAPT in increasing the risk for FTD-spectrum and Alzheimer's diseases. Hum Mol Genet. 2012;21(15):3500–12.

Coppola G, Karydas A, Rademakers R, Want Q, Baker M, Hutton M, Miller BL, Geschwind DH. Gene expression study on peripheral blood identifies progranulin mutations. Ann Neurol. 2008:64:92–6.

Cruts M, Gijselinck I, van der Zee J, Engelborghs S, Wils H, Pirici D, Rademakers R, Vandenberghe R, Dermaut B, Martin JJ, van Duijn C, Peeters K, Sciot R, Santens P, De Pooter T, Mattheijssens M, Van den Broeck M, Cuijt I, Vennekens K, De Deyn PP, Kumar-Singh S, Van Broeckhoven C. Null mutations in progranulin cause ubiquitin-positive frontotemporal dementia linked to chromosome 17q21. Nature. 2006; 442(7105);920–4.

Dange T, Smith D, Noy T, Rommel PC, Jurzitza L, Cordero RJ, Legendre A, Finley D, Goldberg AL, Schmidt M. Blm10 protein promotes proteasomal substrate turnover by an active gating mechanism. J Biol Chem. 2011;286(50):42830–9.

DeJesus-Hernandez M, Mackenzie IR, Boeve BF, Boxer AL, Baker M, Rutherford NJ, Nicholson AM, Finch NA, Flynn H, Adamson J, Kouri N, Wojtas A, Sengdy P, Hsiung GY, Karydas A, Seeley WW, Josephs KA, Coppola G, Geschwind DH, Wszolek ZK, Feldman H, Knopman DS, Petersen RC, Miller BL, Dickson DW, Boylan KB, Graff-Radford NR, Rademakers R. Expanded GGGGCC hexanucleotide repeat in noncoding region of C9ORF72 causes chromosome 9p-linked FTD and ALS. Neuron. 2011;72:245–56.

Delacourte A, Defossez A. Alzheimer's disease: Tau proteins the promoting factors of microtubule assembly, are major components of paired helical filaments. J Neurol Sci. 1986;76(2–3):173–86.

Deng HX, Chen W, Hong ST, Boycott KM, Gorrie GH, Siddique N, Yang Y, Fecto F, Shi Y, Zhai H, Jiang H, Hirano M, Rampersaud E, Jansen GH, Donkervoort S, Bigio EH, Brooks BR, Ajroud K, Sufit RL, Haines JL, Mugnaini E, Pericak-Vance MA, Siddique T. Mutations in UBQLN2 cause dominant X-linked juvenile and adult-onset ALS and ALS/dementia. Nature. 2011;477(7363):211–5.

Feany MB, Dickson DW. Neurodegenerative disorders with extensive tau pathology: a comparative study and review. Ann Neurol. 1996;40:139–48.

Fecto F, Yan J, Vemula SP, Liu E, Yang Y, Chen W, Zheng JG, Shi Y, Siddique N, Arrat H, Donkervoort S, Ajroud-Driss S, Sufit RL, Heller SL, Deng HX, Siddique T. SQSTM1 mutations in familial and sporadic amyotrophic lateral sclerosis. Arch Neurol. 2011;68 (11):1440–6.

Finch N, Baker M, Crook R, Swanson K, Kuntz K, Surtees R, Bisceglio G, Rovelet-Lecrux A, Boeve B, Petersen RC, Dickson DW, Younkin SG, Deramecourt V, Crook J, Graff-Radford NR, Rademakers R. Plasma progranulin levels predict progranulin mutation status in frontotemporal dementia patients and asymptomatic family members. Brain. 2009;132(Pt 3):583–91.

Finch N, Carrasquillo MM, Baker M, Rutherford NJ, Coppola G, Dejesus-Hernandez M, Crook R, Hunter T, Ghidoni R, Benussi L, Crook J, Finger E, Hantanpaa KJ, Karydas AM, Sengdy P, Gonzalez J, Seeley WW, Johnson N, Beach TG, Mesulam M, Forloni G, Kertesz A, Knopman DS, Uitti R, White CL 3rd, Caselli R, Lippa C, Bigio EH, Wszolek ZK, Binetti G, Mackenzie IR, Miller BL, Boeve BF, Younkin SG, Dickson DW, Petersen RC, Graff-Radford NR, Geschwind DH, Rademakers R. TMEM106B regulates progranulin levels and the penetrance of FTLD in GRN mutation carriers. Neurology. 2011;76:467–74.

Finley D. Misfolded proteins driven to destruction by Hul5. Nat Cell Biol. 2011;13(11):1290–2.

Fung HC, Evans J, Evans W, Duckworth J, Pittman A, de Silva R, Myers A, Hardy J. The architecture of the tau haplotype block in different ethnicities. Neurosci Lett. 2005;377(2):81–4.

Gass J, Cannon A, Mackenzie IR, Boeve B, Baker M, Adamson J, Crook R, Melquist S, Kuntz K, Petersen R, Josephs K, Pickering-Brown SM, Graff-Radford N, Uitti R, Dickson D, Wszolek Z, Gonzalez J, Beach TG, Bigio E, Johnson N, Weintraub S, Mesulam M, White CL 3rd, Woodruff B, Caselli R, Hsiung GY, Feldman H, Knopman D, Hutton M, Rademakers R. Mutations in progranulin are a major cause of ubiquitin-positive frontotemporal lobar degeneration. Hum Mol Genet. 2006;15:2988–3001.

Gennatas ED, Cholfin JA, Zhou J, Crawford RK, Sasaki DA, Karydas A, Boxer AL, Bonasera SJ, Rankin KP, Gorno-Tempini ML, Rosen HJ, Kramer JH, Weiner M, Miller BL, Seeley WW. COMT Val158Met genotype influences neurodegeneration within dopamine-innervated brain structures. Neurology. 2012;78(21):1663–9.

Geschwind DH, Robidoux J, Alarcón M, Miller BL, Wilhelmsen KC, Cummings JL, Nasreddine ZS. Dementia and neurodevelopmental predisposition: cognitive dysfunction in presymptomatic subjects precedes dementia by decades in frontotemporal dementia. Ann Neurol. 2001;50:741–746.

Ghetti B, Gambetti P. Comparative immunocytochemical characterization of neurofibrillary tangles in experimental maytansine and aluminum encephalopathies. Brain Res. 1983; 276(2):388–93.

Gold M, Lorenzl S, Stewart AJ, Morimoto BH, Williams DR, Gozes I. Critical appraisal of the role of davunetide in the treatment of progressive supranuclear palsy. Neuropsychiatr Dis Treat. 2012;8:85–93.

Gray DA, Woulfe J. Lipofuscin and aging: a matter of toxic waste. Sci Aging Knowledge Environ. 2005;2005(5):re1.

Grobmyer SR, Barie PS, Nathan CF, Fuortes M, Lin E, Lowry SF, Wright CD, Weyant MJ, Hydo L. Reeves F, Shiloh MU, Ding A. Secretory leukocyte protease inhibitor, an inhibitor of neutrophil activation, is elevated in serum in human sepsis and experimental endotoxemia. Crit Care Med. 2000;28(5):1276–82.

Guan L, Disney MD. Recent advances in developing small molecules targeting RNA. ACS Chem Biol. 2012 Jan 20; 7(1):73–86. Guidelines for the molecular genetics predictive test in Huntington's disease. International Huntington Association (IHA) and the World Federation of Neurology (WFN) Research Group on Huntington's Chorea. Neurology. 1994;44:1533–6.

Hong M, Zhukareva V, Vogelsberg-Ragaglia V, Wszolek Z, Reed L, Miller BI, Geschwind DH, Bird TD, McKeel D, Goate A, Morris JC, Wilhelmsen KC, Schellenberg GD, Trojanowski JQ, Lee VM. Mutation-specific functional impairments in distinct tau isoforms of hereditary FTDP-17. Science. 1998;282:1914–17.

Hosler BA, Siddique T, Sapp PC, Sailor W, Huang MC, Hossain A, Daube JR, Nance M, Fan C, Kaplan J, Hung WY, McKenna-Yasek D, Haines JL, Pericak-Vance MA,

Horvitz HR, Brown RH Jr. Linkage of familial amyo-trophic lateral sclerosis with frontotemporal dementia to chromosome 9q21-q22. JAMA. 2000;284:1664–9.

Hsiung GYR, Fok A, Feldman HH, Rademakers R, Mackenzie IRA. rs5848 polymorphism and serum pro-granulin level. J Neurol Sci. 2011;300(1–2):28–32.

Hu F, Padukkavidana T, Vægter CB, Brady OA, Zheng Y, Mackenzie IR, Feldman HH, Nykjaer A, Strittmatter SM. Sortilin-mediated endocytosis determines levels of the frontotemporal dementia protein, progranulin. Neuron. 2010;68(4):654–67.

Huey ED, Ferrari R, Moreno JH, Jensen C, Morris CM, Potocnik F, Kalaria RN, Tierney M, Wassermann EM, Hardy J, Grafman J, Momeni P. FUS and TDP-43 genetic variability in FTD and CBS. Neurobiol Aging. 2012;33(5):1016.e9–17.

Hutton M, Lendon CL, Rizzu P, Baker M, Froelich S, Houlden H, Pickering-Brown S, Chakraverty S, Isaacs A, Grover A, Hackett J, Adamson J, Lincoln S, Dickson D, Davies P, Petersen RC, Stevens M, de Graaff E, Wauters E, van Baren J, Hillebrand M, Joosse M, Kwon JM, Nowotny P, Che LK, Norton J, Morris JC, Reed LA, Trojanowski J, Basun H, Lannfelt L, Neystat M, Fahn S, Dark F, Tannenberg T, Dodd PR, Hayward N, Kwok JB, Schofield PR, Andreadis A, Snowden J, Craufurd D, Neary D, Owen F, Oostra BA, Hardy J, Goate A, van Swieten J, Mann D, Lynch T, Heutink P. Association of missense and 5'-splice-site mutations in tau with the inherited dementia FTDP-17. Nature. 1998;393:702–5.

Johnson JO, Mandrioli J, Benatar M, Abramzon Y, Van Deerlin VM, Trojanowski JQ, Gibbs JR, Brunetti M, Gronka S, Wuu J, Ding J, McCluskey L, Martinez-Lage M, Falcone D, Hernandez DG, Arepalli S, Chong S, Schymick JC, Rothstein J, Landi F, Wang YD, Calvo A, Mora G, Sabatelli M, Monsurrò MR, Battistini S, Salvi F, Spataro R, Sola P, Borghero G; ITALSGEN Consortium, Galassi G, Scholz SW, Taylor JP, Restagno G, Chiò A, Traynor BJ. Exome sequenc-ing reveals VCP mutations as a cause of familial ALS. Neuron. 2010;68:857–64.

Kao AW, Eisenhut RJ, Martens LH, Nakamura A, Huang A, Bagley JA, Zhou P, de Luis A, Neukomm LJ, Cabello J, Farese RV Jr, Kenyon C. A neurodegenerative disease mutation that accelerates the clearance of apoptotic cells. Proc Natl Acad Sci U S A. 2011;108(11):4441–6.

Kfoury N, Holmes BB, Jiang H, Holtzman DM, Diamond MI. Trans-cellular propagation of Tau aggregation by fibrillar species. J Biol Chem. 2012;287(23):19440–51.

Khan BK, Woolley JD, Chao S, See T, Karydas AM, Miller BL, Rankin KP. Schizophrenia or neurodegenera-tive disease prodrome? Outcome of a first psychotic episode in a 35-year-old woman. Psychosomatics. 2012;53:280–4.

Khan BK, Yokoyama JS, Takada LT, Sha SJ, Rutherford NJ, Fong JC, Karydas AM, Wu T, Ketelle RS, Baker MC, Hernandez MD, Coppola G, Geschwind DH, Rademakers R, Lee SE, Rosen HJ, Rabinovici GD, Seeley WW, Rankin KP, Boxer AL, Miller BL. Atypical, slowly progressive behavioural variant fron-totemporal dementia associated with C9ORF72 hexa-nucleotide expansion. J Neurol Neurosurg Psychiatry. 2012;83:358–64.

Kiyohara C, Miyake Y, Koyanagi M, Fujimoto T, Shirasawa S, Tanaka K, Fukushima W, Sasaki S,

Tsuboi Y, Yamada T, Oeda T, Miki T, Kawamura N, Sakae N, Fukuyama H, Hirota Y, Nagai M; Fukuoka Kinki Parkinson's Disease Study Group. APOE and CYP2E1 polymorphisms, alcohol consumption, and Parkinson's disease in a Japanese population. J Neural Transm. 2011;118(9):1335–44.

Kosik KS, Joachim CL, Selkoe DJ. Microtubule-associated protein tau (tau) is a major antigenic component of paired helical filaments in Alzheimer disease. Proc Natl Acad Sci U S A. 1986;83(11):4044–8.

Kosik KS, Shimura H. Phosphorylated tau and the neu-rodegenerative foldopathies. Biochim Biophys Acta. 2005;1739(2–3):298–310.

Kwiatkowski TJ Jr, Bosco DA, Leclerc AL, Tamrazian E, Vanderburg CR, Russ C, Davis A, Gilchrist J, Kasarskis EJ, Munsat T, Valdmanis P, Rouleau GA, Hosler BA, Cortelli P, de Jong PJ, Yoshinaga Y, Haines JL, Pericak-Vance MA, Yan J, Ticozzi N, Siddique T, McKenna-Yasek D, Sapp PC, Horvitz HR, Landers JE, Brown RH Jr. Mutations in the FUS/TLS gene on chromosome 16 cause familial amyotrophic lateral sclerosis. Science. 2009;323,1205–8.

Le Ber I, Camuzat A, Hannequin D, Pasquier F, Guedj E, Rovelet-Lecrux A, Hahn-Barma V, van der Zee J, Clot F, Bakchine S, Puel M, Ghanim M, Lacomblez L, Mikol J, Deramecourt V, Lejeune P, de la Sayette V, Belliard S, Vercelletto M, Meyrignac C, Broeckhoven C, Lambert JC, Verpillat P, Campion D, Habert MO, Dubois B, Brice A; French research network on FTD/FTD-MND. Phenotype variability in progranulin mutation carriers: a clinical, neuropsychological, imag-ing and genetic study. Brain. 2008;131(Pt 3):732.46.

Lindquist SG, Braedgaard H, Svenstrup K, Isaacs AM, Nielsen JE; FReJA Consortium. Frontotemporal dementia linked to chromosome 3 (FTD-3)—current concepts and the detection of a previously unknown branch of the Danish FTD-3 family. Eur J Neurol. 2008;15:667–70.

Mandelkow EM, Mandelkow E. Biochemistry and cell biology of tau protein in neurofibrillary degenera-tion. Cold Spring Harb Perspect Med. 2012;2(7): a006247.

Merner ND, Girard SL, Catoire H, Bourassa CV, Belzil VV, Rivière JB, Hince P, Levert A, Dionne-Laporte A, Spiegelman D, Noreau A, Diab S, Szuto A, Fournier H, Raelson J, Belouchi M, Panisset M, Cossette P, Dupré N, Bernard G, Chouinard S, Dion PA, Rouleau GA. Exome Sequencing Identifies FUS Mutations as a Cause of Essential Tremor. Am J Hum Genet. 2012;91(2):313–9.

Millecamps S, Boillée S, Le Ber I, Seilhean D, Teyssou E, Giraudeau M, Moigneu C, Vandenberghe N, Danel-Brunaud V, Corcia P, Pradat PF, Le Forestier N, Lacomblez L, Bruneteau G, Camu W, Brice A, Cazeneuve C, Leguern E, Meininger V, Salachas F. Phenotype difference between ALS patients with expanded repeats in C9ORF72 and patients with mutations in other ALS-related genes. J Med Genet. 2012;49:258–63.

Miller TM, Cleveland DW. Has gene therapy for ALS arrived? Nat Med. 2003;9(10):1256–7.

Min SW, Cho SH, Zhou Y, Schroeder S, Haroutunian V, Seeley WW, Huang EJ, Shen Y, Masliah E, Mukherjee C, Meyers D, Cole PA, Ott M, Gan L. Acetylation of tau inhibits its degradation and contributes to tauopathy.

Acetylation of tau inhibits its degradation and contributes to tauopathy. Neuron. 2010;67:953–66.

Mosca L, Lunetta C, Tarlarini C, Avemaria F, Maestri E, Melazzini M, Corbo M, Penco S. Wide phenotypic spectrum of the TARDBP gene: homozygosity of A382T mutation in a patient presenting with amyotrophic lateral sclerosis, Parkinson's disease, and frontotemporal lobar degeneration, and in neurologically healthy subject. Neurobiol Aging. 2012;33(8):1846.e1–4.

Münch C, Rosenbohm A, Sperfeld AD, Uttner I, Reske S, Krause BJ, Sedlmeier R, Meyer T, Hanemann CO, Stumm G, Ludolph AC. Heterozygous R1101K mutation of the DCTN1 gene in a family with ALS and FTD. Ann Neurol. 2005;58(5):777–80.

Myers AJ, Pittman AM, Zhao AS, Rohrer K, Kaleem M, Marlowe L, Lees A, Leung D, McKeith IG, Perry RH, Morris CM, Trojanowski JQ, Clark C, Karlawish J, Arnold S, Forman MS, Van Deerlin V, de Silva R, Hardy J. The MAPT H1c risk haplotype is associated with increased expression of tau and especially of 4 repeat containing transcripts. Neurobiol Dis. 2007;25(3):561–70.

Narvid J, Gorno-Tempini ML, Slavotinek A, Dearmond SJ, Cha YH, Miller BL, Rankin K. Of brain and bone: the unusual case of Dr. A. Neurocase. 2009;15(3):190–205.

Petkau TL, Neal SJ, Milnerwood A, Mew A, Hill AM, Orban P, Gregg J, Lu G. Feldman HH, Mackenzie IR, Raymond LA, Leavitt BR. Synaptic dysfunction in progranulin-deficient mice. Neurobiol Dis. 2012;45(2):711–22.

Piedrahita D, Hernández I, López-Tobón A, Fedorov D, Obara B, Manjunath BS, Boudreau RL, Davidson B, Laferla F, Gallego-Gómez JC, Kosik KS, Cardona-Gómez GP. Silencing of CDK5 reduces neurofibrillary tangles in transgenic Alzheimer's mice. J Neurosci. 2010;30(42):13966–76.

Poorkaj P, Bird TD, Wijsman E, Nemens E, Garruto RM, Anderson L, Andreadis A, Wiederholt WC, Raskind M, Schellenberg GD. Tau is a candidate gene for chromosome 17 frontotemporal dementia. Ann Neurol. 1998;43(6):815–25.

Rademakers R, Baker M, Gass J, Adamson J, Huey ED, Momeni P, Spina S, Coppola G, Karydas AM, Stewart H, Johnson N, Hsiung GY, Kelley B, Kuntz K, Steinbart E, Wood EM, Yu CE, Josephs K, Sorenson E, Womack KB, Weintraub S, Pickering-Brown SM, Schofield PR, Brooks WS, Van Deerlin VM, Snowden J, Clark CM, Kertesz A, Boylan K, Ghetti B, Neary D, Schellenberg GD, Beach TG, Mesulam M, Mann D, Grafman J, Mackenzie IR, Feldman H, Bird T, Petersen R, Knopman D, Boeve B, Geschwind DH, Miller B, Wszolek Z, Lippa C, Bigio EH, Dickson D, Graff-Radford N, Hutton M. Phenotypic variability associated with progranulin haploinsufficiency in patients with the common 1477C-->T (Arg493X) mutation: an international initiative. Lancet Neurol. 2007;6:857–68.

Renton AE, Majounie E, Waite A, Simón-Sánchez J, Rollinson S, Gibbs JR, Schymick JC, Laaksovirta H, van Swieten JC, Myllykangas L, Kalimo H, Paetau A, Abramzon Y, Remes AM, Kaganovich A, Scholz SW, Duckworth J, Ding J, Harmer DW, Hernandez DG, Johnson JO, Mok K, Ryten M, Trabzuni D, Guerreiro RJ, Orrell RW, Neal J, Murray A, Pearson J,

Jansen IE, Sondervan D, Seelaar H, Blake D, Young K, Halliwell N, Callister JB, Toulson G, Richardson A, Gerhard A, Snowden J, Mann D, Neary D, Nalls MA, Peuralinna T, Jansson L, Isoviita VM, Kaivorinne AL, Hölttä-Vuori M, Ikonen E, Sulkava R, Benatar M, Wuu J, Chiò A, Restagno G, Borghero G, Sabatelli M; ITALSGEN Consortium, Heckerman D, Rogaeva E, Zinman L, Rothstein JD, Sendtner M, Drepper C, Eichler EE, Alkan C, Abdullaev Z, Pack SD, Dutra A, Pak E, Hardy J, Singleton A, Williams NM, Heutink P, Pickering-Brown S, Morris HR, Tienari PJ, Traynor BJ. A hexanucleotide repeat expansion in C9ORF72 is the cause of chromosome 9p21-linked ALS-FTD. Neuron. 2011;72:257–68.

Roberson ED, Scearce-Levie K, Palop JJ, Yan F, Cheng IH, Wu T, Gerstein H, Yu GQ, Mucke L. Reducing endogenous tau ameliorates amyloid beta-induced deficits in an Alzheimer's disease mouse model. Science. 2007;316(5825):750–4.

Rohrer JD, Warren JD. Phenotypic signatures of genetic frontotemporal dementia. Curr Opin Neurol. 2011;24(6):542–9.

Ryan CL, Baranowski DC, Chitramuthu BP, Malik S, Li Z, Cao M, Minotti S, Durham HD, Kay DG, Shaw CA, Bennett HP, Bateman A. Ryan CL, Baranowski DC, Chitramuthu BP, Malik S, Li Z, Cao M, Minotti S, Durham HD, Kay DG, Shaw CA, Bennett HP, Bateman A. Progranulin is expressed within motor neurons and promotes neuronal cell survival. BMC Neurosci. 2009;10:130.

Schaeffer V, Goedert M. Stimulation of autophagy is neuroprotective in a mouse model of tauopathy. Autophagy. 2012;8(11):1686–7.

Schaeffer V, Lavenir I, Ozcelik S, Tolnay M, Winkler DT, Goedert M. Stimulation of autophagy reduces neurodegeneration in a mouse model of human tauopathy. Brain. 2012;135(Pt 7):2169–77.

Seelaar H, Rohrer JD, Pijnenburg YA, Fox NC, van Swieten JC. Clinical, genetic and pathological heterogeneity of frontotemporal dementia: a review. J Neurol Neurosurg Psychiatry. 2011;82:476–86.

Sha S, Takada LT, Rankin KP, Yokoyama JS, Rutherford NJ, Fong JC, Khan B, Karydas A, Baker MC, DeJesus-Hernandez M, Pribadi M, Coppola G, Geschwind DH, Rademakers R, Lee SE, Seeley W, Miller BL, Boxer AL. Frontotemporal dementia due to C9ORF72 mutations: Clinical and imaging features. Neurology. 2012;79:1002–11.

Sleegers K, Brouwers N, Van Broeckhoven C. Role of progranulin as a biomarker for Alzheimer's disease. Biomark Med. 2010;4(1):37–50.

Smith KR, Damiano J, Franceschetti S, Carpenter S, Canafoglia L, Morbin M, Rossi G, Pareyson D, Mole SE, Staropoli JF, Sims KB, Lewis J, Lin WL, Dickson DW, Dahl HH, Bahlo M, Berkovic SF. Strikingly different clinicopathological phenotypes determined by progranulin-mutation dosage. Am J Hum Genet. 2012;90:1–6.

Spillantini MG, Bird TD, Ghetti B. Frontotemporal dementia and Parkinsonism linked to chromosome 17: a new group of tauopathies. Brain Pathol. 1998;8:387–402.

Spillantini MG, Murrell JR, Goedert M, Farlow MR, Klug A, Ghetti B. Mutation in the tau gene in familial multiple system tauopathy with presenile dementia. Proc Natl Acad Sci U S A. 1998;95(13):7737–41.

Takada LT, Pimentel MLV, DeJesus-Hernandez M, Fong JC, Yokoyama JS, Karydas A, Thibodeau MP, Rutherford NJ, Baker MC, Lomen-Hoerth C, Rademakers R, Miller BL. Frontotemporal dementia in a Brazilian kindred with the *C9ORF72* mutation. Arch Neurol. 2012 Sep 1;69(9):1149–53..

Tanji K, Zhang HX, Mori F, Kakita A, Takahashi H, Wakabayashi K. p62/sequestosome 1 binds to TDP-43 in brains with frontotemporal lobar degeneration with TDP-43 inclusions. J Neurosci Res. 2012;90(10):2034–42.

Tapia L, Milnerwood A, Guo A, Mills F, Yoshida E, Vasuta C, Mackenzie IR, Raymond L, Cyander M, Jia W, Bamji SX. Progranulin deficiency decreases gross neural connectivity but enhances transmission at individual synapses. J Neurosci. 2011;31(31):11126–32.

Todd PK, Paulson HL. RNA-mediated neurodegeneration in repeat expansion disorders. Ann Neurol. 2010;67(3):291–300.

Toh H, Chitramuthu BP, Bennett HP, Bateman A. Structure function and mechanism of progranulin: the brain and beyond. J Mol Neurosci. 2011;45(3):538–48.

Vilariño-Güell C, Wider C, Soto-Ortolaza AI, Cobb SA, Kachergus JM, Keeling BH, Dachsel JC, Hulihan MM, Dickson DW, Wszolek ZK, Uitti RJ, Graff-Radford NR, Boeve BF, Josephs KA, Miller B, Boylan KB, Gwinn K, Adler CH, Aasly JO, Hentati F, Destée A, Krygowska-Wajs A, Chartier-Harlin MC, Ross OA, Rademakers R, Farrer MJ. Characterization of DCTN1 genetic variability in neurodegeneration. Neurology. 2009;72:2024–8.

Vossel KA, Bien-Ly N, Bernardo A, Rascovsky K, Karydas A, Rabinovici GD, Sidhu M, Huang EJ, Miller BL, Huang Y, Seeley WW. ApoE and TDP-43 neuropathology in two siblings with familial FTLD-motor neuron disease. Neurocase. 2012 Apr 18. [Epub ahead of print]

Ward ME, Miller BL. Potential Mechanisms of Progranulin-deficient FTLD. J Mol Neurosci. 2011;45:574–82.

Watts GD, Thomasova D, Ramdeen SK, Fulchiero EC, Mehta SG, Drachman DA, Weihl CC, Jamrozik Z, Kwiecinski H, Kaminska A, Kimonis VE. Novel VCP mutations in inclusion body myopathy associated with Paget disease of bone and frontotemporal dementia. Clin Genet. 2007;72:420–6.

Weingarten MD, Lockwood AH, Hwo SY, Kirschner MW. A protein factor essential for microtubule assembly. Proc Natl Acad Sci U S A. 1975;72(5):1858–62.

Wolozin BL, Pruchnicki A, Dickson DW, Davies P. A neuronal antigen in the brains of Alzheimer patients. Science. 1986; 232(4750):648–50.

Yan J, Deng HX, Siddique N, Fecto F, Chen W, Yang Y, Liu E, Donkervoort S, Zheng JG, Shi Y, Ahmeti KB, Brooks B, Engel WK, Siddique T. Frameshift and novel mutations in FUS in familial amyotrophic lateral sclerosis and ALS/dementia. Neurology. 2010;75:807–14.

Zhang B, Carroll J, Trojanowski JQ, Yao Y, Iba M, Potuzak JS, Hogan AM, Xie SX, Ballatore C, Smit AB, Lee VM, Brunden KR. The microtubule-stabilizing agent, apothilone D, reduces axonal dysfunction, neurotoxicity, cognitive deficits, and Alzheimer-like pathology in an interventional study with aged tau transgenic mice. J Neurosci. 2012;32(11):3601–11.

Zhou J, Gennatas ED, Kramer JH, Miller BL, Seeley WW. Predicting regional neurodegeneration from the healthy brain functional connectome. Neuron. 2012;73:1216–27.

Zhu J, Nathan C, Jin W, Sim D, Ashcroft GS, Wahl SM, Lacomis L, Erdjument-Bromage H, Tempst P, Wright CD, Ding A. Conversion of proepithelin to epithelins: roles of SLPI and elastase in host defense and wound repair. Cell. 2002;111(6):867–78.

Chapter 9

FTD Reflections on Psychology and Philosophy

EMOTIONS

THE SELF

FREE WILL

RELIGIOUS BELIEFS

PSYCHOLOGY
Social and Emotional Functioning
Executive Control

von ECONOMO NEURONS

REFERENCES

Frontotemporal dementia (FTD) is a neurological disorder that offers profound insights into the human condition. There is much to learn from the study of patients with FTD that can help to inform our conceptualization of what makes us uniquely human, what binds us to other people, what freedom we have in decision making and behavior, and what parts of the brain support the concepts of the self, creativity, religion, and philosophy. Additionally, a disorder that selectively attacks circuits in the frontal and anterior temporal lobes has much to teach us about the cognitive and psychological functions of these regions. Indeed, the anatomic substrates of behavioral variant of FTD (bvFTD) and semantic variant of primary progressive aphasia (svPPA) are unique, facilitating understanding of frontoinsular and anterior

temporal lobe circuits. This chapter discusses these topics by emphasizing specific examples of how FTD illuminates and challenges modern philosophical and psychological constructs.

EMOTIONS

James and Lange's theories suggest that an emotional experience begins when we feel the activation of our autonomic system. This activation involves multiple organs and can range from the sensation of an accelerating or slowing of our heart rate to the contractions of our stomach. James comments,

> Common sense says, we lose our
> fortune, are sorry and weep; we meet

a bear, are frightened and run; we are insulted by a rival, are angry and strike. The hypothesis here...says that this order of sequence is incorrect...and that the more rational statement is that we feel sorry because we cry, angry because we strike, afraid because we tremble....Without the bodily states following on the perception, the latter would be purely cognitive in form, pale, colorless, destitute of emotional warmth. (James 1890; Ellsworth 1994)

Much has been learned about the organization of the brain since James proposed his imaginative, and still influential theories regarding the brain (James 1907). We now understand that the physiological changes that accompany emotion are relayed by specific pathways in the spinal cord to centers in the brainstem, thalamus, and cortex that are responsible for processing this information and for connecting it to regions in the frontal and temporal lobes that then integrate this emotion-laden data with higher-order knowledge structures and valuation systems (Craig 2009) (Figure 9–1).

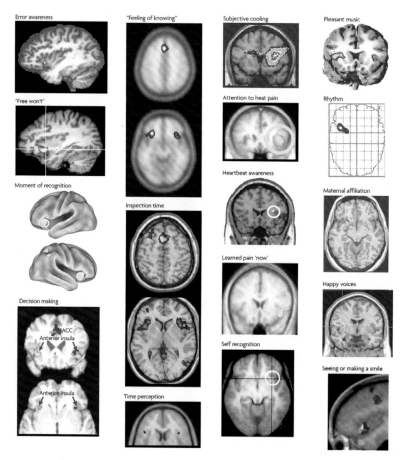

Figure 9–1. A summary of imaging results showing activation of the anterior insular cortex (AIC) during particular tasks and emotions highlighted in the text. The two right-hand columns contain images from different studies that found predominantly unilateral activation; images in the two left-hand columns show mostly bilateral activation. Stimuli that activate the right AIC are generally arousing to the body (for example, pain). The left AIC is activated mainly by positive and affiliative emotional feelings. For example, activation of the left AIC was reported in mothers viewing photos of their own child; greater activation of the left than of the right AIC was associated with both maternal and romantic love; activation of the left AIC was reported while subjects were either seeing or making a smile; activation of the left AIC was found while subjects attended to happy voices; activation of the left AIC was associated with hearing pleasant music; selective activation of the left AIC was observed in subjects experiencing joy; and selective activation of the left AIC in females was found that correlated with self-reported orgasm ratings. ACC, anterior cingulate cortex. (Craig 2009.)

Additionally, the cortical systems involved with triggering the output from the autonomic nervous system are much better understood (Saper 2002).

Although the idea that peripheral autonomic sensations drive our emotions has been largely rejected, a more modern interpretation of James-Lange would hold that emotions take place through the limbic brain structures. What happens next is that the feeling of these experiences is subsequently interpreted, identified, and reexperienced as "fear," "anger," "disgust," or "happiness." FTD offers fascinating data that supports the more modern conceptualization of James-Lange's theory.

Dr. Robert Levenson, Professor of Psychology at the University of California at Berkeley, is an innovative scientist who has pioneered the study of emotion in the laboratory. His quantitative research on the reactions of the autonomic system and the face to emotional stimuli (Levenson 2003) has led to significant discoveries about aging, marriage, and relationships. He has demonstrated that the emotional system remains intact, and in some ways strengthened, in association with normal aging (Sze et al. 2012). Additionally, in pioneering work on marriage he evaluated 73 couples between 1983 and 1987 and was able to predict those couples likely to dissolve their relationships based on a combination of autonomic and emotional measures (Levenson et al. 1993).

In his studies on the physiological profile of emotion in FTD, Dr. Levenson has systematically probed the affective systems of FTD patients and other neurodegenerative conditions at the levels of perception and autonomic responsivity as well as facial expression and other behavioral outputs (Levenson et al. 2008).

Patients studied in his laboratory are observed in a variety of structured paradigms that are designed to stimulate and quantify emotional perception, reaction, and regulation. While in the laboratory, patients observe scenes from movies that have been chosen to elicit specific emotions. These scenes have been extensively validated with healthy controls, and they predictably trigger emotions including sadness, fear, disgust, happiness, pride, and embarrassment (Levenson 2003).

While these films are shown, the subjects' facial movements, eye movements, and autonomic responses are measured. After viewing the film, subjects are asked to describe what happened in the film, how the characters in the movies felt, and how they themselves felt while watching the movie.

Additionally, patients are placed in embarrassing situations, like being subjected to a loud, unexpected noise or watching recordings of themselves singing karaoke. Finally, the patient and their caregiver are asked to describe an area of conflict between them and the discussion is recorded, as are their autonomic responses allowing the systematic analysis and measurement of a real-world conflict.

In his comprehensive assessment of FTD, Dr. Levenson and his colleagues have reported that low-level emotional processing is relatively preserved in FTD, but there are extensive deficits in more complex cortically mediated aspects of emotion perception, regulation, and output (Sturm et al. 2008). Reactivity to threat is intact. When a loud noise is made behind the patient, a strong defensive reaction occurs that includes elevated heart rate, increased galvanic skin response (GSR), and raising of the shoulders in a protective posture (Sturm et al. 2006). Similarly, in at least some of the emotion-triggering paradigms, patients show preservation of autonomic output. Yet, despite the intactness of the peripheral autonomic nervous system (and its connections to and from the brain), it does not protect the patients from profound deficits in the experience and expression of emotions (Levenson & Miller, 2007).

Many deficits in the FTD patients have been quantified within the laboratory that help to explain the behavioral alterations in FTD. For example, when patients watch a videotape of themselves singing the song "My Girl," signs of embarrassment that occur in healthy people (such as blushing, covering the eyes and giggling) are absent (Sturm et al. 2008). This paradigm shows that the FTD patients' abilities to self-reflect and realize that they have participated in an activity that is silly and then to feel the self-conscious emotion of embarrassment, are impaired.

There are widespread implications for this specific emotional scotoma in FTD. Unable to self-reflect on the appropriateness of their behavior, FTD patients go through life acting in ways that embarrass their loved ones and injure their social status. They eat off of other people's plates in restaurants, compete seriously with little children in games like checkers or tag, walk in public while inappropriately dressed (or even with no clothes at all), sexually solicit their pastors or rabbis, touch little children, and urinate in public without concern or distress (Miller et al. 1997; Miller et al. 2001).

Other components of emotion lead to this disruption of self-conscious emotion. The higher-order cortical brain systems responsible for the perception and feeling of other people's emotions slowly degenerate, and these deficits can be quantified in the laboratory. Perceiving that someone is sad or disgusted in movies is beyond the capability of many patients, and they describe a patient who is disgusted as happy, or a patient who is sad as happy (Rosen et al. 2002; Rosen et al. 2004; Rosen et al. 2006; Werner et al. 2007). Detecting sarcasm and lies also becomes impaired (Shany-Ur et al. 2012), diminishing that patient's ability to understand what others are communicating. Similarly, in many instances these patients lose the ability to experience normal emotions. What should make them disgusted or sad no longer does (Eckart et al. 2012). Further exacerbating these deficits, the semantic knowledge about how to behave is being lost.

The laboratory demonstrates that the normal autonomic responses, seen in controls while watching emotions experiencing the emotions of others, disappear (Werner et al. 2007). Virginia Sturm at UCSF has demonstrated that the severity of this autonomic and behavioral impairment correlates very strongly with the volume of the anterior cingulate, a region involved with initiating visceral and motor responses that accompany emotion (Sturm et al. 2011). Similarly, Rosen and colleagues have shown that fear conditioning is impaired, correlating strongly with loss of tissue in the orbitofrontal cortex (Hoefer et al. 2008).

The strongest anatomic correlate of diminished perception of emotion is decreased volume in the right anterior temporal lobe and amygdala (Rosen et al. 2002; Rosen et al. 2006) (Figure 9–2), while diminished empathy in FTD strongly correlates with diminished volume of the right anterior temporal lobe, right orbitofrontal-insular cortex, and right ventral striatum (Rankin et al. 2006) (Figure 9–3).

These studies have helped to define the specific emotional circuits that go awry in FTD, particularly in behavioral variant of FTD

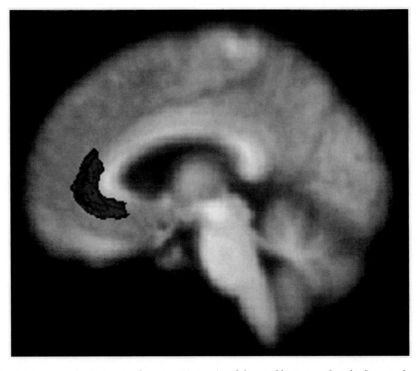

Figure 9–2. Right pregenual anterior cingulate cortex (pACC) as delineated by Freesurfer. The figure is the composed of a standardized average MRI coregistered with average regions representing the pACC (dark gray). (Sturm et al. 2012.)

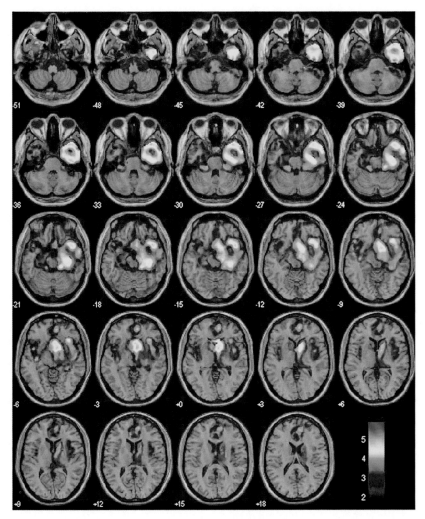

Figure 9–3. Continuous, unthresholded map of t-scores for empathy total score analysis across all diagnostic groups, superimposed on a normal control template image (SPM2: single_subj_T1.mnc). The figure represents axial slices taken every 3 mm from z = −51 to z = +18. t-Scores range from 2.00 (blue–black) to 5.91 (red), and include slices from all three clusters containing significant voxels in the analysis. (Rankin et al. 2006.)

(bvFTD) and in patients with selective right frontal and anterior temporal lobe degeneration. Perception of others' emotions is impaired due to degeneration of a right frontotemporal insular circuit. Additionally, degeneration of anterior cingulate region diminishes the brain's ability to generate autonomic signals that help with the "feeling" associated with a real emotion. Hence, the systematic study of FTD both enriches and expands the constructs surrounding the James-Lange theory, while adding a layer of understanding to how we experience emotion.

THE SELF

The self has been defined as "the total, essential or particular being of a person" and includes "the essential qualities distinguishing one person from another." The neuroanatomical constituents of these "essential qualities" are unknown. How and where we represent the self represents a fundamental question in modern philosophy and neuroscience (James 1907).

In a 2001 paper we described seven FTD patients in whom there were dramatic alterations in well-established components of their prior self (Miller et al. 2001). These patients changed long-standing political or religious ideologies and patterns of dress, style, and eating.

One dramatic example of this alteration in self was a woman who developed multiple personality disorder and flipped back and forth between a socially conservative, well-behaved, and well-dressed individual to a more liberal and verbally profane person who spoke her mind in a crude fashion, shifted from a taste in French food to fast food, and began to dress in t-shirts. She called this new persona "Skippy." These alternating shifts in her sense of self occurred before she was diagnosed with FTD and occurred in the setting of relatively spared language and memory (Miller et al. 2001).

Other patients that we described in this paper changed their political views from conservative to liberal, their religion from Protestant to Catholic, their fashion style from elegant to crude, or their taste in food from sophisticated to simple. In six of the seven patients the most prominent site of neurodegeneration was in the right frontal lobe, and these subjects had relative sparing of the left frontal and anterior temporal regions as well as the parietal cortex.

These patients represent an interesting model for thinking about what are the anatomic constituents of the self. They maintained language and semantic constructs that represent a critical component of their sense of self and the constructs around which it was anchored. Yet, their emotional attachments to these self-constructs weakened as the disease progressed.

By the time that we reach middle-age, most people are strongly attached to their philosophical, religious, and political ideologies and their styles of dress, but these patients easily changed well-established loyalties to a specific ideology, religion, style of dress, or eating. The emotional feelings that attached these people to the philosophical components of the self were gone. In many ways, these people had developed a new self, one that was removed from all of the loyalties of the old self.

These cases suggest a division of labor between the two hemispheres, in which the left hemisphere stores verbal and conceptual concepts relevant to the self, but in which the importance of these concepts to the self are anchored by processes in the right hemisphere.

The contemporary philosopher Derek Parfit, inspired by Buddhist conceptions of the self, has argued that the self is not separate from our thoughts and experiences, but is instead constituted by connections between them (Parfit 1973). When these links are weakened or broken, as seen in patients with FTD, it may make sense to think of the patient as a new self distinct from the previously healthy person.

Parfit has written about moral responsibility in a changing self, imagining a prisoner who, when he was younger, had committed a violent crime. Over many years this person changes and becomes compassionate, caring, and nonviolent. For this person Parfit suggests that we might think of this person's life as divided into earlier and later selves.

FTD brings up similar questions of responsibility as the disease alters the fundamental aspects of the human core, while diminishing the ability of that core to behave in a socially acceptable or responsible manner (see "Free Will," below). Physicians who look after patients with FTD are frequently asked by legal authorities to comment on behaviors committed by the patient that would never have happened if the right frontoinsula had not degenerated. Luckily, these crimes are almost always non-violent and cause minor impact on the society (Miller et al. 1997). Typically, I argue that the patient has lost their ability to control their behavior and plea for leniency. The previous self is irreversibly changed.

FREE WILL

FTD restrains the potential of the individual and drives the human being to highly stereotyped behaviors, specific personality profiles, and profound dissociations from knowing and doing. Human beings' frontal and anterior temporal lobes help to make us a highly adaptable species that can take salient information from the internal and external environment and quickly revise constructs about the world from this information (Fuster, 1997).

FTD prevents these subtle, continuous adaptations and keeps the patients fixed to stereotyped, previously learned behaviors that are driven by internal and external signals. In some instances, there is a pathological rigidity and inflexibility, and they behave in a highly predictable inflexible manner. Yet, simultaneously, in other ways the patient becomes less strongly connected to loyalties.

Environmental dependency (Lhermitte 1986) and imitation and utilization behavior (Lhermitte et al. 1986) are common features of patients with frontal disorders. FTD leads patients to mimic the behaviors of others or to respond predictably and inflexibly to stimuli in their environment (Ikeda 2008). A proneness to environmental dependency can mean that if the spouse eats ice cream, the patient eats ice cream; if someone walks out the door, the FTD patients follows; or when a phrase is uttered to them, they often repeat it. Repetitive TV watching has also been reported in FTD (Shin et al. 2012).

Similarly, utilization behavior is common, and if a glass of water is present the FTD patient is likely to drink from it, or if a hammer and nail is placed in front of the patient he may hit the nail. Hence the highly rich and complex possible responses to what happens in the world are simplified, and the patient becomes highly dependent on programmed motor responses to whatever he or she sees in the environment.

Antisocial behaviors become predictable, as the patient now responds in a stereotyped fashion to internal signals of hunger, sexual drive, urinary frequency, or anger (Hull 2011), even if these symptoms occur in a setting where these behaviors are normally inhibited. For example, the patient may be unable to inhibit their desire to eat food, leading predictably to weight gain (Woolley et al. 2007, Piguet et al. 2011), or a patient may watch pornography in front of children, hopelessly unable to inhibit this desire. Motor habits, and external stimuli overwhelm the patients and dictate their responses, overriding the ability to adapt behaviors appropriately to the proper context. Patients become guided by stereotyped previously learned behaviors, and lose the ability to adapt to a complex environment. It is common to see patients who know what they should do, or even want to do, but are unable to respond appropriately (Miller et al. 1997). A patient with diabetes may continue to eat large amounts of sweets, even though they know that this behavior will worsen their physical illness. Being able to state correctly that they shouldn't drive through stoplights or drive too fast does not prevent a patient from doing so. The ability to change, adapt, and dictate our own responses erodes and eventually vanishes.

Viewing this loss of control over behavior generates at least some potential answers regarding free will in humans. Does FTD prove that the frontal lobes are critical for a flexible repertoire of responses to challenges in the environment? Definitely, yet the loss of this flexibility does not really tell us whether or not free will truly exists prior to the onset of FTD. Given that the frontal lobes increase the complexity of responses that are possible in humans compared to other species, FTD diminishes this flexibility and thereby slowly decimates and eventually eliminates an individual's free will. As the disease progresses there is little left in adaptability beyond highly predictable and stereotyped stimulus-response behaviors.

RELIGIOUS BELIEFS

One of the remarkable aspects of FTD is how it can change philosophical or religious beliefs in patients (Edwards-Lee et al. 1997; Miller et al. 2001). When this change is seen, it is almost always in patients whose disease involves the right hemisphere.

Patients with right temporal lobe degeneration often present a fascinating constellation of decreased empathy, intensification of philosophical beliefs and rigidity, and excessive moralism in their relationships with others (Edwards-Lee et al. 1997; Perry et al. 2001; Rankin et al. 2006). In patients with selective degeneration of the right anterior temporal lobe, one often sees fanatical, rigid, and unbending adherence to ideas, both religious and political. This fanaticism is made even less appealing by the fact that the patients seem to lose their ability to feel empathy for others. By contrast, patients with predominantly right frontal disease (as is described previously in this chapter) have a propensity to lose the connection to previously held beliefs.

For example, one of our patients began to spend many hours in church and became angry on a Sunday when the community placed sandbags at the river to protect the town from flooding rather than joining him in church. Similarly, he became angry when his wife cried in front of the neighbors when she injured her finger, thinking that public displays of emotion were wrong. When his wife suffered from headaches he would tell her that her pain was

God's punishment for her sins. This rigid cold personality disorder accompanied by religious fanaticism is reminiscent of the quote from Edna St. Vincent Millay, "I love humanity, but I hate people."

It is tempting to hypothesize that historical figures with a reputation for fanaticism and indifference to suffering like Pol Pot, Osama bin Laden, Joseph Stalin, or Adolf Hitler had deficiencies in this right anterior temporal, orbitofrontal, and ventral striatal circuit that led them to the unfeeling and cruel policies (Figure 9–4). Yet, we are still far from understanding the anatomical versus environmental substrates of crime, and still farther from applying the underlying data to rational predictions of abhorrent behavior.

By contrast to the intensely rigid and sometimes cruel patient with right anterior temporal lobe degeneration, the pathologically blasé, right frontal patients drift from one philosophy or religion to another, losing interest in previously held ideologies. The person no longer carries the will to pursue ideas or beliefs. By contrast, patients with Alzheimer's disease or the left frontal or temporally dominant forms of FTD tend to show neither pattern of behavior. This suggests that there may be a balance between right frontal and temporal systems regarding the strength of our beliefs.

PSYCHOLOGY

Social and Emotional Functioning

Adolphs defined social functioning as "the ability to construct representations of the relations between oneself and others, and to use those representations flexibly to guide social behavior" (Adolphs et al. 1999). Complex constructs like personality and social conduct are derived from multiple distributed networks of functional circuits. While the study of brain-behavior relationships in social cognition is relatively new, the brain regions considered central to social functioning include the temporal lobes (TLs), the orbitofrontal cortex (OFC), the insula, the dorsomedial frontal cortex (dmPFC), the dorsolateral frontal cortex (dlPFC), and the ventral striatum (Shany-Ur et al. 2011).

THE NONDOMINANT ANTERIOR TEMPORAL LOBE

The nondominant TL is essential for accurate perception and interpretation of social cues. It is central for the recognition of familiar faces and emotional facial expressions, interpreting voice prosody, and understanding a person's intentions and affect from their body posture,

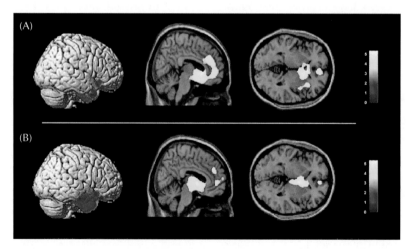

Figure 9–4. **(A)** Main effect of EC score, showing rendered, sagittal (x = 7) and axial (z = 0) views of voxels significantly related to EC score at P < 0.001 uncorrected for multiple comparisons across the whole brain. Maps of significant correlation were superimposed on sections of a normal brain template image (SPM2: single_subj_T1.mnc). The design matrix for this analysis contained only EC score, with sex, age, and TIV included as nuisance covariates, and a t-test was used. **(B)** Main effect of PT score, showing voxels significantly related to PT score at P < 0.001 uncorrected. The design matrix for this analysis contained only PT score, with sex, age, and TIV included as nuisance covariates, and a t-test was used.

gestures, and movements (Cardinal et al. 2002). In two cross-sectional studies, fear recognition was shown to be impaired in bvFTD (Keane et al. 2002; Rosen et al. 2002). A test of identifying vocal emotion yielded similar results: angry and sad voices were poorly identified, but there were additional deficits in recognizing the sounds of happiness or surprise. In patients with svPPA, atrophy in the right anterior temporal cortex tends to be associated with impaired recognition of emotional facial expressions, while the left anterior temporal lobe and parahippocampal regions play an important role in the detection of sarcasm in the voices of others (Shany-Ur et al. 2011).

Work with bvFTD and the right temporal variant of FTD suggest that the right anterior temporal lobe may play a key role in the generation of emotional empathy (Rankin et al. 2006). Focal damage to the right anterior temporal lobe and right frontoinsular cortex diminishes the ability to perceive nonverbal signals and evaluate their communicative intent. If a patient is unable to recognize emotion in a face, it is hard to respond appropriately to the needs of that person. This, in turn, disrupts higher order social cognitive processing that is performed within the frontal lobes.

While previous work has postulated that negative emotions are disproportionately affected by right anterior temporal lobe damage, increasingly our work suggests that decoding complex emotions, whether positive or negative is influenced by right-sided anterior temporal lobe damage. One of the previous problems with previous work, including our own, is that only one positive emotion (happiness) was compared to three negative emotions (anger, sadness, fear). As we have layered on more complexity to the positive emotions (by adding emotions like pride), it appears that the temporal and frontal patients have equally impaired ability with positive emotions.

When a loved one cries, the FTD patient may be indifferent, in part because they do not detect or feel the sadness of others. The ordinarily cautious approach to other people and animals diminishes. Patients may inappropriately approach children, challenge angry people, or even pick up snakes. Encoding the complex social signals that allow us to function and survive as humans eventually disappears.

ORBITOFRONTAL CORTEX: REWARD AND PUNISHMENT

Alteration in our ability to evaluate the reward or punishment value of social information is another important reason why some patients with frontal lobe injury fail to adhere to social norms (Panksepp 1998). Reward and punishment are both strongly mediated by the orbitofrontal cortex (OFC) and anterior insula (O'Doherty et al. 2001; Paulus et al. 2003). In behavioral terms, patients with damage to the OFC, particularly in the right hemisphere, show a pattern of behavioral dyscontrol that may involve making socially inappropriate comments, exhibiting poor manners, and committing theft or infidelity (Rosen et al. 2005).

Disinhibition is a core feature of bvFTD, and a wide variety of studies suggest that disinhibition seems to disproportionately correlate with right orbitofrontal brain volumes (Rosen et al. 2005). The mechanism for the right-sided dominance for behavioral control is unknown, but this seems to also be true in studies of traumatic brain injury.

While many patients aggressively seek out rewards, a process that is mediated by medial OFC, they have serious trouble understanding the potentially punishing consequences of seeking this reward, a function of the lateral OFC and the anterior insula (Paulus et al. 2003). This is in part the reason why patients overeat, smoke, drink, or shop excessively. The signals that ordinarily tell them that their behavior will be punished are dysfunctional.

THE INSULA

The insula is a complex structure with three major histological types of tissue associated with a rostral to caudal (anterior to posterior) progressive decrease in lamination. Regions that lack a layer IV are called agranular, while regions that have only a rudimentary layer IV are called dysgranular. The anterior (rostral) insula is phylogentically old with an agranular cortical structure, the mid portions of the insula are dysgranular, while the posterior (caudal) insula has a six-layered granular cortex (Mesulam & Mufson 1982). The posterior insula is the cortical region responsible for the detection for pain and temperature, the middle insula is where autonomic output is controlled, and the anterior insular is a region that appears to be critical for an emotional awareness of the internal state.

Additionally, Bud Craig has suggested that the anterior insula is a site where higher order cognitive processing about our internal state occurs. While pain activates the contralateral dorsal posterior and mid-insula (right more than left), while subjective experience of pain, or watching a loved one experience pain activates only the anterior insula (right more than left) (AD Craig 2009; Singer et al. 2004).

The insula, particularly the right anterior insula, is devastated in FTD. William Seeley at UCSF has demonstrated that the loss of von Economo neurons layered within the anterior insular cortex and anterior cingulate cortex (Seeley et al. 2006; Kim et al. 2012) is an early and consistent feature of bvFTD (see "Von Economo Neurons," below). Misinterpretation of information from pain pathways and other interoceptive systems is a common in bvFTD. Many patients with bvFTD respond inappropriately to the pain of their loved one, and to their own pain.

Commonly, patients respond in a blunted fashion to the discomfort of their loved ones, whether emotional or physical. Similarly, we have seen patients experience severe burns and ignore skin infections or bone fractures. Loss of disgust leads patients to play with their feces, become indifferent to their own incontinence, collect dead animals, and eat food off of the plates of strangers, or even from garbage cans. Observing these patients' deficits in detecting and experiencing disgust while watching disgusting behavior helps us to understand at a mechanistic level why these behaviors occur (Eckart et al. 2012).

These behaviors are driven by the distorted signaling, and eventually complete loss of function, across the entire insular cortex. More work is needed to better understand the critical but still poorly understood behaviors of FTD as they relate to self-awareness, awareness of others, and the complex behavioral disturbance seen in FTD.

DORSOLATERAL PREFRONTAL CORTEX

The dorsomedial portions of the frontal lobes, including the anterior cingulate, paracingulate, superior frontal gyrus, and frontal pole (Brodmann's area 9/10), appear to be involved in higher-level social cognition. Additionally,

there is increasing evidence that the complex processes of self-monitoring and taking the perspective of others are both highly interdependent and are both mediated by dmPFC structures. Hodges and colleagues (Lough et al. 2006) and Rankin and colleagues (Shany-Ur 2011) have demonstrated marked deficits in tasks of theory of mind in bvFTD. While the anatomy of these changes is complex, dmPFC and dlPFC are extremely important if either cognitive or emotional theory of mind tasks are going to be performed effectively. Additionally, apathy strongly correlates with dmPFC volumes in both bvFTD and in AD.

AMYGDALA AND SUBCORTICAL STRUCTURES

Other aspects of emotional processing occur in subcortical structures, including the amygdala, hypothalamus, the ventral striatum, and multiple regions in the brainstem (Panksepp 1998; Luria 1966). Human and animal studies have revealed that the frontal and temporal lobes, regions that are extensively injured in FTD, interact with these regions.

The amygdala appears crucial for learning the association between a previously neutral stimulus (such as a light or tone, called a conditioned stimulus or CS) and a biologically relevant reward or punishment (e.g., food or shock, both unconditioned stimuli or US) and helps to alter behavior to match these new associations (for an excellent review see Cardinal et al. 2002). In humans, amygdala damage also leads to impaired recognition of specific facial expressions of emotion. Rosen and colleagues have emphasized the atrophy of the amygdala in svPPA and bvFTD.

Another important structure is the nucleus accumbens in the ventral striatum. In an excellent review of factors that mediate sexual drive, stimulant use, and eating, Hull discusses the previous work of Bart Hoebel. Hoebel found that feeding, stimulant drug administration, and electrical stimulation of the lateral hypothalamus all led to increased dopamine release in the nucleus accumbens. Hoebel suggested that dopamine in the nucleus accumbens enhanced motivation while dopamine in the lateral hypothalamus diminished motivated behaviors. Piguet and colleagues and Halabi and colleagues have demonstrated that the hypothalamus (Piguet et al. 2011) and the nucleus accumbens (Halabi et al. 2013) are both attacked in bvFTD. The profoundly, but variably disordered changes in sexual drive (usually diminished, but sometimes increased) (Miller et al. 1995), appetite (usually increased) (Miller et al. 1995), mood (usually normal or enhanced but sometimes diminished), and addictive behaviors (usually increased) are all influenced by the relative balance of function and dysfunction within these structures.

Executive Control

The frontal lobes, which make up 40% of the human cerebral cortex, are greatly expanded in humans compared to nonhuman primates. Far from a monolithic structure with a single purpose, the frontal lobes are divided into multiple structurally, physiologically, and functionally distinct regions with important functions related to movement, motor planning, language, intelligence, working memory, generation, inhibition, alternating sequences, drive, emotion, self-awareness, insight, and personality. Additionally, the frontal lobes have extensive connections with subcortical and other cortical structures. Hence injury to these subcortical structures can lead to frontal lobe syndromes.

Efficient, successful completion of tasks requires the ability to avoid distraction and to maintain mental effort on a given task until it is complete. Patients with frontal lobe damage are often impaired in these functions, leading them to be distractible, disorganized, and very inefficient.

The cognitive functions most commonly attributed to the frontal lobes are higher order or executive processes that involve the organization of more basic cerebral processes to promote efficient task performance and establishment of associations beyond basic representation of incoming sensory information. Some examples of important cognitive functions of the frontal lobes include abstraction, inhibition and facilitating the shifting of cognitive sets. Also, the frontal lobes play a key role in attention, memory (particularly working memory), and language (Miller & Cummings 2007).

The lateral frontal lobe areas mediate conventional executive skills such as planning, sequencing, inhibition, generation, working memory, and abstract reasoning, all of which directly impact our ability to perform complex reasoning about social information (Possin et al. 2009). The capacity to intentionally regulate, organize, and plan our own behavior, as well as to deliberate about the behaviors of others, is partly mediated by these dorsolateral prefrontal cortex (dlPFC) functions. While most patients with bvFTD show deficits in executive control, in very early patients these regions are not yet damaged, and some patients show relatively good executive controls.

In a variety of paradigms ranging from design fluency to the flanker task, we have found that in patients with dementia, the dlPFC is critical for outcomes, particularly the right dlPFC. Rule violations and perseverative errors on tasks of executive control tend to correlate strongly with dlPFC volume in the same way that disinhibition correlates with orbital frontal cortex in bvFTD (Possin et al. 2009).

Often we are required to maintain two or more tasks in mind simultaneously and constantly shift between them. In addition, it is sometimes necessary to suppress the impulse to perform certain tasks in order to reach our goals. These functions are significantly impaired with frontal lobe injury with profound consequences. Many of the functions described above are associated with the dorsolateral portions of the frontal lobes. Generally, verbal tasks disproportionately tap left frontal functions, while visual tasks are more likely to use the right frontal lobe. Inhibition tasks seem to rely on both the dorsolateral and the orbitofrontal region, although perseverative errors tend to be strongly associated with right frontal dysfunction in FTD.

Finally, a variety of disorders with selective subcortical involvement, like progressive supranuclear palsy (PSP), disconnect the frontal lobes from subcortical activation and lead to frontal lobe neuropsychological syndromes (Albert 1974). Hence, a patient with predominantly subcortical damage from a disease like PSP can exhibit the same deficits in executive control or emotional dysregulation as the bvFTD patient (Bak et al. 2010). In our experience, the vast majority of patients with PSP present with behavioral and psychiatric symptoms years prior to developing a motor syndrome.

VON ECONOMO NEURONS

The last topic of this chapter is the von Economo neuron (VEN). These enormous neurons sit in layer 5b of the anterior cingulate and ventral frontoinsular cortex and have a 30% higher concentration in the right frontoinsular regions of the brain than the left. Receptors involved with the modulation of satiety, mood, and affiliation (dopamine-3, serotonin1b and 2b, and vasopressin1a) sit on these neurons. They emerge late in gestation, at approximately 34–38 weeks, peak in total number by 4 years of age and are pruned to the adult number by 8 years of age (Seeley et al. 2006).

One of the most fascinating features of these neurons is that they appear to have emerged phylogenetically in big-brained social species including cetaceans (whales and dolphins) (Butti et al. 2009), elephants (Hakeem et al. 2009), and great apes (Évrard et al. 2012). One of the features that these species have in common is that they all have the capacity to recognize their own face in a mirror (Delfour et al 2001). A variety of roles have been hypothesized for VENs including helping the species to process self-referential information.

Three disorders of social cognition have been associated with changes in the concentration of von Economo neurons, schizophrenia, autism, and FTD. Brüne and colleagues found small reductions in the concentration of these neurons in the right anterior cingulate cortex in a subgroup of schizophrenics with early age of onset (Brüne et al. 2010). Additionally, several studies have found that at least a subset of patients with autism have increased concentration of VENs in the frontoinsular region. Santos and colleagues found that the concentration of VENs was increased in four children with autism compared to three healthy controls (Santos et al. 2011). This outgrowth could have been related to changes in "migration, cortical lamination, and apoptosis." The authors wondered whether these changes were related to the heightened interoceptive sensitivity associated with autism.

Finally, William Seeley at UCSF has linked these neurons strongly to bvFTD. In two seminal studies, Dr. Seeley and colleagues found markedly diminished levels of VENs in the anterior insular and anterior cingulate cortex. Additionally, their concentration was markedly diminished in early-stage cases of bvFTD,

when the adjacent pyramidal layer neurons were normal (Seeley et al. 2006). Work from this laboratory shows that the VEN may be the first neuron to die, setting off a circuit-specific cascade of neurodegeneration (Kim et al. 2012). With time the role of these neurons in social cognition and behavior is likely to be elucidated, in part, through the study of FTD from a clinical to a pathological level.

REFERENCES

Adolphs R. Social cognition and the human brain. Trends Cogn Sci. 1999;3:469–79.

Albert ML, Feldman RG, Willis AL. The "subcortical dementia" of progressive supranuclear palsy. J Neurol Neurosurg Psychiatry. 1974;37(2):121–30.

Bak TH, Crawford LM, Berrios G, Hodges JR. Behavioural symptoms in progressive supranuclear palsy and frontotemporal dementia. J Neurol Neurosurg Psychiatry. 2010;81(9):1057–9.

Brüne M, Schöbel A, Karau R, Benali A, Faustmann PM, Juckel G, Petrasch-Parwez E. Von Economo neuron density in the anterior cingulate cortex is reduced in early onset schizophrenia. Acta Neuropathol. 2010;119(6):771–8.

Butti C, Sherwood CC, Hakeem AY, Allman JM, Hof PR. Total number and volume of Von Economo neurons in the cerebral cortex of cetaceans. J Comp Neurol. 2009;515:243–59.

Cardinal RN, Parkinson JA, Hall J, Everitt BJ, Emotion and motivation: the role of the amygdala, ventral striatum and prefrontal cortex. Neurosci Biobehav Rev. 2002;26:321–52.

Craig AD. How do you feel—now? The anterior insula and human awareness. Nat Rev Neurosci. 2009;10:59–70.

Delfour F, Marten K. Mirror image processing in three marine mammal species: killer whales (orcinus orca), false killer whales (Pseudorca crassidens) and California sea lions (Zalophus californianus). Behav Prcesses. 2001;53 (3):181–90.

Eckart JA, Sturm BE, Miller BL, Levenson. Diminished disgust reactivity in behavioral variant frontotemporal dementia. Neuropsychologia. 2012;50:786–90.

Edwards-Lee T, Miller BL, Benson DF, Cummings JL, Russell GL, Boone K, Mena I. The temporal variant of frontotemporal dementia. Brain. 1997;120(Pt 6):1027–40.

Ellsworth PC. William James and emotion: is a century of fame worth a century of misunderstanding? Psychological Review. 1994;101(2):222–9.

Évrard HC, Forro T, Logothetis NK. Von Economo neurons in the anterior insula of the macaque monkey. Neuron. 2012;74:482–9.

Fuster JM. The Prefrontal Cortex. Philadelphia: Lippincott-Raven; 1997.

Gottman JM, Levenson RW. Marital processes predictive of later dissolution: behavior, physiology, and health. J Pers Soc Psychol. 1992;63(2):221–33.

Hakeem AY, Sherwood CC, Bonar CJ, Butti C, Hof PR, Allman JM. Von Economo neurons in the elephant brain. Anat Rec (Hoboken). 2009;292:242–8.

Halabi C, Halabi A, Dean DL, Wang PN, Boxer AL, Trojanowski JQ, Dearmond SJ, Miller BL, Kramer JH, Seeley WW. Patterns of striatal degeneration in frontotemporal dementia. Alzheimer Dis Assoc Disord. 2013;27:74–83.

Hoefer M, Allison SC, Schauer GF, Neuhaus JM, Hall H, Dang N, Weiner MW, Miller BL, Rosen HJ. Fear conditioning in frontotemporal lobar degeneration and Alzheimer's disease. Brain. 2008;131:1646–57.

Hull EM. Sex, drugs and gluttony: how the brain controls motivated behaviors. Physiol Behav. 2011;104:173–7.

Ikeda M. Symptomatology of fronto-temporal dementia. Rinsho Shinkeigaku. 2008;48(11):1002–4.

James W. The principles of psychology. classics in the history of psychology [online], http://psychclassics. yorku. ca/James/Principles/ (1890).

James W. The energies of men. Science. 1907;25:321–32.

Keane J, Calder AJ, Hodges JR, Young AW. Face and emotion processing in frontal variant frontotemporal dementia. Neuropsychologia. 2002;40:655–65.

Kim EJ, Sidhu M, Gaus SE, Huang EJ, Hof PR, Miller BL, DeArmond SJ, Seeley WW. Selective frontoinsular von Economo neuron and fork cell loss in early behavioral variant frontotemporal dementia. Cereb Cortex. 2012;22:251–9.

Levenson RW, Ascher E, Goodkind M, McCarthy M, Sturm V, Werner K. Chapter 25: Laboratory testing of emotion and frontal cortex. Handb Clin Neurol. 2008;88:489–98.

Levenson RW, Carstensen LL, Gottman JM. Long-term marriage: age, gender, and satisfaction. Psychol Aging. 1993;8(2):301–13.

Levenson RW, Miller BL. Loss of cells—loss of self: frontotemporal lobar degeneration and human emotion. Current Direct Psychol Sci. 2007;16:289–94.

Levenson RW. Blood, sweat and fears: the autonomic architecture of emotion. Ann N Y Acad Sci. 2003;1000:348–66.

Lhermitte F. Human autonomy and the frontal lobes. Part II: Patient behavior in complex social situations: the "environmental dependency syndrome." Ann Neurol 1986;19(4):335–43.

Lhermitte F, Pillon B, Serdaru M. Human autonomy and the frontal lobes. Part I: Imitation and utilization behavior: a neuropsychological study of 75 patients. Ann Neurol. 1986;19(4):326–34.

Lough S, Kipps CM, Treise C, Watson P, Blair JR, Hodges JR. Social reasoning, emotion and empathy in frontotemporal dementia. Neuropsychologia. 2006;44:950–8.

Luria AR. "Brain and conscious experience": a critical notice from the U.S.S.R. of the symposium edited by J. C. Eccles (1966). Br J Psychol. 1967;58:467–76.

Mesulam MM, Mufson E J. Insula of the old world monkey. III: Efferent cortical output and comments on function. J. Comp. Neurol. 1982;212:38–52.

Miller BL, Cummings J. The Human Frontal Lobes, 2nd Edition. New York: Guilford Press; 2007.

Miller BL, Darby A, Benson DF, Cummings JL, Miller MH. Aggressive, socially disruptive and antisocial behavior in frontotemporal dementia. Brit J Psychiatry. 1997;170:150–56.

Miller BL, Darby AL, Swartz JR, Yener GG, Mena I. Dietary changes, compulsions and sexual behavior in frontotemporal degeneration. Dementia. 1995;6(4):195–9.

Miller BL, Mychack P, Seeley W, Rosen, H, Boone KB. Neuroanatomy of the self: evidence from patients with frontotemporal dementia. Neurology. 2001;57:817–21.

O'Doherty J, Kringelbach ML, Rolls ET, Hornak J, Andrews C. Abstract reward and punishment representations in the human orbitofrontal cortex. Nat Neurosci. 2001;4(1):95–102.

Panksepp J. Affective Neuroscience: The Foundations of Human and Animal Emotions. New York: Oxford University Press; 1998.

Parfit, Derek A. Later selves and moral principles. In A. Montefiore (ed.), Philosophy and Personal Relations. London: Routledge and Kegan Paul; 1973:137–69.

Paulus MP, Rogalsky C, Simmons A, Feinstein JS, Stein MB. Increased activation in the right insula during risk-taking decision making is related to harm avoidance and neuroticism. Neuroimage. 2003;19(4):1439–48.

Perry RJ, Rosen HR, Kramer JH, Beer JS, Levenson RL, Miller BL. Hemispheric dominance for emotions, empathy and social behaviour: evidence from right and left handers with frontotemporal dementia. Neurocase. 2001;7(2):145–60.

Piguet O, Petersén A, Yin Ka Lam B, Gabery S, Murphy K, Hodges JR, Halliday GM. Eating and hypothalamus changes in behavioral-variant frontotemporal dementia. Ann Neurol. 2011;69:312–9.

Possin KL, Brambati SM, Rosen HJ, Johnson JK, Pa J, Weiner MW, Miller BL, Kramer JH. Rule violation errors are associated with right lateral prefrontal cortex atrophy in neurodegenerative disease. J Int Neuropsychol Soc. 2009;15:354–64.

Rankin K, Gorno-Tempini ML, Allison S, Stanley CM, Glenn S, Weiner MW, Miller BL. Structural anatomy of empathy in neurodegenerative disease. Brain. 2006;129:2945–56.

Rosen HJ, Allison SC, Schauer GF, Gorno-Tempini ML, Weiner MW, Miller BL. Neuroanatomical correlates of behavioural disorders in dementia. Brain. 2005;128 (Pt 11):2612–25.

Rosen HJ, Pace-Savitsky K, Perry RJ, Kramer JH, Miller BL, Levenson RW. Recognition of emotion in the frontal and temporal variants of frontotemporal dementia. Dement Geriatr Cogn Disord. 2004;17:277–81.

Rosen HJ, Perry RJ, Murphy J, Kramer JH, Mychack P, Schuff N, Weiner M, Levenson RW, Miller BL. Emotion comprehension in the temporal variant of frontotemporal dementia. Brain. 2002;125:2286–95.

Rosen HJ, Wilson MR, Schauer GF, Allison S, Gorno-Tempini ML, Pace-Savitsky C, Kramer JH, Levenson RW, Weiner M, Miller BL. Neuroanatomical correlates of impaired recognition of emotion in dementia. Neuropsychologia. 2006;44:365–73.

Santos M, Uppal N, Butti C, Wicinski B, Schmeidler J, Giannakopoulos P, Heinsen H, Schmitz C, Hof PR. Von Economo neurons in autism: a stereologic study of the frontoinsular cortex in children. Brain Res. 2011;1380:206–17.

Saper CB. The central autonomic nervous system: conscious visceral perception and autonomic pattern generation. Annu Rev Neurosci. 2002;25:433–69.

Seeley WW Carlin D, Allman JM, Macedo MN, Bush C, Miller BL, DeArmond S. Early frontotemporal dementia targets neurons unique to apes and humans. Ann Neurol. 2006;60:660–67.

Shany-Ur, Poorzand P, Grossman SN, Growdon ME, Jang JY, Ketelle RS, Miller BL, Rankin K. Comprehension of insincere communication in neurodegenerative disease: Lies, sarcasm, and theory of mind. Cortex. 2012;48(10):1329–41.

Shin JS, Kim MS, Kim NS, Kim GH, Seo SW, Kim EJ, Heilman KM, Na DL. Excessive TV watching in patients with frontotemporal dementia. Neurocase. 2012 Jul 25. [Epub ahead of print]

Singer T, Seymour B, O'Doherty J, Kaube H, Dolan RJ, Frith CD. Empathy for pain involves the affective but not sensory components of pain. Science. 2004;303:1157–62.

Sturm VE, Ascher EA, Miller BL, Levenson RW. Diminished self-conscious emotional responding in frontotemporal lobar degeneration patients. Emotion. 2008;8:861–69.

Sturm VE, McCarthy ME, Yun I, Madan A, Yuan JW, Holley SR, Ascher EA, Boxer AL, Miller BL, Levenson RW. Mutual gaze in Alzheimer's disease, frontotemporal and semantic dementia couples. Soc Cogn Affect Neurosci. 2011;6:359–67.

Sturm VE, Rosen HJ, Allison S, Miller BL, Levenson RW. Self-conscious emotion deficits in frontotemporal lobar degeneration. Brain. 2006;129 (Pt 9):2508–16.

Sturm VE, Sollberger M, Seeley WW, Rankin KP, Ascher EA, Rosen HJ, Miller BL, Levenson RW. Role of right pregenual anterior cingulate cortex in self-conscious emotional reactivity. Soc Cogn Affect Neurosci. 2012 Mar 20. [Epub ahead of print]

Sze JA, Goodkind MS, Gyurak A, Levenson RW. Aging and emotion recognition: not just a losing matter. Psychol Aging. 2012;27(4):940–50.

Werner KH, Roberts NA, Rosen HJ, Dean DL, Kramer JH, Weiner MW, Miller BL, Levenson RW. Emotional reactivity and emotion recognition in frontotemporal lobar degeneration. Neurology. 2007;69(2):148–55.

Woolley JD, Gorno-Tempini ML, Seeley WW, Rankin K, Lee SS, Matthews BR, Miller BL. Binge eating is associated with right orbitofrontal-insular-striatal atrophy in frontotemporal dementia. Neurology. 2007;69(14):1424–33.

Zakzanis KK. Neurocognitive deficit in fronto-temporal dementia. Neuropsychiatry Neuropsychol Behav Neurol. 1998;11:127–35.

Chapter 10

Treatments

DIAGNOSIS

The first step in the treatment of frontotemporal dementia (FTD) is getting an accurate diagnosis. Although not uncommon, these patients often go undiagnosed by clinicians and radiologists (Suárez et al. 2009) and often are labeled and treated as psychiatric patients (Woolley et al. 2011). Many of the patients sent to our program diagnosed with behavioral variant of FTD (bvFTD) have Alzheimer's disease (AD), another non-FTD neurodegenerative condition, or a primary psychiatric disorder. Additionally, as has been noted previously in this book, as we move toward molecule-based therapies for bvFTD knowing the underlying neuropathology for the bvFTD syndrome will become critical.

bvFTD presents with changes in personality, behavioral problems, executive impairment, or any combination of these signs and symptoms (Rascovsky et al. 2011). The poor decision-making abilities and the behavioral and social inappropriateness of FTD are a source of grief and frustration for caregivers and can endanger the patient and those with whom the patient interacts. While there are no disease-modifying therapies for any of the FTD subtypes, ameliorating symptoms can improve quality of life for both patients and their caregivers.

FTD is associated with a profound breakdown in the emotional system in bvFTD, causing severe impairments in social relationships. Loss of empathy is a core feature of FTD (Rankin et al. 2006), and the basis for this symptom can be broken down and understood at multiple levels. In studies performed in the laboratory of Dr. Robert Levenson at the University of California, Berkeley, the FTD patients show diminished gaze toward loved ones (Sturm et al. 2011), impaired perception of the emotions on others faces (Rosen et al. 2002), decreased emotional reactivity (Werner et al. 2007), decreased embarrassment (Sturm et al. 2008), and decreased reactivity to disgusting movies (Eckart et al. 2012). All of these deficits in emotion regulation lead to severe marital discord and dissatisfaction for the caregiver (Ascher et al. 2010). All of these deficits occur early in the course of the illness and have proven elusive to treatment, yet effective treatments will need to focus on the core features of bvFTD and svPPA that trouble both the patient and their loved ones.

bvFTD: TARGETING SYMPTOMS, EDUCATING THE FAMILY

Typically, treatment begins with discussing the diagnosis and educating the family about the disease. The caregivers need to be informed about the potential issues around the patient's safety and they should be instructed about how to organize strategies to protect the patient's safety (and their own).

Due to the apathy and absence of concern for the consequences of their actions, bvFTD and svPPA patients often represent a danger around the stove, are dangerous as drivers, and cannot look after children (Merrilees et al. 2009). We have frequently heard of bvFTD patients leaving infants or young children unattended, sometimes with near disastrous consequences. One parent dropped off his children aged eight, six and three in the most dangerous neighborhood in Los Angeles, hoping that they would learn to fend for themselves in the modern world. Another was asked to care for her infant grandson and left the child alone for many hours.

Pacing, restlessness, and deficits in impulse control make wandering off unattended a constant concern. One of the first patients that I ever saw went to the bathroom, walked away, and was found two days later, at an 18-mile distance from the hospital. This type of wandering is common, and patients can get lost and become subject to the dangers of their environment.

Often, the bvFTD patient has a diminished response to pain, and we have seen patients suffer from heat stroke, frostbite, injury to nerves, and necrosis of arm muscles due to lack of responsivity to painful stimuli (Carlino et al. 2010). Furthermore, their inability to gauge social situations can lead them to get injured if they wander into dangerous areas. The patient's lack of insight and disinhibition may lead to potentially dangerous behaviors whereby aggressive outbursts by the patient could lead to harm, usually from others reacting to the patient's disinhibition. It is important to encourage caregivers to remove dangerous items such as guns from the home and to eliminate driving if the patient is unsafe.

Perhaps the greatest threat to the patient is that they will anger other people in their environment and get attacked or arrested. Recently, we had a patient inappropriately touch a young woman in a store in front of her boyfriend, nearly leading to a physical fight. Another patient was arrested near a children's park. His repetitive urination and ritualistic shaking of his penis was misinterpreted as public masturbation in front of children. There are far too many examples of how patients with bvFTD end up in the legal system rather than being treated for their medical condition (Miller et al. 1997: Mendez et al. 2005). Recognition of this potential to exhibit behaviors that can or do lead to arrest is the first step toward preventing this tragic complication that can occur in bvFTD and svPPA.

Comorbid movement problems are particularly problematic with bvFTD phenotypes because the patients may have profound deficits in their insight into these problems. The patient with a bvFTD syndrome associated with PSP-like movement abnormalities is particularly problematic because their propensity to fall is associated with the desire to walk and unconcern about the consequences of walking. The patients who develop swallowing problems will still blithely place large amounts of food into their mouths, exacerbating the existing problem, and will need very close attention when they are eating (Langmore et al. 2007). Rarely is it possible to place a feeding tube into a patient with FTD-ALS due to the likelihood that the patient will pull the tube.

svPPA: TARGETING SYMPTOMS, EDUCATING THE FAMILY

svPPA often presents with marked language impairment, in the form of a loss of memory for words or a loss of word meaning. These patients are aware of their anomia, which is a source of significant frustration for many of them. svPPA patients often obsess over their language problem, and it can be a cause for extremely low self-esteem. It is common to see them hit their heads and say, "nothing is there." Targeting the aphasia with speech and language therapy can sometimes be extremely helpful in convincing the svPPA individual that they are doing something to combat their illness.

Conversely, these same patients often lack insight into their behavioral problems, a deficit that troubles their loved ones much more than does the anomia (Rosen et al. 2006; Rosen et al. 2011). Right-sided temporal cases present with deficits in knowledge about people and with loss of empathy that are profoundly troubling to the family (Rankin et al. 2006). As the temporal variant of FTD progresses it spreads out into the regions attacked in bvFTD. Therefore, many of the behavioral problems seen in bvFTD eventually emerge in svPPA including disinhibition, obsessive collecting, loss of empathy for loved ones, apathy, bad decision-making, and overeating.

svPPA and right temporal patients are particularly prone to deficits in fear and recognition of the emotions of others (Rosen et al. 2002). Therefore, these individuals can approach extremely angry people or animals. One of my

patients was repetitively bitten by a neighborhood dog but continued to approach and pet the animal. Similarly, I have had two patients with this variant of FTD pick up rattlesnakes and one actually approached a mountain lion. Placing of nonfood items into the mouth can lead to death. Understanding these risks helps the FTD caregiver set up an environment that protects the patient from himself and from outside threats.

nfvPPA: TARGETING SYMPTOMS AND EDUCATING THE FAMILY

nfvPPA, typically involves changes in fluency or word finding difficulty. These patients are well aware of their deficits and can be the first one to notice the aphasia. Mood disorders are common, but not invariable, in these patients and many will require therapies focused around the speech and mood.

While there are many nfvPPA patients who do not develop features of bvFTD, some do as the illness progresses, and such patients require the same behavioral attention as bvFTD individuals as the disease spreads into the right frontal regions. Parkinsonian features are common in this subtype of FTD, and patients may briefly benefit from a target on these sets of symptoms.

LATE STAGES OF FTD

All of the FTD clinical subtypes eventually reach a stage when the patient has difficulty with speech, swallowing, and movement and an inability to recognize their loved ones. Bedridden and unable to move due to either parkinsonian features or motor neuron disease, many of these patients need to be moved to chronic care facilities or hospice, not more aggressive care. Helping the family expect and understand this late stage of FTD is extremely important.

EARLY INTERVENTIONS

Nonpharmacological forms of therapy should be initiated first for the management of inappropriate or aggressive behavior. This includes discussing tolerance for disruptive but nondangerous behavior with the caregivers. While many of the behaviors of bvFTD may be unpleasant, making intelligent decisions about those that can be treated or are life-threatening is an important component of effective caregiving (Merrilees et al. 2010). For example, while overeating or only eating certain foods or exhibiting bad manners such as eating with the hands or licking a plate, may be mildly distressing to the family, none of these behaviors represents a threat to the patient.

A medical alert bracelet for the patient and a note or card explaining the patient has a disease can be extremely helpful and will help to convert threatening situations. Distraction is an excellent way to deal with irrational requests or to help alter behaviors. Sometimes food can be used to convince patients to do things that they don't want to do. Nutrition is an ongoing push and pull in FTD and requires a balance between not allowing the patient to massively overeat versus allowing the patient to pursue this pleasure.

As with all dementias, patients with FTD may have difficulty explaining that they have pain or other metabolic issues causing a disruption in consciousness. Any abrupt changes in behavior, whether agitation or withdrawal, should be meticulously evaluated, and a broad search for causes should be instituted. Infection, electrolyte imbalance, changes in glucose, constipation, bone fractures, and pain are common reasons for behavioral changes in FTD.

The family and caregivers should be referred to support groups and local chapters that, in addition to providing information and advice, organize respite care (Morhardt 2011). Depression in caregivers is common (even more common than in AD) and leads patients to earlier nursing home placement (Merrilees et al. 2005). The need for a power of attorney cannot be overemphasized, as the patients quickly, if not many years prior to the time of diagnosis, are no longer able to make medical and financial decisions. The behavioral symptoms are often the cause for the institutionalizing patients, so the symptoms need to be addressed and adequately treated.

PHARMACOLOGICAL REVIEW

There are no medications available to cure or delay the progression of FTD, but there are a number of medications available for symptomatic relief (Huey et al. 2006). Medical management includes treatment of concomitant medical conditions including infections, parkinsonian symptoms, seizures, and pain. It is imperative to review all medications that the patient is taking. This includes prescription drugs, nonprescription drugs, social drugs (caffeine, nicotine, alcohol), and/or alternative products (e.g., herbals, vitamins, minerals). Many medically prescribed and over-the-counter medications can exacerbate behaviors or cognitive problems (e.g., high doses of vitamins, stimulants, antidepressants, some antiepileptic medications), so any unnecessary drug should be discontinued. Any medication that the patient is taking should be formally reassessed for whether the dosage is optimal, and the patient should only be taking medications that have a reasonable chance of improving rather than exacerbating the underlying conditions. Often, taking away medications is more effective than adding them.

Selective Serotonin Reuptake Inhibitors (SSRIs)

While there is no known treatment that can delay progression, environmental and pharmacological interventions can help with the behavioral management (Perry et al. 2001, Jicha 2011). Certain behaviors, especially aggression and extreme disruptiveness, and profoundly disturbing delusions will require medications and often a change in the patient's environment.

Patients with FTD show both postsynaptic and presynaptic serotonin defects and this disruption in a major neurotransmitter system can have a significant effect on behavior. Overeating, repetitive motor behaviors, irritability, aggression, alterations in sleep and wake cycles, and impulsivity can all occur in patients with serotonin deficiency and represent reasonable targets for serotonin boosting (Swartz et al. 1997; Merrilees et al. 2009).

Selective serotonin reuptake inhibitors (SSRIs) have been used with some success in FTD. Swartz and colleagues and Lebert and colleagues were the first to show modest effects on behavior with SSRIs (Swartz et al. 1997; Lebert et al. 2004). Swartz's study was open-label and used a variety of SSRIs, while Lebert and colleagues used Trazodone. Similarly, 30 mg of citalopram followed by a 6-week open-label study of up to 40 mg of citalopram from the group in Toronto, Canada, showed significant decreases in the Neuropsychiatric Inventory total score with improvements in disinhibition, irritability, and depression scores over the 6 weeks (Herrmann et al. 2012). Another 14-month, open-label study with paroxetine showed modest efficacy for behavior (Moretti et al. 2003). By contrast, Deakin and colleagues in Cambridge, England, did not find improvements, and these authors also reported mild but negative effects on cognition related to sedation (Deakin et al. 2004).

The SSRIs can be tried as a therapy for the compulsions, ritualistic behaviors, carbohydrate cravings, anxiety, irritability, and sleep disturbance in patients with FTD. The side effects with these compounds are tolerable for most patients with far fewer side effects than the atypical antipsychotics.

We tend to start on low doses of SSRIs or serotonin-norepinephrine reuptake inhibitors (SNRIs) and slowly increase the dosage. SNRIs may be slightly more alerting, while traditional SSRIs can be chosen if slight sedation is desired. The agitation side effect of fluoxetine makes this SSRI less appealing, and the seizure potential of buproprion has led us to avoid this SNRI.

Atypical Antipsychotics

Low doses of atypical antipsychotics such as quetiapine, olanzepine, or risperidone can be used for agitation, aggression, or psychotic behavior. In the Clinical Antipsychotic Trials of Intervention Effectiveness (CATIE) study of antipsychotics for AD patients with psychotic symptoms there was a low likelihood of efficacy (approximately 19%) and a high side-effects profile (Schneider et al. 2006). Therefore the potential benefit of the sedating effect of antipsychotics must be weighed against the potential risks, and all of these medications have a "black box" warning due to their potential for precipitating diabetes, cerebrovascular adverse events, and even mortality. Furthermore, the influence of these compounds on movement and swallowing is always a reason to use only when absolutely necessary and to begin therapy with low doses.

Typical antipsychotics are associated with extrapyramidal side effects and usually should be avoided, since patients with FTD, even those without obvious movement difficulties, have very significant basal ganglia atrophy (Halabi et al. 2013). Many of these individuals are on the way to either parkinsonism or ALS. Medications for behavioral symptoms should start at a low dose and then subsequently be titrated slowly based on the patient's response and the presence of adverse effects. Additionally, it is important to consider tapering these patients off atypical antipsychotics once the behavioral stresses for which they were used have stabilized.

Acetylcholinesterase Inhibitors (AChEIs)

Although one open-label trial with rivastigmine showed mild efficacy (Moretti et al. 2004), there is little data to support the use of acetylcholinesterase inhibitors in managing symptoms of FTD. Furthermore, there are some FTD patients in whom these compounds exacerbate irritability, agitation, and disinhibition. The cholinesterase compounds are particularly worrisome in FTD patients with motor neuron disease as they can lead to increased oral secretions.

The best explanation for their lack of effectiveness in FTD is that the cholinergic system, in particular the cholinergic neurons in the cortex, is relatively spared in FTD (Wood et al. 1983). In fact, in my opinion, an extremely positive response to a cholinesterase inhibitor sometimes means that the patient suffers not from FTD but rather from another disorder that is associated with a cholinergic deficit such as Parkinson's disease dementia, dementia with Lewy bodies, or AD.

NMDA-Receptor Antagonist

Memantine, an NMDA-receptor antagonist, is approved for the treatment of AD. While a small open-label study with memantine showed mild efficacy (Boxer et al. 2009), the results of two multicenter studies, one in Europe (Vercelletto et al. 2011) and one in the United States (Boxer et al. 2009), have both been negative. With that said there are occasional patients with agitation in whom memantine offers a good safety profile and can be considered.

Dextromethorphan Hydrobromide and Quinidine Sulfate for Pseudobulbar Affect

Many patients with FTD-ALS develop uncontrolled episodes of intense laughter or crying, so-called pseudobulbar affect. These episodes are usually triggered by real emotional triggers but the patient's ability to suppress the emotional response is diminished, leading to an intense physiological response (Olney et al. 2011). Recently the combination of dextromethorphan hydrobromide and quinidine sulfate marketed as Nuedexta is effective for helping the patient control these spells (Olney & Rosen 2010) and should be considered in patients with troubling or disabling episodes of pseudobulbar affect.

Valproic Acid

Valproic acid and derivatives (divalproex sodium) have been touted for aggressive behavior and for impulse control in individuals diagnosed with AD, although in placebo-controlled studies valproic acid displayed little or no benefit (Tariot et al. 2011). While there may be anecdotal stories of patients with FTD in whom valproic acid and related drugs have shown efficacy, there is no convincing data for the use of these compounds in FTD.

Gabapentin

Gabapentin has also been reported to be helpful in managing behavioral problems in a few case reports, although there is no strong data supporting its use in the treatment of FTD. We cannot recommend the use of this compound in bvFTD, and the side effects of fatigue, weight gain, and drowsiness can exacerbate the symptoms of these patients.

Oxytocin

Elizabeth Finger (Finger 2011) has recently proposed the use of oxytocin as a potential therapy for the emotional deficits in FTD. It is now recognized that oxytocin, a neuropeptide produced in the supraoptic and paraventricular nuclei of the hypothalamus, plays an important role in social cognition and prosocial behavior. No degenerative disorder has such a negative impact on these aspects of behavior as does FTD.

In a placebo-controlled study (Jesso et al. 2011) there was a mild effect on the Neuropsychiatric Inventory and on some tests of emotional recognition. While unlikely to have a large impact on this illness, oxytocin has potential to have mild efficacy for some of the emotional changes seen with bvFTD, and these studies represent an intelligent and targeted effort toward treating the antisocial aspects of this disorder.

NONPHARMACOLOGICAL THERAPIES

Individualized exercise programs can have a positive impact on functional performance in persons with mild to moderate dementia and can be helpful for patients with FTD (and their caregivers). Adequate sleep may reduce behavioral problems, and it is important to encourage caregivers to aggressively make certain that they maintain a good sleep-wake cycle. The disrupted sleep of dementia patients can have a profoundly negative effect on their caregivers (Merrilees et al. 2009). Recognizing and treating concomitant illnesses or infections can also improve behavioral problems.

There have been no systematic efforts to try cognitive-behavioral therapy (CBT) for bvFTD, although there have been limited efforts in FTD; it is possible that for patients with mild disease such approaches might be modestly effective. This is particularly true for gene carriers who can be diagnosed very early in their illness.

Similarly, there is almost no data on music therapy or art therapy for FTD patients, although we believe that there are many dementia patients in whom creative activities can be fruitful and emotionally satisfying (Flaherty 2011). In particular, patients with left-brain degeneration have a propensity for visual creativity and can produce remarkable products (Miller & Hou 2004). Yet, a one-size-fits-all approach is not possible, and one patient may respond to music while another may do better with painting or sculpture.

COMPLEMENTARY AND ALTERNATIVE MEDICINE

Many individuals also use nonprescription and herbal medical foods or alternative approaches, such as acupuncture, for symptoms related to bvFTD. To date, however, there is no evidence that any of these approaches have any efficacy for bvFTD or related disorders. In fact, the lack regulation of medical food and herbal medicines can mean that these approaches are more toxic than therapeutic. Additionally, there are many patients who take a multitude of over-the-counter medications, with toxic drug–drug interactions and can be extremely expensive, despite no legitimate data supporting their use. Sadly, the use of cholinesterase inhibitors and memantine is common in FTD, despite little evidence for efficacy (Hu et al. 2010).

LANGUAGE IMPAIRMENT

While there are not useful medications to help with language impairment, nfavPPA and early svPPA and bvFTD warrant a speech pathology assessment and intervention. There is an emerging literature to suggest that all of the progressive aphasia subtypes respond to speech and language therapy that is tailored around their own particular strengths and deficits (Rapp et al. 2009, Bonner et al. 2009, Henry et al. 2013). In svPPA, speech is normal, and the therapy should focus around learning words that are commonly used in day-to-day activities. By contrast, nfvPPA patients often benefit from help with speech and language output. Maintaining adequate communication can decrease frustration and give the patient a better sense of mastery of their aphasia. Many of our patients find speech therapy a highly gratifying and effective intervention, although there are still no large placebo-controlled studies with any of the aphasic variants of FTD.

FUTURE TREATMENTS

There is a paucity of randomized, placebo-controlled data on most symptomatic treatments for FTD and related conditions. The development of animal models of FTD where new compounds can be tested has greatly facilitated the drug development effort in FTD while facilitating a better understanding of the underlying pathophysiology of these conditions (Lee & Trojanowski 2001, Vossel & Miller 2008). This is a source of optimism, and there are many serious drug development efforts going on across the world.

As with AD, treatment of FTD is moving from a neurotransmitter-based symptomatic methodology to a molecule-based prevention approach. Hence, therapies will require recognition of the underlying molecules participating in the neurodegenerative process, and targeting these molecules. Because of the molecular and probably etiological diversity of FTD therapies, it is unlikely that a single "one compound fits all" approach will be possible. Currently, the major efforts to treat FTD have focused around developing therapies for syndromes caused by abnormal processing of tau, progranulin, TDP-43, FUS, and *C9ORF72*.

Tau

As has been described in previous chapters, CBD, PSP, and argyrophilic grain disease (AGD) are all 4R tauopathies, while Pick's disease is a 3R tauopathy. Until recently, most of treatment efforts have focused around tau-stabilizing compounds. Because abnormally phosphorylated tau is considered a toxic form of tau, efforts to prevent phosphorylation of tau have received significant attention. GSK-β is a kinase that is responsible for the phosphorylation of tau, and the initial efforts to treat tauopathies have tried GSK-β inhibitors.

Lithium works on this enzyme and has been considered as a potential therapy for PSP and AD disease. Even though relatively low doses of this compound were used, lithium proved too toxic to pursue in a small study sponsored by the National Institutes of Health. Another GSK-β inhibitor, Tideglusib (Nypta-R), did not show efficacy in a large, placebo-controlled study.

More recent efforts have focused on a tau-stabilizing compound called davunetide (NAP), an eight-amino-acid compound derived from activity-dependent neuroprotective protein by Ilana Gozes (Gozes 2011). A 300-person placebo-controlled trial for PSP was completed but failed to show efficacy.

Another compound that has generated considerable interest is the microtubule-stabilizing compound epothilone D, developed for dementia by Kurt Brunden, John Trojanowski, and Virginia Lee. This compound is microtubule-stabilizing, reduces axonal degeneration, and stabilizes cognitive function in an aged tauopathy mouse (Zhang et al. 2012). This compound is being considered as a potential treatment for both AD and the FTLD-related tauopathies.

Finally, a derivative of methylene blue (Rember) has been developed by Dr. Claude Wischik in Scotland as a potential tau-modifying compound through his company *TauRx*. The potential efficacy of methylene blue on tau was recently reviewed (Schirmer et al. 2011). While the mechanism of action for methylene blue appears to be tau-stabilizing, it may also work by increasing proteasome activity (Medina et al. 2011). Trials for both AD and bvFTD were planned with Rember in 2012.

As is described in the previous chapters 6, 7, and 8, with the realization that tau propagates from one cell to the next (Kfoury et al. 2012), the greatest excitement for therapies has focused around monoclonal antibodies, or drugs that suppress tau expression. If these types of molecules could be delivered in the relatively early stages of disease in patients with tau mutations, PSP, CBD, or Pick's disease, achieving a positive outcome seems very possible.

Progranulin

Progranulin mutations lead to a slowly progressive neurodegenerative condition that attacks frontoinsular cortex and the basal ganglia. Unlike the other forms of FTLD, where an increase in a toxic protein causes neurodegeneration, in this form of FTLD a deficiency in the progranulin protein is the cause for neurological syndrome. Many of these mutations work via nonsense-mediated decay, so that the protein coming from the mutated gene is never produced (Ward & Miller 2011). In some ways this is an ideal molecular mechanism to explore because the peripheral levels (and possibly cerebrospinal fluid levels) of progranulin can be used as a way to judge the efficacy of a new medication. One issue that still needs to be worked through is the variability of peripheral and central measures with or without treatment.

Two research groups, one centered at the University of California, San Francisco (UCSF; The Consortium for Frontotemporal Dementia), and the other led by Dr. Christian Haass in Munich, Germany, have discovered compounds that boost the production of progranulin. In one study led by Joachim Herz at the University of Texas, Dallas (Cenik et al. 2011), it was found that the histone deacetylase (HDAC) inhibitor vorinostat approximately doubled progranulin levels. While vorinostat does not easily pass the blood-brain barrier, there are other HDAC inhibitors that do, and they are now being seriously considered for a trial for progranulin gene carriers.

Additionally, Li Gan, also part of the Consortium for Frontotemporal Dementia Research, found that nimodipine, a highly lipid soluble calcium channel blocker that easily crosses the blood-brain barrier, also elevated progranulin expression (personal communication). Similar to HDAC inhibitors, a trial with nimodipine is also being considered for progranulin carriers.

Finally, Dr. Haass (Capell et al. 2011) showed that four selective inhibitors of vacuolar ATPase (bafilomycin A1, concanamycin A, archazolid B, and apicularen A) elevate intracellular and secreted GRN. Additionally, they discovered that other alkalizing drugs, including chloroquine, bepridil, and amiodarone, also stimulated progranulin production. While these compounds are relatively toxic in the dosages that would be needed to treat progranulin deficiency, they too offer new strategies for progranulin elevation and the correction of haploinsufficiency.

TDP-43, FUS, *C9ORF72*

TDP-43, FUS, and *C9ORF72* represent the most recently discovered molecules associated with FTLD and a mutation in each of these molecules can lead to an FTLD syndrome with or without ALS. Both TDP-43 and FUS represent DNA- and RNA-binding proteins that regulate gene expression, while the normal function of *C9ORF72* remains unknown.

Both TDP-43 and FUS leave the nucleus in the setting of FTLD, and the loss of their normal function within the nucleus appears to be a likely mechanism of action in both the genetic and sporadic forms of FTD-ALS. One potential link in mechanism between TDP-43, FUS, and *C9ORF72*, is that with *C9ORF72* abnormal aggregates of the RNA can be found within the nucleus and may cause disease by binding to and preventing the normal function of specific nuclear genes.

Therapies for these different genes and molecules is likely to be difficult, although anti-oligonucleotide methods and possibly RNA silencing via small molecules are two exciting approaches that could be applied to the treatment of these molecular mechanisms in FTD and ALS. It is encouraging that Matt Disney has shown some initial success in the RNA silencing approach to one RNA-mediated neurodegenerative disorder, myotonic dystrophy (Disney et al. 2010).

CONCLUSIONS

Only recently have investigators begun to think about the treatment of FTD and the number of centers that have expertise in the diagnosis of FTD is limited. Similarly, the pharmaceutical industry has to date only exhibited limited interest in investing in the treatment of FTD, in part because FTD is less frequent than AD. Another impediment to the treatment of FTD is the fact that there are a diverse number of molecular mechanisms for the clinical phenotypes of bvFTD, svPPA, and nfvPPA, and it is still not possible to readily separate out tau, TDP-43, and FUS in the clinic.

Yet, Adam Boxer from UCSF has established a clinical trials network for FTD, and there is a growing interest in these disorders from the pharmaceutical industry. One advantage of the FTD disorders is that they offer a relatively pure form of neurodegenerative disease, unlike AD, where many patients have multiple molecules including Aβ, tau, α-synuclein, and TDP-43 contributing to the disease. Additionally, many of the FTD clinical syndromes move more quickly than AD, allowing for shorter trials with smaller numbers of subjects. We hope and expect that there will slow but steady progress against each of the FTLD-related molecular subtypes and look forward to the time when these disorders are preventable.

REFERENCES

Ascher EA, Sturm VE, Seider BH, Holley SR, Miller BL, Levenson RW. Relationship satisfaction and emotional language in frontotemporal dementia and Alzheimer disease patients and spousal caregivers. Alzheimer Dis Assoc Disord. 2010;24(1):49–55.

Bei Hu, Ross L, Neuhaus J, Knopman D, Kramer J, Boeve B, Caselli RJ, Graff-Radford N, Mendez MF, Miller BL, Boxer AL. Off label medication use in frontotemporal dementia. Am J Alzheimers Dis Other Demen. 2010;25(2):128–33.

Bonner MF, Vesely L, Price C, Anderson C, Richmond L, Farag C, Avants B, Grossman M. Reversal of concreteness effect in semantic dementia. Cogn Neuropsychol. 2009;26:568–79.

Boxer AL, Lipton AM, Womack K, Merrilees J, Neuhaus J, Pavlic D, Gandhi A, Red D, Martin-Cook K, Svetlik D, Miller BL. An open label study of memantine treatment in three subtypes of frontotemporal lobar degeneration. Alzheimer Dis Assoc Disord. 2009;23:211–7.

Capell A, Liebscher S, Fellerer K, Brouwers N, Willem M, Lammich S, Gijselinck I, Bittner T, Carlson AM, Sasse F, Kunze B, Steinmetz H, Jansen R, Dormann D, Sleegers K, Cruts M, Herms J, Van Broeckhoven C, Haass C. Rescue of progranulin deficiency associated with frontotemporal lobar degeneration by alkalizing reagents and inhibition of vacuolar ATPase. J Neurosci. 2011;31(5):1885–94.

Carlino E, Benedetti F, Rainero I, Asteggiano G, Cappa G, Tarenzi L, Vighetti S, Pollo A. Pain perception and tolerance in patients with frontotemporal dementia. Pain. 2010;151(3):783–9.

Cenik B, Sephton CF, Dewey CM, Xian X, Wei S, Yu K, Niu W, Coppola G, Coughlin SE, Lee SE, Dries DR, Almeida S, Geschwind DH, Gao FB, Miller BL, Farese RV, Posner BA, Yu G, Herz J. Suberoylanilide hydroxamic acid (vorinostat) up-regulates progranulin transcription: rational therapeutic approach to frontotemporal dementia. J Biol Chem. 2011;286(18):16101–8.

Deakin JB, Rahman S, Nestor PJ, Hodges JR, Sahakian BJ. Paroxetine does not improve symptoms and impairs cognition in frontotemporal dementia: a double-blind randomized controlled trial. Psychopharmacology (Berl). 2004;172:400–8.

Disney MD, Lee MM, Pushechnikov A, Childs-Disney JL. The role of flexibility in the rational design of modularly assembled ligands targeting the RNAs that cause the myotonic dystrophies. Chembiochem. 2010;11(3):375–82.

Eckart JA, Sturm VE, Miller BL, Levenson RW. Diminished disgust reactivity in behavioral variant frontotemporal dementia. Neuropsychologia. 2012;50(5):786–90.

Finger EC. New potential therapeutic approaches in frontotemporal dementia: oxytocin, vasopressin and social cognition. J Mol Neurosci. 2011;45:696–701.

Flaherty A. Brain illness and creativity. Can J Psychiatry. 2011; 56:142–43.

Gozes I. NAP (davunetide) provides functional and structural neuroprotection. Curr Pharm Des. 2011;17(10):1040–4.

Halabi C, Halabi A, Dean DL, Wang PN, Boxer AL, Trojanowski JQ, Dearmond SJ, Miller BL, Kramer JH, Seeley WW. Patterns of striatal degeneration in frontotemporal dementia. Alzheimer Dis Assoc Disord. 2013;27(1):74–83.

Henry ML, Meese MV, Truong S, Babiak MC, Miller BL, Gorno-Tempini ML. Treatment for apraxia of speech in nonfluent variant primary progressive aphasia. Behav Neurol. 2013;26(1–2):77–88.

Herrmann N, Black SE, Chow T, Cappell J, Tang-Wai DF, Lanctot KL. Serotonergic function and treatment of behavioral and psychological symptoms of frontotemporal dementia. Am J Geriatr Psychiatry. 2012;20(9):789–9.

Huey ED, Putnam KT, Grafman J. A systematic review of neurotransmitter deficits and treatments in frontotemporal dementia. Neurology. 2006;66:17–22.

Jesso S, Morlog D, Ross S, Pell MD, Pasternak SH, Mitchell DG, Kertesz A, Finger EC, The effects of oxytocin on social cognition and behaviour in frontotemporal dementia. Brain. 2011;134:2493–501.

Jicha GA, Nelson PT. Management of frontotemporal dementia: targeting symptom management in such a heterogeneous disease requires a wide range of therapeutic options. Neurodegener Dis Manag. 2011;1:151–56.

Kfoury N, Holmes BB, Jiang H, Holtzman DM, Diamond MI. Trans-cellular propagation of tau aggregation by fibrillar species. J Biol Chem. 2012;287(23):19440–51.

Langmore SE, Olney RK, Lomen-Hoerth C, Miller BL. Dysphagia in patients with frontotemporal lobar dementia. Arch Neurol. 2007;64(1):58–62.

Lebert F, Stekke W, Hasenbroekx C, Pasquier F. Frontotemporal dementia: a randomised, controlled trial with trazodone. Dement Geriatr Cogn Disord. 2004;17:355–9.

Lee VM, Trojanowski JQ. Transgenic mouse models of tauopathies: prospects for animal models of Pick's disease. Neurology. 2001;56:S26–30.

Medina DX, Caccamo A, Oddo S. Methylene blue reduces aβ levels and rescues early cognitive deficit by increasing proteasome activity. Brain Pathol. 2011;21(2):140–9.

Mendez MF, Chen AK, Shapira JS, Miller BL. Acquired sociopathy and frontotemporal dementia. Dement Geriatr Cogn Disord. 2005;20(2–3):99–104.

Merrilees J, Hubbard E, Mastick J, Miller BL, Dowling GA. Rest-activity and behavioral disruption in a patient with frontotemporal dementia. Neurocase. 2009;15:515–26.

Merrilees J, Klapper J, Murphy J, Lomen-Hoerth C, Miller BL. Cognitive and behavioral challenges in caring for patients with frontotemporal dementia and amyotrophic lateral sclerosis. Amyotroph Lateral Scler. 2010;11:298–302.

Merrilees J, Miller BL. Comparing Alzheimer's disease and frontotemporal lobar degeneration: implications for long-term care. Ann Longterm Care. 2005;12:37–40.

Miller BL, Darby A, Benson DF, Cummings JL, Miller MH. Aggressive, socially disruptive and antisocial behavior in frontotemporal dementia. Brit J Psychiatry. 1997;170:150–56.

Miller BL, Hou CE. Portraits of artists: emergence of visual creativity in dementia. Arch Neurol. 2004;61(6):842–4.

Moretti R, Torre P, Antonello RM Cattaruzza T, Cazzato G, Bava A. Rivastigmine in frontotemporal dementia: an open label study. Drugs Aging. 2004;21(14):931–7.

Moretti R, Torre P, Antonello RM, Cazzato G, Bava A. Frontotemporal dementia: paroxetine as a possible treatment of behavior symptoms. A randomized, controlled, open 14-month study. Eur Neurol. 2003;49:13–9.

Morhardt D. Accessing community-based and long-term care services: challenges facing persons with frontotemporal dementia and their families. J Mol Neurosci. 2011;45:737–41.

Olney N, Rosen H. AVP-923, a combination of dextromethorphan hydrobromide and quinidine sulfate for the treatment of pseudobulbar affect and neuropathic pain. Drugs. 2010;13:254–65.

Olney NT, Goodkind MS, Lomen-Hoerth C, Whalen PK, Williamson CA, Holley DE, Verstaen A, Brown LM, Miller BL, Kornak J, Levenson RW, Rosen HJ. Behaviour, physiology and experience of pathological laughing and crying in amyotrophic lateral sclerosis. Brain. 2011;134(Pt 12):3455–66.

Perry RJ, Miller BL. Behavior and treatment in frontotemporal dementia. Neurology. 2001;56:S46–51.

Rankin KP, Gorno-Tempini ML, Allison SC, Stanley CM, Glenn S, Weiner MW, Miller BL. Structural anatomy of empathy in neurodegenerative disease. Brain. 2006;129:2945–56.

Rapp B, Glucroft B. The benefits and protective effects of behavioural treatment for dysgraphia in a case of primary progressive aphasia. Aphasiology. 2009;23:236–65.

Rascovsky K, Hodges JR, Knopman D, Mendez MF, Kramer JH, Neuhaus J, van Swieten JC, Seelaar H, Dopper EG, Onyike CU, Hillis AE, Josephs KA, Boeve BF, Kertesz A, Seeley WW, Rankin KP, Johnson JK, Gorno-Tempini ML, Rosen H, Prioleau-Latham CE, Lee A, Kipps CM, Lillo P, Piguet O, Rohrer JD, Rossor MN, Warren JD, Fox NC, Galasko D, Salmon DP, Black SE, Mesulam M, Weintraub S, Dickerson BC, Diehl-Schmid J, Pasquier F, Deramecourt V, Lebert F, Pijnenburg Y, Chow TW, Manes F, Grafman J, Cappa SF, Freedman M, Grossman M, Miller BL. Sensitivity of revised diagnostic criteria for the behavioural variant of frontotemporal dementia. Brain. 2011;134:2456–77.

Rosen HJ, Allison SC, Ogar JM, Amici S, Rose K, Dronkers N, Miller BL, Gorno-Tempini ML. Behavioral features in semantic dementia vs other forms of progressive aphasias. Neurology. 2006;67(10):1752–6.

Rosen HJ, Perry RJ, Murphy J, Kramer JH, Mychack P, Schuff N, Weiner M, Levenson RW, Miller BL. Emotion comprehension in the temporal variant of frontotemporal dementia. Brain. 2002;125 (Pt 10):2286–95.

Rosen HJ. Anosognosia in neurodegenerative disease. Neurocase. 2011; 17:231–41.

Schirmer RH, Adler H, Pickhardt M, Mandelkow E. "Lest we forget you—methylene blue…". Neurobiol Aging. 2011;32(12):2325.e7–16.

Schneider LS, Tariot PN, Dagerman KS, Davis SM, Hsiao JK, Ismail MS, Lebowitz BD, Lyketsos CG, Ryan JM, Stroup TS, Sultzer DL, Weintraub D, Lieberman JA; CATIE-AD Study Group. Effectiveness of atypical antipsychotic drugs in patients with Alzheimer's disease. N Engl J Med. 2006;355:1525–38.

Sturm VE, Ascher EA, Miller BL, Levenson RW. Diminished self-conscious emotional responding in frontotemporal lobar degeneration patients. Emotion. 2008;8(6):861–9.

Sturm VE, McCarthy ME, Yun I, Madan A, Yuan JW, Holley SR, Ascher EA, Boxer AL, Miller BL, Levenson RW. Mutual gaze in Alzheimer's disease, frontotemporal and semantic dementia couples. Soc Cogn Affect Neurosci. 2011;6:359–67.

Suárez J, Tartaglia MC, Vitali P, Erbetta A, Neuhaus J, Laluz V, Miller BL. Characterizing radiology reports in patients with frontotemporal dementia. Neurology. 2009;73(13):1073–4.

Swartz JR, Miller BL, Lesser IM, Darby AL. Frontotemporal dementia: treatment response to serotonin selective reuptake inhibitors. J Clin Psychiatry. 1997;58:212–6.

Tariot PN, Schneider LS, Cummings J, Thomas RG, Raman R, Jakimovich LJ, Loy R, Bartocci B, Fleisher A, Ismail MS, Porsteinsson A, Weiner M, Jack CR Jr, Thal L, Aisen PS; Alzheimer's Disease Cooperative Study Group. Chronic divalproex sodium to attenuate agitation and clinical progression of Alzheimer disease. Arch Gen Psychiatry. 2011;68(8):853–61.

Vercelletto M, Boutoleau-Bretonnière C, Volteau C, Puel M, Auriacombe S, Sarazin M, Michel BF, Couratier P, Thomas-Antérion C, Verpillat P, Gabelle A, Golfier V, Cerato E, Lacomblez L; French research network on Frontotemporal dementia. Memantine in behavioral variant frontotemporal dementia: negative results. J Alzheimers Dis. 2011;23:749–59.

Vossel KA, Miller BL. New approaches to the treatment of frontotemporal lobar degeneration. Curr Opin Neurol. 2008;21:708–16.

Ward ME, Miller BL. Potential mechanisms of progranulin-deficient FTLD. J Mol Neurosci. 2011; 45:574–83.

Werner KH, Roberts NA, Rosen HJ, Dean DL, Kramer JH, Weiner MW, Miller BL, Levenson RW. Emotional reactivity and emotion recognition in frontotemporal lobar degeneration. Neurology. 2007;69(2):148–55.

Wood PL, Nair NP, Etienne P, Lal S, Gauthier S, Robitaille Y, Bird ED, Palo J, Haltia M, Paetau A. Lack of cholinergic deficit in the neocortex in Pick's disease. Prog Neuropsychopharmacol Biol Psychiatry. 1983;7(4):725–7.

Woolley JD, Khan BK, Murthy NK, Miller BL, Rankin KP. The diagnostic challenge of psychiatric symptoms in neurodegenerative disease: Rates of and risk factors for prior psychiatric diagnosis in patients with early neurodegenerative disease. J Clin Psychiatry. 2011;72:126–33.

Zhang B, Carroll J, Trojanowski JQ, Yao Y, Iba M, Potuzak JS, Hogan AM, Xie SX, Ballatore C, Smith AB 3rd, Lee VM, Brunden KR. The microtubule-stabilizing agent, epothilone D, reduces axonal dysfunction, neurotoxicity, cognitive deficits, and Alzheimer-like pathology in an interventional study with aged tau transgenic mice. J Neurosci. 2012;32(11):3601–11.

Index